KETO LIVING
Day by Day

An inspirational guide to the ketogenic diet,
with 130 deceptively simple recipes

KRISTIE H. SULLIVAN, PhD
Foreword by Andreas Eenfeldt, MD

VICTORY BELT PUBLISHING INC.
LAS VEGAS

This book is dedicated to my people—those with metabolic dysfunction
who have endured a lifetime struggle with obesity.

If you've ever been told:

"eat less, move more"

"push away from the table"

"you have such a pretty face, if only you'd just lose weight."

If you've ever struggled with endless hunger . . .

If you've ever been referred to a dietician or nutritionist . . .

If you've ever prayed that the largest size in the store might fit . . .

If you've ever worried about the size of the airplane seat or the auditorium seat . . .

If you've failed every diet known, then this book is dedicated to YOU.

Like the brave woman in my "before" pictures, may you have the courage
to try one more time, one more day.

First Published in 2018 by Victory Belt Publishing Inc.

Copyright © 2018 by Kristie Sullivan

ISBN-13: 978-1-628602-72-2

Cover Design by Charisse Reyes

Interior Design by Justin-Aaron Velasco

Illustrations by Charisse Reyes and Elita San Juan

Cover Photography by Hayley Mason and Bill Staley

Photography by Kristie Sullivan and Jenny Lowder

Printed in Canada

TC 0118

Contents

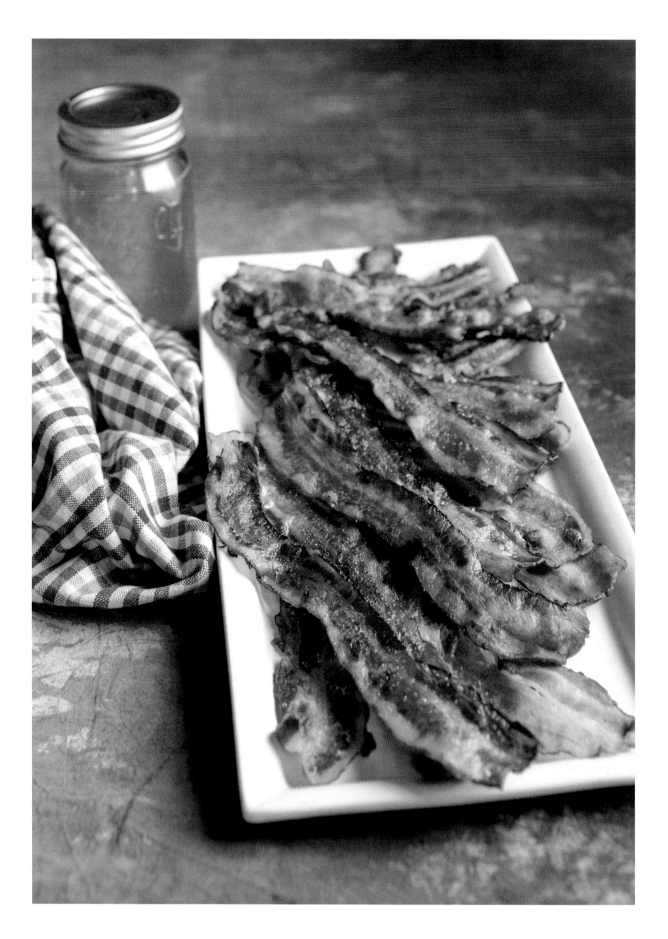

Foreword

Have you heard about the keto diet? Probably you have, because it's exploded in popularity in recent years. Also, you're holding a book about keto, so likely you're interested.

With all these people claiming to have lost weight effortlessly and improved their health dramatically, it can feel like the latest new fad diet. But it's not. For one thing, it's far from new. Similar diets—other strict low-carb diets—have been successfully used for at least 150 years for weight loss and a number of health conditions, like type 2 diabetes.

The recurring popularity likely has a simple explanation: it simply works. Modern science proves it, with study after careful study showing keto resulting in more effective weight loss than other diets, better blood sugar control, better blood pressure, and (perhaps surprisingly) a common improvement in the cholesterol profile. This suggests that keto could even be very healthy for people's hearts. A study of a similar low-carb, high-fat diet even found a reduction in atherosclerosis in people's blood vessels.

This obviously doesn't mean that every human needs to be on a keto diet to be healthy. Far from it. Keto is just a tool, and a very powerful one. It can be a good first option for people who want to get rid of excess weight without hunger, reverse type 2 diabetes or pre-diabetes, normalize high blood pressure or other connected disorders, and potentially control a few other common health issues, like migraine, PCOS, and IBS.

Many people use keto diets simply for the effect on how they feel: less hunger, more stable energy all through the day, more mental clarity, less need for snacking. People often spontaneously start skipping snacks and the occasional meal altogether because the uncontrollable hunger just isn't there anymore. This can result not only in weight loss, but also in lots of time and money saved.

There is, however, one problem: A keto diet isn't simple to do, especially not when living in a society where sugar and other processed carbohydrates are available everywhere, at any moment, tasting great and costing almost nothing. A society where eating refined carbs every few hours is considered normal and where diabetes type 2 and obesity have become normalized. Most Americans are now obese or overweight, and more than half of all Americans born today are predicted to end up with type 2 diabetes during their lives.

Living the way most people do is likely to lead you down the same path of excess weight and disease. And living differently from other people can be hard. That's where this book could be life-changing. Kristie Sullivan has completely transformed her own life using a keto diet and shares her amazing story in this book. She knows how to do it, and even more importantly, she knows how to inspire and empower other people to do the same thing.

From her vibrant Facebook community of over 150,000 people to her popular YouTube channel with millions of views, people around the world have come to rely on Kristie's warmth and guidance to help them succeed. During the last year, she's also been an important contributor to our site, DietDoctor.com, inspiring people to improve their lives using a keto diet. And now, with this book, she can do the same thing for you.

Are you just starting out, or do you want new inspiration to keep going? Do you want to make keto simple, cooking delicious meals with inexpensive and easy-to-find ingredients? This book supplies simple instructions and all the recipes and meal plans you need to get started with keto living.

But this book doesn't just contain what you need to make keto simple. You'll also get the hard-earned practical tips and the emotional support that can be equally important for your success, supporting you through the challenges that may arise. Pick up this book for day-by-day inspiration from Kristie Sullivan. You couldn't ask for a better guide on your journey.

Andreas Eenfeldt, MD
Founder & CEO, Diet Doctor

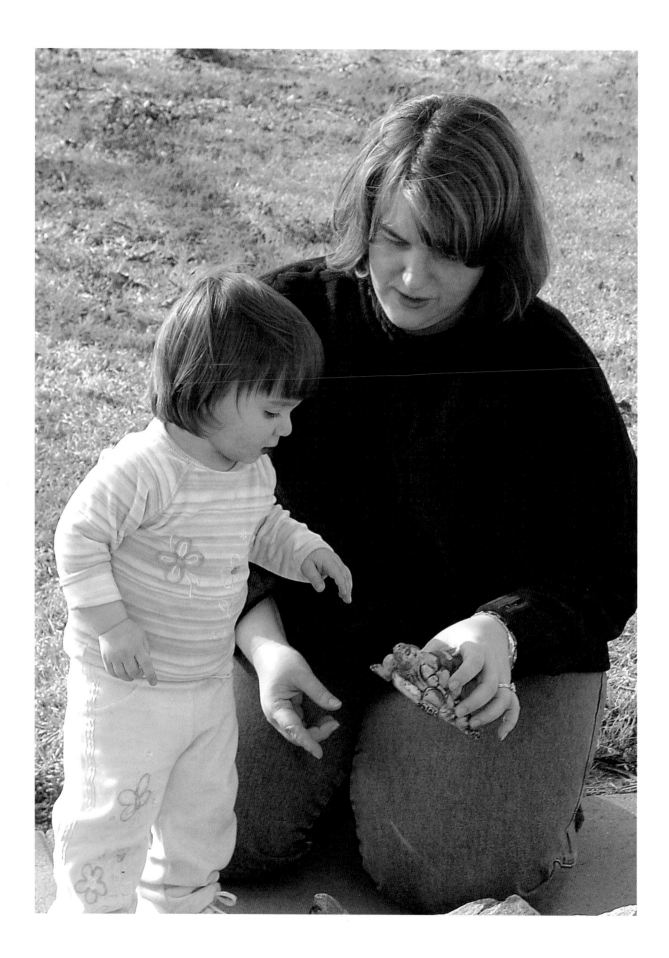

Introduction:

My Story

We've all been there: We get fed up with our clothing size or disgusted by recent photos of ourselves. Sometimes it's the reality check of a doctor's appointment or stepping on the scale to the biting reality that our weight is out of control. We vow that this time is going to be different. We muster resolve from our desperation and despair. In that moment, we would sell our souls for a solution. We make promises that we have never been able to keep. We are going to take control: we will eat the right foods; we will exercise every single day; we will lose weight. Sometimes that resolve lasts until after lunch. It might last more than twenty-four hours. When we are really feeling stubborn and committed, it might survive for two to three weeks, but the hunger is always there, along with miserable feelings of deprivation. We see others enjoying their food and their lives, but we are counting and weighing and measuring and dreaming of a time when we might be able to eat and not be hungry.

Between the ages of eighteen and forty-five, I went from overweight to obese to morbidly obese and back to overweight at least four times. When I was a sophomore in college, I went on a calorie-restricted diet. I'm not sure anyone realized how little I was eating. I remember sitting in a McDonald's with a grilled chicken salad with maybe a teaspoon of dressing and eating only a third of it. Even though I was starving, I worried that I was eating too much. As I tossed the bulk of that tiny salad in the trash, the disordered eater in me was relieved that I had disposed of it before devouring the entire thing along with the plastic bowl it came in! But somewhere a rational voice inside me dared to wonder, "Is this really a healthy way to live?" That same voice wondered whether the people I was eating with were the least bit concerned that the tiny amount of salad I'd eaten was my entire food intake for the day. Did they not notice, or were they, too, so desperate for me to lose weight that they were silently applauding my efforts?

Perhaps they didn't notice my disordered eating, but they did notice my weight loss. When I went home for a family gathering that fall, my relatives were thrilled to see me "skinny." I even wore a belt with my skirt, which they had never seen me do. At a size 18, I was the slimmest most of them had ever seen me. I was embarrassed by the attention. It had taken me about four months to lose the weight, and then came the holidays. By the end of my sophomore year, I was no longer able to wear that skirt or belt, and I had ballooned back to my size-22 clothes.

In my senior year, the diet resolution hit me once more. I had a boyfriend who insisted that our relationship would be perfect if I just lost weight, and I was dumb enough to believe him. I begged my mother for money to enroll in a physician-assisted weight-loss program. She agreed, and I plunked down money that she didn't have to spare. The program was low-fat and low-carb. I was so committed that I even lobbied the dean of students to have the school cafeteria prepare special meals for me. Ninety-nine percent of my lunches and dinners were comprised of boiled chicken breast with broccoli—no butter, no seasoning. I sometimes put a tablespoon of shredded low-fat cheese on my plate. Twenty-eight years later, I still remember how good that splurge of low-fat cheese tasted! The diet plan instructed me to avoid salt and even listed celery as a forbidden food because it was too salty.

I followed that physician-assisted plan for about four months without ever seeing a physician. I exercised the entire time. The sharp pangs of hunger were at least temporarily dulled by the "success" of weight loss.

When I graduated from college, I was a svelte size 14 and was able to purchase two linen skirts for job interviews. Even though it was one of the few times I didn't need plus sizes, I was still being told that I wasn't thin enough. I didn't enjoy being that smaller size because I was still considered fat. When I stopped the ridiculously expensive and impossible low-carb, low-fat physician-assisted diet, I continued counting calories, but the weight slowly crept back.

Eventually (and mercifully), I lost about 175 pounds in the form of a self-centered ex-boyfriend, but I was devastated. I spent a whole year mourning our breakup, trying to diet, and eventually giving up. My focus turned to my full-time job and to graduate school. Not only did I work long hours, but the graduate program in which I was enrolled was a three-hour drive from my home. With no Internet yet invented, I was a "distance learner" in every sense of the word! Those commutes were punctuated with fast-food drive-through meals. I kept candy in the car as well because it helped me "stay awake." Each semester I bought boxes of candy and diet soft drinks from a warehouse club. As you might expect, my weight spiraled out of control. By the time I finished my master's degree three years later, I weighed more than 300 pounds.

Not only was it difficult for me to find clothing that fit, but the clothing I did find was often expensive. As a size 26/28, I could shop only in specialty stores that carried plus sizes. I also needed wide-width shoes in a size ten or eleven—the last sizes on the rack. Personal hygiene became difficult, and I started experiencing back pain.

Eventually, I changed jobs, which required me to move farther from family and friends. While I had always worked long hours, I was even more socially isolated and pretty miserable overall. One night while watching television, I saw a commercial for weight-loss surgery. I learned that the Roux-en-Y gastric bypass procedure was still new, but a medical school three hours to the east offered the surgery. I never thought twice about whether it was the right option for me. I was beyond desperate. I weighed 313 pounds and stood barely 5'2" at the time of my first appointment there. When I saw that number on the scale, I gasped.

Maybe it was the 313-pound reality check. Maybe it was because my thirtieth birthday was just a few years away and I feared I would never get married. Maybe it was complete and utter desperation, but I decided to move forward with gastric bypass surgery.

The program required all sorts of medical tests as well as a psychological evaluation. The psychologist asked whether I had at least three people locally who visited me in my home. I lied and said yes. The memory stands out because I realized it was a marker of good health, and I had failed. I was too embarrassed to admit how socially isolated I was, but wise enough to know that the situation needed to change.

A year after the surgery, I had lost more than 125 pounds and had begun working out at a hospital-affiliated fitness center. Even though I hated exercise—hated the workout clothing, hated the time spent at the gym, and especially hated the sweating—I liked getting closer to a "normal" weight. Approximately a year and a half after the surgery, I reached my lowest weight ever—178 pounds—and was wearing a size 14. I was on the cusp of plus-sized clothing; whether I could wear a misses' size depended on the style. For the most part, I shopped in the women's petite section, which offered smaller cuts of plus-sized clothing, because I feared being unable to wear the largest regular sizes in the trendier stores. Once again, I didn't quite fit.

It was at that time that I met the love of my life. I noticed him the moment I walked into the room—blond hair, blue eyes, broad shoulders, a kind smile, and an air of confidence. He wasn't my type at all! I doubted if he would even consider dating a fat girl, but I knew I wanted to speak to this man whom I found charming, even from across the room.

We were participating in a professional development program, working for different employers. This statewide leadership program required an initial two-day retreat, a meeting once a month for six months, and then another two-day retreat to conclude the one-year program. Thirty minutes into the first day, we were asked to participate in an icebreaker. Before I could even leave my seat, I was startled to find the fella of my dreams standing in front of me. Later I learned that I had caught *his* eye when I entered the room. Our day was busy, and it wasn't until after an after-dinner meeting that I had a chance to really speak to him. Okay, I confess, I nearly jumped into his path as he was leaving the meeting room. "Excuse me . . ." turned into a three-hour conversation in which we shared our life's passions and dreams for the future. Everything about him seemed perfect. Except his girlfriend. The fact that I was also dating someone at the time was impertinent.

We spent the following day sitting together when we could, and we exchanged contact information before departing for home. I had not even left the driveway of the retreat center when I called my dearest friend and nearly shouted, "I met the man I'm going to marry and the father of my children!" I spent the next 20 miles describing him tip to top and inside out. When I finally took a breath, she asked, "But you said he has a girlfriend?" Without hesitation, I replied, "Yes, poor girl. I feel sorry for her. It's only a matter of time." My confidence surprised even me, but I had met this man's heart, and I knew that I loved it. My prayer on the day that I met him (November 5, 1998) was, "Lord, let him be the one. If he isn't the one, then please let him have the same heart. He can be shorter, taller, fatter, or thinner, but Lord, please let him have that same heart."

Neither of us is certain when we had our first date, but David and I were married in March 2002. I wore a size-20 wedding dress, which mortified me. I weighed about 190 pounds. I know my weight because as we planned our honeymoon, we were considering activities with a 200-pound weight limit. I worried that I wouldn't be able to do some of those activities, such as ride a mule into the Grand Canyon or enjoy a hot air balloon ride over Sedona, because of my weight, but I did not want to admit that to David.

After the honeymoon, we settled into a new routine, with David completing graduate school and beginning a new job and me in graduate school while working full-time. We were busy, but I loved him, and I showed that love in one of the best ways I knew: food. We celebrated with food. We connected with friends and family over food. I loved to eat. David loved to eat. I loved feeding others. David loved being cared for in that way. It was not a healthy form of love, though; we both gained enormous amounts of weight from all my cooking combined with our busy lifestyles.

We decided to try Weight Watchers. I starved even though I ate all my points every day, and I resented that David was allowed nearly twice as many points as I was. Each week I made a huge batch of low-fat taco soup because it was low in points. How I came to despise that soup! David did well on Weight Watchers, even though he drank at least four points per day in Pepsi, while I stuck to water and lost half the amount he did.

Eventually, I became pregnant. Welcome to french fries and Krispy Kreme doughnuts! When that pregnancy ended in a miscarriage, we consoled ourselves with food—I more so than he. A miscarriage is a very private grief. There were days when food was the only "friend" who understood what I was going through.

Thankfully, I became pregnant again quickly, and we were thrilled. Carbohydrates seemed to keep morning sickness at bay, so I ate nearly every waking hour. I weighed nearly 250 pounds when our daughter, Grace, was born eight weeks premature. I had been in the hospi-

tal on bed rest for two weeks prior to her birth, and David had kept me supplied with peanut M&Ms, milkshakes, and cheeseburgers from our favorite fast-food place. Because of my girth and her prematurity, there were acquaintances who did not even realize I was pregnant until after I was hospitalized.

As a mom, I tried to give Grace the best nutrition I could, and I dutifully followed the pediatrician's advice for weaning. Our daughter had Goldfish Crackers and O-shaped cereal to help develop her fine motor skills. As soon as she caught up on the preemie growth charts, we began feeding her low-fat whole-grain foods. We restricted juice and switched to skim milk. As she grew, though, her appetite seemed to match her mother's. I worried. Pediatricians warned us. We tried to restrict food, and I made an extra effort to buy low-fat dairy and to provide five servings of fruits and vegetables a day. All three of us continued to gain weight.

Three years later, our son, Jonathan, was born ten weeks early. He was healthy until his fifth day of life, when he was diagnosed with necrotizing enterocolitis (NEC), a horrific illness that can afflict the intestines of preemies. He was rushed to an NICU three hours from our home to be near a pediatric surgeon who eventually removed 75 percent of Jonathan's large intestine. We spent two months in the hospital while our son underwent multiple surgeries. Between the stress and never wanting to leave his side, I dropped to 225 pounds and a size 20. I remember only because folks commented on how great I looked despite enduring some of the most difficult days of my life.

By the time our son started kindergarten, my weight had climbed to over 260 pounds again. My size-22 pants were often too tight, and I had begun wearing some size-24 clothes. I also began having significant back pain from conditions related to scoliosis.

In short, my back is a mess. My chart lists spondylolisthesis, stenosis, arthritis, and some Latin words I cannot even pronounce. There is a second curvature above the section where my spine was fused in 1984. The curve is also twisting. My neurologist told me, "No good

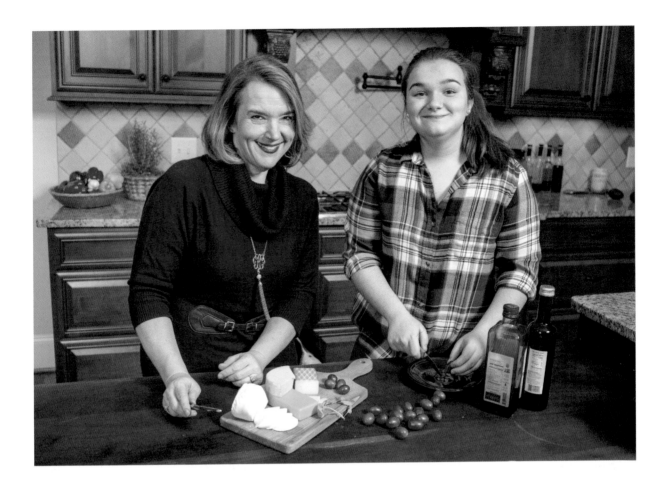

surgeon is gonna operate on you. Our goal for you is pain management." At the pain management clinic to which I was referred, the anesthesiologist called in his colleagues and exclaimed, "You gotta see this!"

I began epidural steroid injections in the summer of 2012. My pain management program included three prescription medications and two over-the-counter meds. I purchased 500-tablet bottles of ibuprofen because I was taking an average of more than six pills per day.

The pain was mostly in my lower back but radiated through my hips and down my legs. Walking any real distance was not only painful but also resulted in my becoming winded and sweaty. Some days I waited until I got to work to put on makeup because I sweated so much just walking into the building. I used a desk that could be raised to alleviate my back pain; nonetheless, at the end of the day, the pain was often so severe that just preparing dinner left me in

tears. As soon as the meal was ready, David would help me to bed. He offered me his forearms and walked backward while I used him as a walker. We joked about getting me an actual walker, wondered if we should purchase disability insurance, and built our new house to accommodate a wheelchair. I was in my early forties.

Even though I had accomplished many of my life's goals, I was unhappy. I could not do the things that mattered most to me. My children didn't have the mother I thought they deserved. Instead of me walking them upstairs and tucking them into bed, they kissed me goodnight and then went upstairs for their daddy to tuck them in. Back pain kept me from climbing the stairs most nights.

The kids began to accept that "Mommy's back hurts" and "Mommy can't go for a walk." I couldn't chase them on the playground, nor could I carry them when they were little. I stayed behind when they went for hikes or played with their dad. I was the mom who couldn't. Even when I volunteered at their schools, I worried that their classmates would make fun of my weight. I worried that I would embarrass them.

Memorial Day weekend of 2013 was a turning point. A close colleague's daughter was getting married. It was a beautiful celebration. Everyone looked elegant and graceful—except for me. I wore a size-24 pink polyester suit with three-quarter-length sleeves. It was the only thing I could find to wear that was remotely appropriate. The day of the outdoor wedding was very hot, and most of the women wore fitted sleeveless dresses. They were older than I was, and they looked fabulous. I could have been the grandmother of the bride given how I was dressed and how I moved. I was too self-conscious to enjoy myself. I wondered if my husband wished he were there with a truly beautiful woman of whom he could be proud.

After that weekend, I vowed that life would be different. I lay in bed thinking of how my children were being robbed of the mother they deserved. Other mothers were active and wore stylish clothes and did things with their kids. I held them back because "Mommy can't." My husband also deserved more. Because of my back pain, he often did more than his fair share of the cleaning and caring for the children. I was not the partner I wanted to be. While he never complained about my weight, I worried that he too was embarrassed by me. I imagined him with a different wife, one who could be everything he needed—attractive, smart, funny, and a better caregiver for our children. If I couldn't be who they needed, then I decided I would no longer hold them back. They were better off without me. It was a desperate time as I imagined a new wife for my husband and a new mother for my kids.

As I lay there and decided that I would do this or die trying, I thought about everything I had accomplished. I had a PhD and was respected in my career. None of my four grandparents had even finished high school; two were unable to read. Not only was I a first-generation college student, but I had earned my PhD while working full-time in a demanding job and raising two kids. I had bought my first house when I was just twenty-six years old, working two jobs, and completing my master's degree. Whenever anyone told me I couldn't do something that I was determined to do, my response was, "Watch me."

Yet here I was, obese in spite of a lifetime of dieting. I never wanted to be obese, and I had followed every diet and medical intervention ever known. I had even failed at gastric bypass surgery! My hopelessness was rooted in wondering, "What is wrong with me? Why can't I do this? I've overcome many hurdles to accomplish so much, but I cannot manage my weight." My resolve was unparalleled, and I knew that if I could not lose weight this time, I was irreparably broken. My resolve was rooted in "I will not live like this."

I did the only thing I knew to do to lose weight. I did what doctors and nutritionists had been telling me to do for more than forty years: restrict calories and exercise. With my phone app at the ready, I allowed myself 1,200 low-fat calories per day. The first week was miserable. I lost 7 or 8 pounds, but I suffered. My family suffered. The hunger led to grumpiness and an obsession with food that dictated every minute of my days, but I persisted into the next week, obsessing over every morsel. Despite the hunger and humiliation, I went to the gym.

At the end of week two, the weight loss stopped. In spite of a second week of starvation and workouts, the number on the scale was right where it had been the previous week. Panic, fear, and desperation dogged me. What if I couldn't do it? I read journal articles and searched for supplements that might help with weight loss. "Eat less, move more" was the only solution offered by "reliable" medical websites.

One morning when I was feeling especially vulnerable, I dropped the children off at school and started my drive to work. I was tired of searching for solutions. I remembered that a friend from church had talked about losing a significant amount of weight, so I called her. The words rushed out: "What am I doing wrong? I can't live like this!" She listened and then came back with a calm and thoughtful response that changed my life:

"It isn't always about the calories."

Huh? No one had ever said that to me before. She mentioned a book by a fella named Gary Taubes and suggested that I read it. The book was delivered to me on June 19, 2013. Two days later, I pointed at a meal plan in the back of the book and told my husband, "I'm going to do this." David followed my finger and read, "No sugar, no starch. No bread? No potatoes? No pasta? No way!" The man who had counted points with me, eaten endless bowls of low-fat taco soup, and endured diet soft drinks and cakes made with applesauce drew a line in the sand. "Good luck with that," he said. "You can do it, but I'm not going to."

David saw yet another diet that I would try for a week or two and then abandon. He was right to doubt me. It sounded absurd! How could anyone give up bread and pasta and potatoes? This new diet even disallowed carrots! Let's not hop on that crazy train. What my husband did not know was that his wife had just read her story. The book recommended by my friend, *Why We Get Fat,* was the first book I'd ever read that helped me understand, "There's nothing wrong with you. What's wrong is the dietary advice you've been given. You're eating the wrong foods." Taubes commiserated with me. He understands that no one wants to be obese or hungry. He points out that prisoners are starved as a form of punishment. He notes that a lumberjack is hungrier than a tailor, so when the obese are told to eat less and move more, their appetites increase because of the increase in exercise. It wasn't my resolve that was broken, but my approach.

When Taubes describes the role of insulin and hunger hormones, he is describing my experience with food. Maybe I wasn't irreparably broken, weak, or food addicted; maybe my metabolic hormones had been working against me, and the "healthy" foods I was told to eat were making the obesity worse. If this fella was right, then this diet could be the answer to my issues with weight. I had to try. I had nothing else.

The eating plan outlined in the appendix of Taubes' book was contributed by Dr. Eric Westman, an obesity researcher and clinician at Duke University. Duke is a well-respected institution, so I trusted that this diet was safe. I called my friend who had recommended the book and confided to her that I was going to try Taubes' approach. She said another magical thing—"Even one little Hershey's Kiss can throw you off plan"—as she cautioned me that this diet only works if you are very strict about it. Maybe those words resonated because I was desperate, but they became a commandment to me. This plan *had* to work, and if I did not follow it 100 percent, it wouldn't.

I committed to a two-week trial period. I would give it 100 percent for two solid weeks. If Westman and Taubes were wrong, I would know . . . but what if they were right?

It was June 21, 2013, and at that point I didn't even know what a ketogenic diet was. I wouldn't figure that out until sometime in late 2013 or early 2014. I had no clue about macronutrients. I didn't care that this new diet was anti-inflammatory. I was fighting to lose weight, and I was willing to die trying.

Dr. Westman said to count carbs, so I did. His basic plan includes a list of foods to avoid, so I avoided those foods. As I continued cooking for my family, I served meals that included a meat that we all could enjoy—not breaded, but fried, roasted, baked, or stewed—along with one low-carb vegetable, like a salad or green beans, and a second starchy side that I didn't eat but my family liked, such as rice, potatoes, or pasta. By the third day without high-carb foods, I felt good.

Without my realizing it, my hunger had diminished. I was enjoying a particularly busy but productive day at work when I felt the first pangs of hunger. I looked up from the papers I was standing over and glanced at the clock. It was after 3:00 p.m.! Breakfast had been over seven hours earlier! I had heard of people missing meals because they were busy, but that had never, ever happened to me. The occasion was so momentous that I stopped working and called my best friend. "You aren't going to believe this!" I shouted at her, "but I forgot to eat

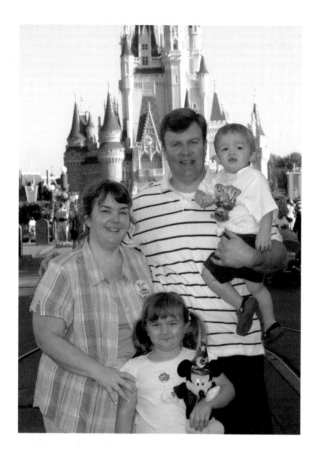

then you will never know whether it works." I reminded myself, "Choose you. Remember the wedding. Remember the pink polyester suit you wore. Remember that David deserves more; the children deserve more." I bargained with the cravings: "Just two weeks. Can't you let me give this plan just two weeks?" Instead of driving to the store, I drove home, but the cravings persisted. They seemed to holler at me, "If we don't get a chocolate chip cookie, someone is gonna get hurt!"

That night I ate a keto meal, but I still craved a cookie. The week before, I had created a Pinterest board of low-carb foods. Looking for a compromise, I searched for a low-carb cookie recipe. My pantry was not well stocked for low-carb baking, but I found a very simple recipe for peanut butter cookies, and I had every ingredient in my kitchen. I decided to make those cookies even though I felt conflicted. Part of me worried that the treat would throw me off plan; another part worried that *not* having the treat would throw me off plan. As I mixed the dough, I promised myself that I would eat only two cookies. If the scale went up the next day, I would know that the cookies had been a bad idea.

Eating those two cookies was one of those moments in life that I will never forget. As I savored the first warm bite, I thought, "If I can eat this cookie and still lose weight, then I can do this for the rest of my life." The following day, I woke to a 2-pound weight loss. That was at the end of June 2013, and I've been eating this way ever since.

Now, after losing more than 100 pounds, what I once thought of as a diet is now my lifestyle. Barring the emergence of new medical information, this is how I will eat for the rest of my life. I now understand that conventional nutrition advice had me eating all the foods that were wrong for my body. After a lifetime of struggle, I am eating the best foods of my life and wearing the smallest clothes. My family is active. We hike. We canoe. We kayak. I can go upstairs to tuck in the kids and tell them to clean their rooms. (Somehow, they don't appreciate that.) I no longer take medications for

lunch!" She knew my lifelong battle with weight. We often marveled at how others might forget a meal, but we commiserated that it would never be us. I had experienced an otherworldly event!

Throughout that week, I simply was not hungry very often. When I was hungry, I enjoyed bacon and full-fat cheese. Small portions satisfied me. My clothes were getting loose. What sorcery was this? Taubes and Westman were on to something. My body *liked* this way of eating. For the first time in my life, I was not hungry every waking minute, and I was losing weight while eating really good food.

The diet seemed pretty easy until toward the end of the second week, when cravings hit hard. Visions of chocolate chip cookies took over my brain. The desire was so strong that I imagined myself driving to the grocery store, purchasing some cookies, and eating the entire bag. An internal battle raged. I begged myself, "Two weeks. Just two weeks. 100 percent on plan. Even one little Hershey's Kiss can throw you off plan." I pleaded with myself, "If you don't give this 100 percent for two weeks, back pain, but I do keep the last giant ibuprofen bottle in my medicine cabinet. Ironically, the expiration date is 2013—the year I began my ketogenic lifestyle. It serves as a reminder of the person I used to be: a woman who was in physical pain and who suffered emotionally because of her physical limitations. When people hear what I eat, they often ask, "Don't you miss bread?" I smile and remember those medications. I remember all the times I told my children, "No, Mommy can't." And I respond with confidence, "Not even a little. I have a life now that is so much better without bread. I no longer wear plus-sized clothes. I no longer take pain medications. I hike and kayak when I want to. I can ride a bike! Why would I miss bread?"

Nearly every day, I am amazed at how much better my life is without high-carb foods. Those foods that I thought were healthy or comforting or celebratory were really poisoning my body. Now I enjoy amazing energy and freedom from pain. I don't struggle, but I see others struggle. When I grocery shop, I see people buying imitation butter, low-fat dairy products, and other low-calorie foods. Their struggle is obvious to me because it was my struggle, too. In restaurants, I can't help but notice overweight people debating whether to do the "right" thing and pass up high-fat entrees in favor of a salad. When they are offered the option of a booth or a table, I recognize the glimmer of fear that they won't fit in the booth. I've sat with friends who lament weight gain or high blood glucose readings and resign themselves to taking medications while following the same nutritional advice that made me sick and obese. My heart hurts for them.

I share my story because I know the struggle. I know what it's like to search for plus-sized clothing and pray that the largest size fits. I have been that person who eats very little in front of others but then binges in the privacy of her own kitchen. In the drive-through, I have ordered two soft drinks so the cashier would not suspect that all the food was for me. I have skipped parties because I was ashamed of my weight and embarrassed to face friends whom I desperately wanted to see, but whom I did not want to see me. I have been that woman on the airplane squeezed between two people silently groaning over their misfortune of sitting next to the fat lady whose body squishes over and under the armrests and into their seats. I've been among those who lament that bath towels and restaurant portions are too small. My journey has taken me to a very different landscape. The views are magnificent now, and I want to show you how different life can be.

Friends who were familiar with my lifelong struggle began asking me to share my "diet" with them. Because I had been active in Facebook support groups, I decided to start a small, closed group just for family and friends. The group was open only to people I knew in real life and their friends. I intended to use the group to share recipes and tips. Some friends requested videos, so I began sharing those from time to time. At some point, my brother suggested that I post my videos on YouTube. I laughed at him, wondering why on earth I would want to do that. Over time, though, the storage space on my phone began to fill up, so I decided to use YouTube to store the videos and make them easily accessible to my friends and family. When I created my channel, I casually asked my husband, "What should I call this?" He suggested, "Cooking Keto with Kristie." I typed that as the name and uploaded my first video. Within two months, I had more than a thousand subscribers, even though I had not promoted the channel. People who had "met" me in other online groups asked to join my private group. Eventually, I agreed to open the group to others, but I was adamant that I would limit membership to 5,000 people.

An odd thing happens when you share your story: people listen. The closed Facebook group grew, and the number of YouTube subscribers doubled and then tripled. Folks who enjoyed the recipes I was sharing began asking me to put my recipes into a cookbook. I never set out to write a cookbook, but I self-published my first one in February 2017. It was not very well done. I took most of the photos with my cell phone. Group members and followers even pitched in to help me take the last thirty images. I sent each person a recipe, and he or she would make it, snap a photo, and send it to me to use in the book. With their help, I published *Journey to Health: A Journey Worth Taking,* which became an Amazon bestseller, much to my surprise! The success of that book was due to the sweet support of those who had shared in my journey—those whose own "before" photos looked a lot like mine. Those precious souls joined me on the journey because they desperately needed answers, too.

Publishing that book opened up many new opportunities. I began working with leaders in the low-carb community, including Dr. Eric Westman, whose "no sugar, no starch" eating plan saved my life, and Dr. Andreas Eenfeldt, the Swedish physician who founded *The Diet Doctor,* the number-one low-carb website in the world. While others were asking me to collaborate to make money, Dr. Eenfeldt invited me to "help empower people to change their lives." Working with him and the Diet Doctor team has been the highlight of my life. In addition to weekly blog posts, I work with his video production team on ketogenic cooking videos.

The obese girl who never had a date in high school and skipped her senior prom, the gastric bypass candidate who lied about having three local friends to visit her, now has over half a million followers on social media. She has people messaging her to share their stories or to say, "I'm praying for you." The woman who wore the frumpy polyester suit to a summer wedding now has a little black dress that she loves to wear with heels that she never could have worn before.

In June 2013, I decided to lose weight or die trying. My resolve, the advice of a sweet friend, and a whole lotta prayer not only helped me, but empowered me to help others. I regret that I missed being active when my children were young. I miss being thirty. I miss the carefree lifestyle that my husband and I enjoyed when we were dating, and I miss being able to read without reading glasses. But, my dear friends, I do *not* miss bread!

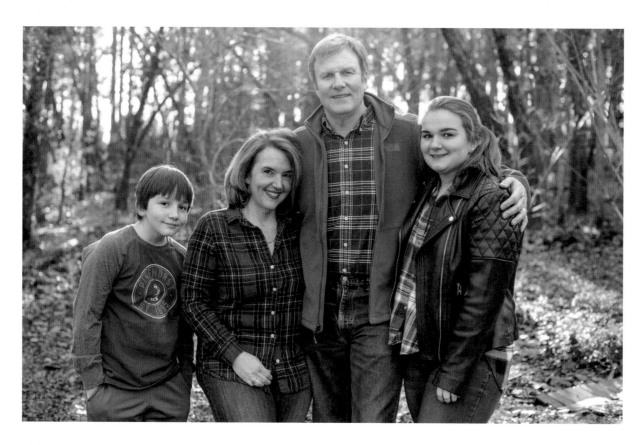

PART I:

All About Keto

Clearly, the ketogenic diet saved my life, but I had to learn the what, why, and how to make it a lifestyle. What is keto, why does it work, and how do you continue restricting carbs long term?

Whenever I learn something new, there seem to be two versions: the technical textbook version and then the real-life implementation. For example, when I took driver's education many, many years ago, the instructor told us that when stopping at a stop sign, we should align the car's front bumper with the post of the stop sign. After that lesson, when I was practicing my driving with my father, I stopped well ahead of an intersection and aligned my front bumper with the stop sign. Then I had to creep forward to check for traffic before crossing. My dad was concerned that I had stopped, rolled forward, and then stopped again. A seasoned driver, he asked, "What are you doing? Why did you stop so far back?" I explained the textbook instructions we were given, and I will never forget his response: "That's crazy! If you do that, someone will run into the back of your car. You don't need to stop that far back and then stop a second time. You pull up to the edge of the intersection where you can see, and then you go when it's safe." He was right. There was the classroom instruction and then the practical reality of how to stay safe at a stop sign.

When learning to follow a ketogenic lifestyle, you will find textbook explanations of how to count macros, detailed lists of "acceptable" and "not acceptable" foods, and lengthy chapters about the science of low-carb eating. While all that is useful, in this book I've chosen to focus on very practical information to help you implement keto each day. For example, knowing that one serving of cauliflower has 5 grams of carbohydrate is useful, but how much is a serving? What does a standard serving size *look* like? (See page 31 for the answer.)

Also, if you encounter conflicting information about how much fat, protein, or carbohydrate you should be eating, how do you know whom to trust? The short answer is that you should trust your own body, and in this part I've included some useful tips for determining which macros are best for *you*. Moreover, eating keto isn't temporary. Just as students need to develop good habits for a lifetime of safe driving, developing good meal planning and shopping habits will serve you well over the long term. Even if you despise the notion of meal planning, there are some simple things that you can do to ensure your success each week.

Lastly, an important part of making keto sustainable is navigating the journey in the "real world" when you're eating with friends and family, celebrating holidays or milestones, or simply eating in restaurants. Coping with these day-to-day challenges is often easier when you have concrete examples to follow. Part I offers sensible solutions to common challenges that you're likely to encounter when you're learning to eat differently.

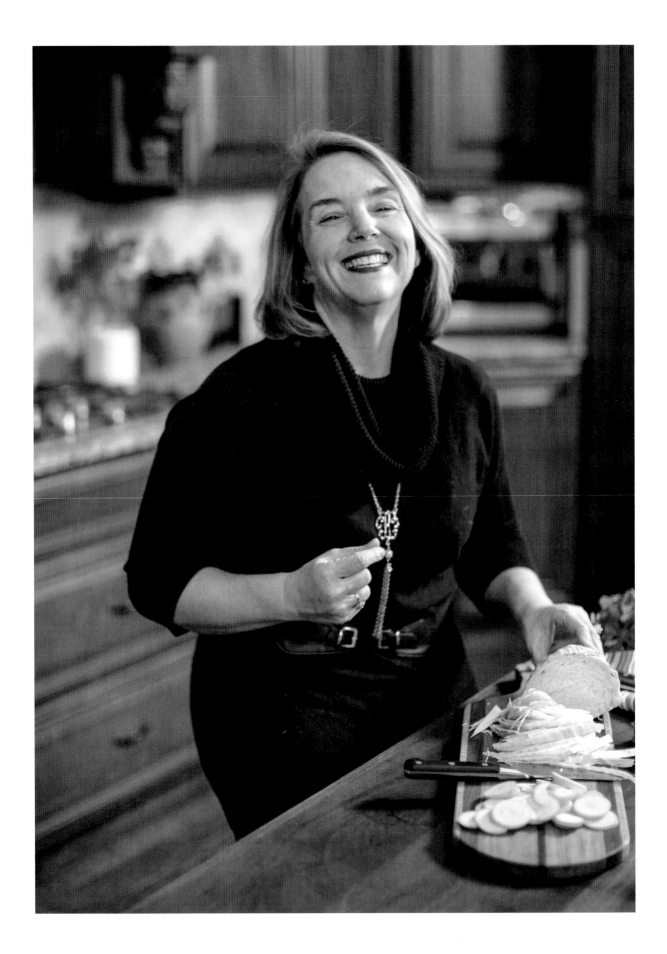

Chapter 1

How to Keto

"But why, Mom?" My children were born asking why. "Why won't you let us run through the mud puddle?" "Why can't we wear shorts in the winter?" "Why can't we buy everything we want?" Even though it's exhausting, David and I have always made the extra effort to explain to them why we won't allow something. Our hope is that they will learn to see that playing in a mud puddle is perfectly acceptable when you're at home where you can take a bath and put on clean clothes, but not a good idea when you're at a park and expect to ride home in Mom's clean car. As the children have grown, understanding why and how we, as parents, make decisions has helped them learn to make decisions for themselves. Because we know we can't be with them all the time and we want to see them grow into happy adults, we try to empower them with knowledge. Similarly, knowing "how to keto" will empower you.

Why a Ketogenic Diet Helped Me

I often refer to my experience of following a ketogenic diet as a journey. In the beginning, my primary "destination," or goal, was not better health; instead, I was desperate to lose weight. Somewhere along the way, though, I discovered that being morbidly obese was not the problem, but a symptom of poor overall health. Instead of treating the symptom, I had to understand the underlying issues that had caused the obesity. When I addressed those issues, the obesity resolved itself. As you consider keto, you may be looking for a way to lose weight. As you do, you too are likely to discover that weight loss is a wonderful side benefit to better overall health.

Quite simply, a ketogenic diet helped me because, as my dear friend said, "It ain't always about the calories." For decades, doctors and nutritionists told me to restrict calories. I was instructed to eat less and move more. If only I could control my eating and exercise, then I would be thin, be beautiful (I had "such a pretty face"), and live happily ever after.

To control calories, I avoided high-fat foods like bacon and full-fat dairy. My main sources of "nourishment" were wheat breads, crackers, and pretzels. I chose low-fat cheese and skim milk, and I nearly always ate my veggies with little or no added fat. My diet was naturally high in carbohydrates, moderate in protein, and very low in fat—exactly the opposite of what my body has thrived on since I started eating a ketogenic diet.

I was doing everything wrong in spite of trying desperately to get it right. Admittedly, I followed various low-fat and low-calorie diets intermittently. Because of constant hunger and feelings of deprivation, I rarely sustained any of these diets for more than six months at a time. Each failure left me feeling worse about myself and wondering what was wrong with me. Why couldn't I lose weight? I thought I must be weak, undisciplined, and/or suffering from a food addiction.

I've never met anyone who truly enjoys being obese. Obesity, and especially morbid obesity, is miserable. Physically keeping up with others is difficult. Going to dinner with friends is fraught with worrying over whether you will fit into a booth, ordering what others think you should eat rather than what you really want, and eating small portions in front of others only to indulge in a second meal later when you are alone because, yet again, you're hungry. You decline invitations to the movies or the theater because the seats might be too small to accommodate you. You avoid any activity that requires walking more than a short distance because you know that you will be out of breath, sweating, and anxious about others noticing all that you cannot do.

When you withdraw physically, you have less in common with other people; therefore, you may have a difficult time connecting or "fitting" socially. Being different can negatively impact your friendships. And there you are, alone in front of the refrigerator, looking for your fifth snack of the day just before bedtime.

Although I was morbidly obese and ate frequently, I was nearly always hungry. Until keto. The first three days of strictly following a ketogenic diet were the first days of my life when I wasn't hungry nearly every waking moment. The lack of appetite was striking. I was eating less food, yet my hunger had abated. How was this possible?

The magic had nothing to do with how many calories I was taking in. I was no longer hungry because my body was able to use the energy I was providing it, along with the energy from my own fat stores. The fat that had been locked in my cells was finally being released because my insulin levels were falling. My blood glucose (or blood sugar) was controlled because I was eating lots of fat, moderating protein, and severely restricting carbohydrates. As I stopped giving my body glucose (that is, carbohydrates), my body produced less insulin.

Insulin is a hoarder hormone that causes fat to be stored rather than used. Could *that* have been the root of my hunger? I was storing excess energy from food as fat, yet high levels of circulating insulin were keeping that energy locked away in my fat cells. I was obese yet still starving because my body could not use that stored energy.

As I ate high-fat and limited carbs, my blood glucose remained stable. I no longer experienced hypoglycemia, or low blood glucose. My body released less insulin. When I followed a low-fat diet, the carb-heavy foods I was eating raised my blood glucose levels. In order to metabolize that glucose, my body released insulin. The high levels of insulin caused fat to be stored rather than used. The less fat and the more carbs I ate, the less able my body was to use the energy, and that energy was stored as fat instead. I was fatter and hungrier as a result of having stored energy that I couldn't use.

High-carb meals also made my blood sugar levels fluctuate dramatically. The extreme highs triggered a cascade of insulin and other hormones, which resulted in extreme lows. The roller coaster of glucose metabolism resulted in inflammation, mood swings, and, yes, more hunger. While I was doing everything I was told to do on low-fat diets, I was actually making my body sicker. By eating small, frequent meals, as I was told to do to manage my hypoglycemia and boost my metabolism, I was keeping my blood glucose and circulating insulin high. Again, I was doing everything wrong when I was *trying* to do everything right.

At the time, I had no idea that I suffered from metabolic dysfunction. After all, I had normal-weight friends who ate the same low-fat granola bars, yogurt, and fresh fruit for breakfast; wore normal-sized clothing; and needed to eat only three meals per day. It became clear that while some people can metabolize carbohydrates efficiently, my body cannot. In their groundbreaking 2011 book *The Art and Science of Low Carbohydrate Living*, Stephen Phinney and Jeff Volek call this being "carbohydrate intolerant." When I limited my intake of total carbs to less than 20 grams per day, my body could efficiently metabolize the fat and protein I ate and then used my energy reserves as it needed to. Thus my blood glucose and hunger were effectively managed with my having done little more than choose bacon over bagels.

Even though I was obese for forty years, not one of my doctors ever tested my fasting insulin to look for insulin resistance, a hallmark of metabolic dysfunction. Insulin resistance occurs when the body doesn't respond to insulin signals even though the pancreas may be overproducing insulin in response to high blood glucose levels. It's as if the pancreas is trying to shout over a loud television by turning up the volume of insulin, yet the liver, muscles, and fat cells cannot hear or respond to the insulin that is being released in an attempt to lower blood glucose. Insulin resistance is often a precursor to diabetes and other serious health issues. Not one doctor had ever considered that I wasn't simply gorging on pastries twenty-four hours a day. They just reiterated at every visit that my weight was a problem, told me that I should lose weight, and then offered me the standard "move more, eat less" (and less fat) dogma.

I was a strong-willed, well-educated professional who despised being obese. Had their advice worked, why wouldn't I have followed it? If a low-fat diet was right for my body, why was it so difficult for me to follow? Why didn't it work for me? I would have done anything to lose weight, yet I could not succeed. With every failure, I questioned myself, when I should have been questioning the dietary advice I had been given.

What We Know About Food

In general, food is comprised of three macro-nutrients: fat, protein, and carbohydrate. Each one is metabolized differently, which simply means that the body's process for using the energy from each macronutrient varies.

Of those three macronutrients, carbohydrate is digested the most easily and is processed as sugar (glucose or fructose). Because carbs provide quick energy, they impact blood glucose faster than protein or fat, causing a spike in blood glucose after a meal. With that rise in blood glucose, the body must release insulin to bring it back down. As I said earlier, insulin is a hoarder hormone that stores excess glucose as body fat. Glucose can be stashed away in cells as fat but cannot be released from cells in the form of glucose. Once glucose is stored as fat, it can only be burned as fat through a process called *lipolysis.*

The second macronutrient is protein, which provides the body with essential amino acids. Protein is metabolized more slowly than carbo-hydrates, but it also elicits an insulin response. While carbs typically have the biggest impact on blood glucose within one hour of eating, large amounts of protein cause blood glucose to peak around two hours after a meal. Protein is the least efficient source of energy for the body because it must be converted to glucose before it can be used for fuel.

Fat is the third macronutrient. It provides essential fatty acids and carries fat-soluble vita-mins, like vitamin D, to cells. Of the three mac-ronutrients, fat impacts blood glucose the least. While fat is a very good fuel for the body, the body will use carbohydrate (glucose) first if it is available.

The body can use either fat or carbohy-drate as its primary source of fuel. If you fol-low a standard American diet based on the USDA's MyPlate model, then your body is pri-marily using glucose (from carbohydrates) for fuel. If you choose to follow a ketogenic diet that restricts carbs, your body will use fat for fuel instead. While there are several benefits to using fat as your primary energy source, one of the main advantages is that blood glucose is kept stable, resulting in lower insulin levels, which allows body fat to be released from cells. When you burn fat for fuel, the energy that is used is in the form of ketones (or ketone bod-ies), hence the name "ketogenic diet."

A person is considered to be "in keto-sis" when he or she is burning fat (more

Macronutrient Impact on Blood Glucose

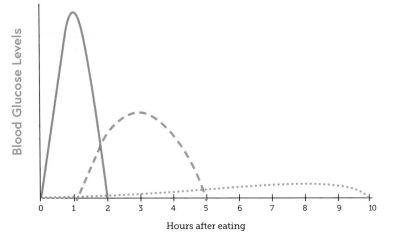

Blood Glucose Levels (y-axis)

Hours after eating (x-axis): 0 1 2 3 4 5 6 7 8 9 10

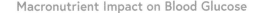

——— **90% to 100% of Carbohydrate Is Converted to Glucose.**
Carbohydrate causes blood glucose to peak 1 hour after eating. In healthy individuals, it returns to baseline 2 hours after eating.

– – – **50% of Protein Is Converted to Glucose.**
Protein impacts blood glucose to a lesser extent than carbohydrate; a high-protein meal causes blood glucose to peak 2 to 3 hours after eating.

· · · · · · **10% of Fat Is Converted to Glucose.**
Fat has a minimal impact on blood glucose when eaten with moderate protein and very little carbohydrate.

specifically, ketone bodies) for fuel. When the body is consistently starved of glucose over time, it adjusts to using fat, becoming "fat-adapted." For most people, it takes at least three weeks of consistent carbohydrate restriction to become fat-adapted. The first step is to eat very-low-carb and high-fat meals. Eating high-fat is especially important in the beginning as your body transitions from burning primarily glucose to burning fat. When you follow a ketogenic diet, you intentionally restrict carbohydrates at each meal, relying instead on high-fat, moderate-protein meals to keep your blood glucose stable. One way to determine the impact of a meal is to measure your blood glucose before eating (fasting), one hour postprandial (after eating), and again two hours postprandial. Ideally, your blood glucose should remain relatively unchanged one and two hours after eating. If it rises by more than fifteen points, then your body will have to release insulin to address the excess glucose.

In people who have type 2 diabetes or are insulin resistant, blood glucose remains high on a high-carb diet. In the case of type 2 diabetes, blood glucose can become uncontrolled because the beta cells of the pancreas produce less and less insulin. Blood glucose that consistently stays above 140 mg/dl causes significant inflammation and can result in organ damage. Type 1 diabetes is a condition in which the body does not make insulin at all. Both type 1 and type 2 diabetics have found that following a ketogenic diet can keep blood glucose stable and can help manage the disease. If you have been diagnosed with diabetes, please work with a medical professional to manage your medications when you begin a ketogenic diet. See pages 382 and 383 for a list of resources that might be helpful to you.

The following chart demonstrates the effects that meals with different macronutrient compositions are likely to have on blood glucose. Note that the high-carb meal affects blood glucose quickly and causes a surge of insulin. High levels of circulating insulin result in increased fat storage. The meal with more protein has a less-immediate impact on blood glucose; however, high protein still raises blood glucose and therefore insulin. The high-fat meal with moderate protein and very low carbs is the least likely to raise blood glucose. Keeping blood glucose stable and keeping levels of circulating insulin low allows for the release of stored fat from cells. When stored fat is used, hunger levels drop because your body is using stored fat for energy and doesn't need food to fuel it. The advantages of lower levels of circulating insulin include not only burning body fat and reducing hunger, but also lowering levels of inflammation throughout the body.

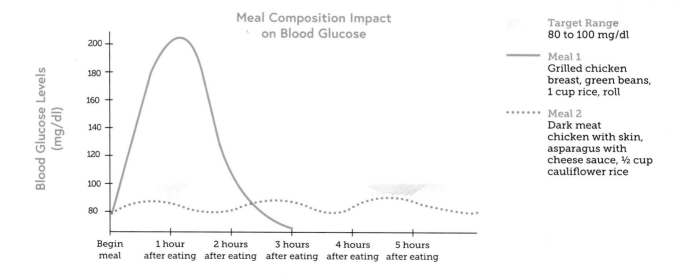

Meal Composition Impact on Blood Glucose

Blood Glucose Levels (mg/dl)

Target Range
80 to 100 mg/dl

Meal 1
Grilled chicken breast, green beans, 1 cup rice, roll

Meal 2
Dark meat chicken with skin, asparagus with cheese sauce, ½ cup cauliflower rice

Meal Composition

Although people on a ketogenic diet tend not to worry too much about counting calories, we do calculate the ratios of macronutrients in our meals based on the percentage of calories coming from each macronutrient.

By definition, on a classic ketogenic diet, roughly 75 percent of calories come from fat, 20 percent from protein, and 5 percent from carbohydrates. We think of these ratios as 75/20/5. Some people following certain medical protocols, such as those used to manage epilepsy or cancer, follow ratios with a higher fat target, such as 80 percent fat, 15 percent protein, and 5 percent carbohydrates, or 80/15/5. There are also less-restrictive ketogenic ratios that use 70 percent fat, 25 percent protein, and 5 percent carbohydrates, or 70/25/5.

Finding the ratio that works best for you can be a process of trial and error. Some people report achieving and staying in ketosis with fat as low as 60 percent, protein as high as 30 percent, and carbohydrates lower than 10 percent. Your ideal ratio depends on your metabolic health, age, gender, activity level, and other factors. A young male who is metabolically healthy, has a lean body mass, and exercises regularly, for example, can generally eat higher ratios of protein and carbohydrates than an older female with metabolic dysfunction who lives a sedentary lifestyle.

All that being said, many people find a safe zone by sticking to ketogenic ratios of 70 percent or more calories from fat, fewer than 25 percent from protein, and fewer than 5 percent from carbohydrate. The exact percentages are less important than simply following a ketogenic diet consistently and sticking close to these ratios in every meal or snack.

In practical terms, what does it mean to get 75 percent of your calories from fat, 20 percent from protein, and 5 percent from carbohydrates? Keep in mind that 1 gram of fat equals 9 calories, whereas 1 gram of protein or carbohydrate equals 4 calories. Gram for gram, fat naturally contributes a higher proportion of calories. To illustrate, suppose we have a meal that is made up of 40 grams of fat, 25 grams of protein, and 5 grams of carbohydrate.

Classic Ketogenic Ratios

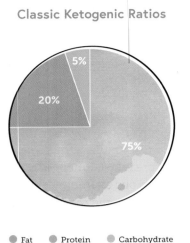

5%

20%

75%

● Fat   ● Protein   ● Carbohydrate

40 grams of fat contribute 360 calories:

40 grams of fat x 9 calories per gram = 360 calories

25 grams of protein contribute 100 calories:

25 grams of protein x 4 calories per gram = 100 calories

5 grams of carbohydrate contribute 20 calories:

5 grams of carbohydrate x 4 calories per gram = 20 calories

So the total calories in our meal is 480 (360 + 100 + 20). Fat makes up 360 of those 480 calories, or 75 percent. Protein makes up 100 of those 480 calories, or 20.8 percent. Carbohydrate makes up 20 of those 480 calories, or 4.2 percent. These ratios are nearly perfect and should keep your blood glucose stable and keep hunger at bay for four to six hours or longer.

You may be wondering what kinds of foods have these kinds of ratios. One of my favorite meals—for breakfast, lunch, or dinner—is a simple and delicious example of just how easy it is to create a ketogenic meal. A ¼-pound hamburger made with 80/20 (or 80 percent lean) ground beef, topped with two strips of bacon, one sunny-side-up egg, two slices of tomato, and a tablespoon of mayonnaise, is a perfect keto meal. The ratios are 75 percent calories from fat (46.6 grams), 23 percent from protein (31.7 grams), and 2 percent from carbs (2.6 grams).

With the carbs this low, you could top your burger with a few sliced jalapeños, a leaf or two of lettuce, or a few slices of peeled cucumber.

Using the USDA Food Composition Database and the nutrition labels on the specific products I purchase, here is the macronutrient breakdown for the ingredients in this meal:

Food	Weight	Carbs	Protein	Fat	Cal from Carbs	Cal from Protein	Cal from Fat
¼-pound hamburger patty	4 ounces	0g	19.4g	22.6g	0	78	203
2 strips bacon	0.6 ounce	0g	5.8g	7g	0	23	63
1 large egg	1.8 ounces	0.4g	6g	5g	2	24	45
2 slices tomato, about ½ inch thick	1.9 ounces	2g	0.5g	0g	8	2	0
1 tablespoon mayonnaise	0.5 ounce	0g	0g	12g	0	0	108
Totals		2.4g	31.7g	46.6g	10	127	419

¼-Pound Burger with Bacon, Egg, Mayo, and Tomato

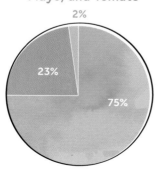

2%

23%

75%

● Fat ● Protein ● Carbohydrate

With 75 percent of calories from fat and just 2 percent from carbohydrates, this balanced ketogenic meal is likely to keep blood glucose stable. Protein remains moderate at 23 percent. If you wanted to reduce the amount of protein, you could omit the egg.

If you don't want to worry about calculating the percentage of calories coming from each macronutrient, you can use a simple formula that begins with number of grams of carbohydrate in a given meal. I find that I need to restrict carbs to fewer than 7 grams per meal in order to keep my blood glucose stable and remain in ketosis. I count total carbohydrates—that is, I do not subtract fiber from the carb count to calculate net carbs.

If you want to use this formula, you'll need to determine your personal carbohydrate target for each meal. Most people remain in ketosis when they eat 7 or fewer grams of carbs per meal. You may choose to eat as many as 12 grams of carbs per meal; however, when you raise fat and protein proportionally, you will find that you are eating a lot of food—probably more than your body wants. Use the examples below to set your carb threshold per meal. Remember that you can eat more fat than your target, but you want to avoid eating more protein or carbs than your target.

To ensure that your meals follow ketogenic ratios, the number of fat grams in each meal should be a minimum of seven times the number of carbohydrate grams in each meal. The maximum amount of protein you want to eat is five times the amount of carbohydrates.

For example, if your meal has 6 grams of carbohydrate, then you want to aim for a minimum of 42 grams of fat (6 grams of carbs x 7 = 42 grams of fat). To calculate your protein target, multiply the number of grams of carbohydrate by 5. In this example, 6 grams of carbs x 5 = 30; therefore, you would want to eat less than 30 grams of protein.

So your meal would include

- at least 42 grams of fat

- less than 30 grams of protein

- 6 grams of carbohydrate

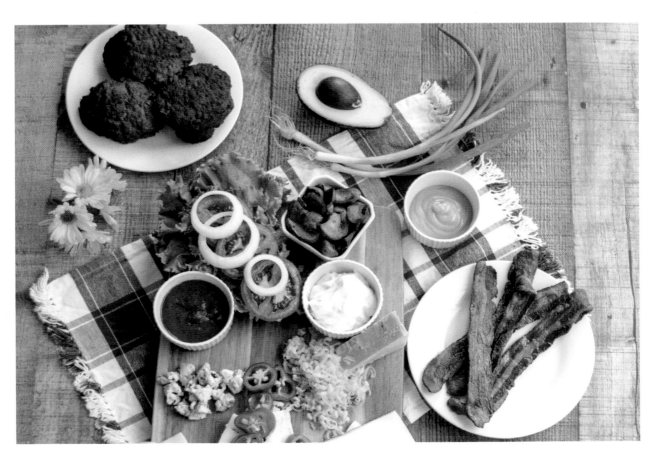

Let's consider another example with lower carbohydrates. Suppose the carbs in your lunch total 3 grams. Therefore, fat should be at least 21 grams (3 grams of carbs x 7 = 21 grams of fat), and protein should be less than 15 grams (3 grams of carbs x 5 = 15 grams of protein). Although hunger is diminished on keto, that is not a very big meal. If you find yourself hungrier than that, simply increase the fat and protein by an equal number of grams. In other words, if you eat an additional 5 grams of protein, increase the fat by 5 grams as well. Doing so would bring the meal to 26 grams of fat, 20 grams of protein, and 3 grams of carbohydrate, with ketogenic ratios of 71 percent fat, 25 percent protein, and 4 percent carbohydrate. If you increased the protein by 10 grams to a total of 25 grams, then you would increase the fat by 10 grams as well, to a total of 31 grams. The meal then would have ratios of 71 percent fat, 26 percent protein, and 3 percent carbohydrate.

Here are a few additional examples of ketogenic meals.

Breakfast can be as simple as eggs cooked in butter, served with bacon (below left). Omitting the butter (below right) would reduce the fat in this meal to 27.5 grams, making fat nearly even with protein. Leaving out the butter also would reduce the calories from fat to 69 percent and increase the calories from protein to 30 percent. Making simple changes to your meal, such as adding butter, coconut oil, or bacon fat, can help you keep your fat ratios high.

Eggs and Bacon with Butter

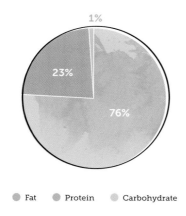

Food	Weight	Carbs	Protein	Fat
2 large eggs	3.5 ounces	0.8g	12g	10g
5 strips bacon	1.4 ounces	0g	14.5g	17.5g
1 tablespoon butter	0.5 ounce	0g	0g	11g
Totals		0.8g	26.5g	38.5g

Eggs and Bacon without Butter

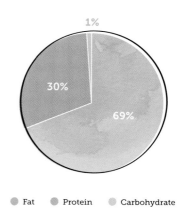

Food	Weight	Carbs	Protein	Fat
2 large eggs	3.5 ounces	0.8g	12g	10g
5 strips bacon	1.4 ounces	0g	14.5g	17.5g
Totals		0.8g	26.5g	27.5g

Although I rarely ate chicken wings before I started eating a ketogenic diet, my family and I enjoy them fairly frequently now. David makes them in the smoker, or I cook them quickly in the oven. Because chicken wings have slightly less fat than protein, we toss them in bacon fat before cooking them and typically serve them with a high-fat homemade dressing like blue cheese or ranch, with just a little bit of celery for crunch. (See page 259 for my Roasted Chicken Wings recipe and page 213 for my Blue Cheese Dressing recipe.) This meal gets 70 percent of its calories from fat, 27 percent from protein, and 3 percent from carbohydrates.

Another of my favorite dinners is salmon with butter and broccoli with homemade Alfredo sauce. Although salmon is a fatty fish that is relatively high in healthy omega-3 fats, the meal still needs the added fats from the butter and Alfredo sauce to maintain ketogenic ratios.

Notice the vegetables that are included in these examples. There is essentially one vegetable side in each meal, and the amount is limited to 3.5 ounces. Traditional diets treat vegetables as "free" foods, so you may never have considered them as a source of carbohydrates. To stay within ketogenic ratios, though, you will need to limit your vegetable intake. Think of vegetables as a vehicle for fat. Not only does fat make the vegetables more palatable, but it also helps you keep your macros balanced. In these examples, the celery is dipped in fatty blue cheese dressing, and the broccoli is smothered in Alfredo sauce.

Chicken Wings with Blue Cheese and Celery

3%
27%
70%

● Fat ● Protein ● Carbohydrate

Food	Weight	Carbs	Protein	Fat
6 chicken wings	5.3 ounces	0g	30g	26g
¼ cup blue cheese dressing	2 ounces	0.8g	4.3g	15.7g
2 stalks celery	3.5 ounces	3g	0.7g	0.2g
Totals		3.8g	35g	41.9g

Salmon with Broccoli, Alfredo, and Butter

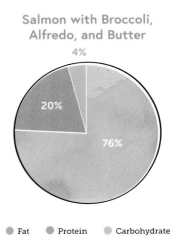

4%
20%
76%

● Fat ● Protein ● Carbohydrate

Food	Weight	Carbs	Protein	Fat
Salmon fillet	3.5 ounces	0g	19.8g	6.3g
3 spears broccoli	3.5 ounces	5.8g	1.2g	0g
½ cup Alfredo sauce	4 ounces	1.3g	10.7g	36.3g
1 tablespoon butter	0.5 ounce	0g	0g	11g
Totals		7.1g	31.7g	53.6g

Portion Sizes

The nutrition information for these meals is accurate only if the portion sizes are kept the same. In the salmon meal, for example, the salmon fillet weighs 3.5 ounces, or about 100 grams. Most salmon fillets that you purchase in stores or order in restaurants are larger. The fillet pictured in the photo below, for example, weighs 4.8 ounces, or about 133.2 grams. If you ate this entire fillet, you would have consumed 26.4 grams of protein and 8.4 grams of fat. The additional 6.6 grams of protein isn't a lot but would push you close to 40 grams of protein for the meal, which would be a lot for me. (Your target ratios might be different.) Please be mindful of portion sizes, especially for carbohydrates and protein.

Using a food scale to educate yourself about portion sizes can be very helpful. Even if you disdain the idea of weighing and measuring food (like I do!), a scale will teach you a lot about serving sizes. On the following pages, I've included some photos of foods weighed in ounces. Keep in mind that 3.5 ounces, equivalent to about 100 grams, is considered a standard serving size. When you look at the carb counts in some vegetables or the amounts of protein in some meats, however, you may find that a full 100-gram serving is too much for you.

When I weigh food, I typically weigh it uncooked. I then use the USDA Food Composition Database or the information on the product's nutrition label to ascertain the macronutrients. If you can, use the nutrition information on the label; otherwise, the USDA database is the most reliable resource I have found.

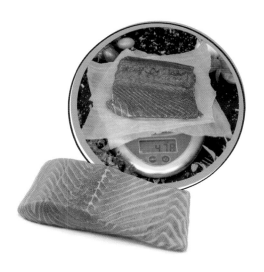

Salmon fillet, 3.5 ounces:
19.8 grams of protein, 6.3 grams of fat

Salmon fillet, 4.8 ounces:
26.4 grams of protein, 8.4 grams of fat

Watch Out for Fractional Carbs!

A word of caution with regard to carbohydrates: Food manufacturers often fail to report fractional carbs. For example, heavy cream has less than 1 gram of carbohydrate per tablespoon, so some nutrition labels list it as 0 grams. The problem comes in when you make a recipe with ½ cup of cream, or when you get heavy-handed and add ¼ cup of cream to your coffee. With carbs estimated at 0.5 gram per tablespoon, ¼ cup (4 tablespoons) of cream has 2 grams of carbohydrate, and ½ cup has 4 grams. When you are limiting carbs to 7 grams per meal, you need to know if you're drinking 2 of those 7 grams!

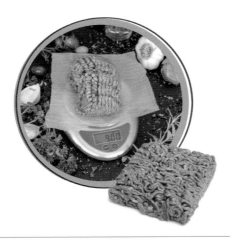

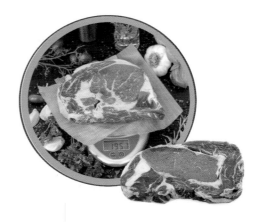

This photo shows 9 ounces of raw ground beef, which is slightly more than two precooked servings. One 4-ounce serving (¼ pound) has 22.6 grams of fat and 19.4 grams of protein.

A rib-eye steak is often my entree of choice when eating out. A 3.5-ounce serving packs 19.5 grams of protein, 11.4 grams of fat, and 1.8 grams of carbs. The photo shows a gorgeous 20-ounce rib-eye steak, which yields more than five standard servings! This entire steak provides 64.6 grams of fat, 110.3 grams of protein, and 9.9 grams of carbohydrates. If I ate even half of it, I would have consumed my entire protein allotment for the day. A more reasonable portion is around 5.5 ounces, or about a quarter of this steak, which would provide about 17 grams of fat, 30 grams of protein, and 2.7 grams of carbohydrates. Yes, meat can have carbs, even without marinades or sugary sauces. You learn that by looking up the nutrition information. Once you make a habit of doing so, you will quickly learn the appropriate serving sizes of the foods you eat often.

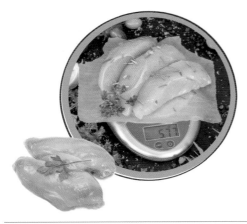

Boneless, skinless chicken breast is high in protein and low in fat. A 3-ounce serving has 19.1 grams of protein and 2.2 grams of fat. The photo shows three chicken breast tenders, which is a typical portion size. But these three tenders weigh 5.7 ounces, which is more than double the amount that many of us should be eating at one time. If you ate all this chicken, you would have eaten 33.5 grams of protein and only 3.9 grams of fat. Because you want to limit protein on a ketogenic diet, you would need to limit other sources of protein in this meal. You would also need to add a fatty sauce or marinade to the chicken and include a high-fat side item, such as broccoli with bacon, cheese, and butter.

Even if you don't weigh or measure your meats, you *do* want to learn appropriate vegetable serving sizes. Carbohydrates from vegetables can add up quickly if you aren't cautious about portion control. While many people think that vegetables can't "make you fat," too much of the wrong vegetables can make it difficult for you to remain in ketosis.

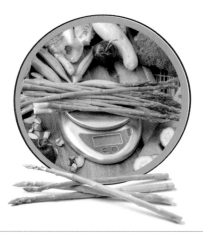

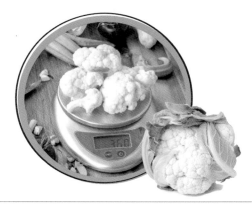

This photo shows about 3.5 ounces of raw asparagus. If you ate this entire amount, you would have eaten 3.9 grams of carbohydrate and 2.2 grams of protein. (Yes, some vegetables have protein, too!) A typical serving size for me is about half this amount, making asparagus a great low-carb option at less than 2 grams of carbs per serving. I like to combine it with other low-carb vegetables in stir-fries, omelets, and frittatas to add flavor and variety without adding a lot of carbs.

Cauliflower is a popular low-carb vegetable. Not unlike cabbage, it is easy to overconsume, especially when riced or pureed. One medium head of cauliflower (5 to 6 inches in diameter) with the inedible portions removed weighs about 20.7 ounces. The entire edible head has 29.2 grams of carbs, 11.3 grams of protein, and 1.7 grams of fat. To keep carbs low, you should get at least six servings from one medium head of cauliflower. The photo shows a 3.6-ounce serving, which has 5 grams of carbs, 0.3 gram of protein, and 0.3 gram of fat.

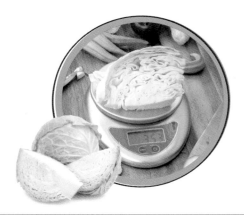

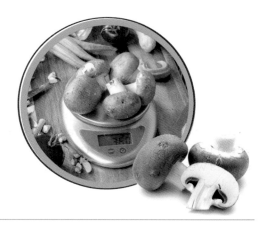

Cabbage is one of those vegetables that, when cooked, reduces quite a bit. While it is low in carbs, portion control is really important. You can see in the photo that a 3.5-ounce serving, which has 1.3 grams of protein and 5.8 grams of carbs, is a small fraction of a medium-sized head of cabbage. For reference, one whole medium head of cabbage (roughly 5¾ inches in diameter) has an estimated 52.7 grams of carbohydrate and 11.6 grams of protein. To keep carbs low, one medium head should yield at least eight servings.

In terms of low-carb value, mushrooms are fantastic! One serving, or about five whole mushrooms, gives you 3.3 grams of carbs, 3 grams of protein, and 0.3 gram of fat. Even better, mushrooms are very filling and tend to absorb fat as they cook. I love to sauté mushrooms in a skillet with plenty of butter or bacon fat. They are also excellent roasted.

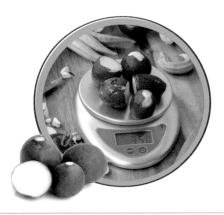

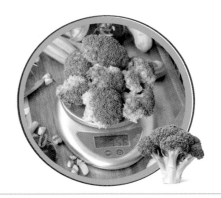

Radishes make a nice substitute for potatoes when roasted or stewed. One serving (roughly five whole radishes) adds only 3.4 grams of carbs, less than 1 gram of protein, and a trace amount of fat to your plate. You can also grate radishes and cook them like hash browns. The longer you cook them and the more fat you add, the better they taste and the healthier they become!

While I've heard it said that no one ever got fat from eating broccoli, the truth is that broccoli does have carbs. If you're carbohydrate intolerant like I am, then eating too much broccoli *can* be a bad thing. One 3.5-ounce serving—approximately seven florets (or three 5-inch spears)—has 6.6 grams of carbs, 2.8 grams of protein, and 0.4 gram of fat. Restaurants often serve double this amount as a side. To manage carb creep, I tend to eat only two small spears and top those with butter, Simple Cheese Sauce (page 199), or Creamy Alfredo Sauce (page 204).

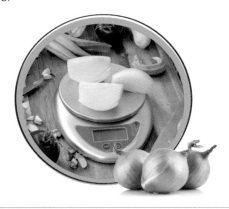

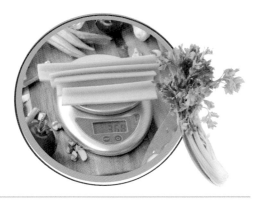

Although I love onions, I often have to remind myself that they pack a lot of natural sugars. Like most vegetables that grow underground, onions are higher in carbs than leafy vegetables. One serving of onions has 9.3 grams of carbs! That is more carbs than I eat in a whole meal. (This serving of onions also has 1 gram of protein and a trace amount of fat.) To keep carbs in check, you could eat only half a serving. Also be aware that cooked onions have less volume than raw onions even though the carb count stays the same; therefore, be very cautious when cooking with onions or including cooked onions on your plate. The carbs can add up quickly!

Celery is considered a classic diet food. While it isn't terribly high in carbs, keep in mind that one serving, or roughly four 6-inch pieces, has 3 grams of carbs, 0.7 gram of protein, and 0.2 gram of fat. Instead of adding peanut butter, which can push you over your carb limit quickly, you might want to dip your celery in a high-fat dressing like blue cheese (page 213) or ranch (page 209).

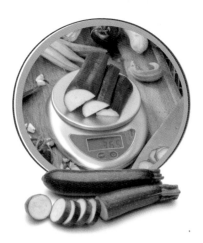

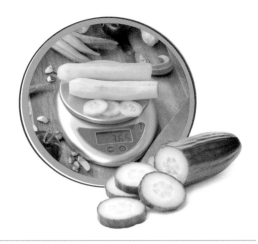

Zucchini is a good low-carb option as long as you keep portions in mind. One serving is about half of one medium-sized zucchini, which gives you 3 grams of carbs, 1.2 grams of protein, and a trace amount of fat. Like cauliflower, the biggest mistake people make with zucchini is boiling it down or shredding it and then losing sight of what constitutes a true serving.

Cucumber is one of my favorites. I love the crisp crunch and fresh, summery taste. One serving has 3.6 grams of carbs, 0.7 gram of protein, and a trace amount of fat. But wait! That's for a cucumber *with* the peel. If you remove the peel, you can have the same amount of cucumber with only 2.2 grams of carbs and 0.6 gram of protein. If you worry about carb creep as I do, then peeling your cucumbers is a wise move.

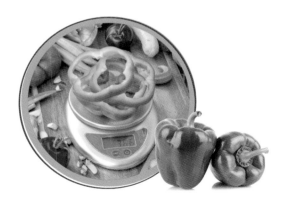

Green bell peppers provide a lot of flavor in small amounts. One serving, which is a lot of bell pepper, has 4.6 grams of carbs, less than 1 gram of protein, and a trace amount of fat. I tend to use just one serving of bell pepper in an entire recipe to add flavor and crunch while minimizing carbs. Keep in mind that red bell peppers (6 grams of carbs) and yellow bell peppers (6.3 grams of carbs) are higher in carbs than green ones.

Determining Your Personal Macronutrient Targets

How do you determine your personal macros? How many carbs can you eat? How much protein is enough for you? How many grams of fat should you eat? That depends. There are dozens of macro calculators available online. Some are tailored to ketogenic ratios and others are not. The primary disadvantage of using a macro calculator is that none of them can account for individual factors such as age, gender, activity level, metabolic health, and lean body mass.

Let's compare me to my longtime friend Bill. I am insulin resistant. I was obese from the time I was three years old until the time I was forty-five. During that forty-two-year span, I was simply overweight for a few years, with several cycles of losing significant amounts of weight, gaining more weight, and losing again. I am a female with a fairly sedentary lifestyle. For me, "working out" is laughing with friends or playing with my family. The only time I run is when I "run to the store." I do well at 20 grams of total carbs per day. More than 7 grams of total carbs in one meal is likely to spike my blood glucose, but it varies by the ingredients in the meal, the time of day, and other factors. I also have hypothyroidism and very low levels of leptin. (Leptin signals to the body as to whether enough fat is stored, regulates hunger, and influences metabolic rate. Low levels of leptin signal that fat stores are low and warn the brain that we are at risk of starvation.) My percentage of body fat is around 25.

Bill is very lean, with roughly 10 percent body fat. He has never been overweight. He spends a minimum of an hour in the gym every single day. He has a desk job but makes an effort to be as active as he can, such as by walking his dog and walking at lunchtime. He is also a competitive athlete. He has no remarkable labs.

Both of us follow a ketogenic diet, but our macro targets are very different. My body is inefficient when it comes to metabolizing food, as evidenced by my issues with leptin, thyroid, insulin resistance, and so on, so I have to be extremely careful with my carb count. Bill's athletic body is highly efficient, so his caloric intake and carbohydrate intake exceed mine. He can safely eat up to 50 grams of total carbs a day. If I ate like he does, I would likely weigh more than 250 pounds again. Even at 30 grams of carbs per day, I get terrible food cravings. Could Bill eat as I do? He could, but he would likely be hungry and lose more weight than he would like. Yet we both follow a ketogenic diet using macros that fit our personal needs.

Through some trial and error, you can find the macros that work best for you. Links to physicians' specific low-carb, high-fat guidelines are included in the Resources section on pages 382 and 383.

Even if you don't aim for specific macro targets at every meal, you still need to be aware of how many grams of carbs, protein, and fat are in the foods you're eating. Before keto, I was one of those people who had never really thought about food in terms of macronutrients. I ate until I felt full, until my plate was clean, or until I had met my calorie limit (if I was on a calorie-restricted diet at the time). On a ketogenic diet, the focus is not on calories, but on macros and hunger. When I put a meal together, I focus primarily on total carbs, keeping them below 7 grams. Next, I try to ensure that the fat grams are higher than the protein grams. Rarely do I weigh or measure food to determine portion sizes now that I intuitively know what a true serving size looks like for most of the foods I eat. Getting a sense of appropriate serving sizes is a really important part of learning how to keep carbs low, fat high, and protein moderate.

If all the math makes your head hurt a little, simply focus on keeping carbohydrates low in the beginning. You can still be successful. In fact, for the first six months, I counted only total carbohydrate grams. I did not calculate ratios, nor did I worry about fat or protein grams. When you restrict your total carbohydrate intake to fewer than 20 grams, your body has no choice but to burn fat, which means that you are in ketosis. The single most important thing you can do is to consistently keep carbs low. You also want to avoid sugar, especially fructose (found in fruit and in foods sweetened with high-fructose corn syrup, such as tomato-based products, salad dressings, dips, and condiments), and eat high fat. Your eating plan can be just that simple.

Exogenous Ketones

Exogenous ketones (also known as ketone supplements) are ketones made outside of the body and ingested, as opposed to the ketones that your body produces when it is burning fat. While there is research showing that exogenous ketones may be therapeutically beneficial for some medical therapies such as cancer and epilepsy, exogenous ketones are not necessary for weight loss. Arguably, exogenous ketones are unnecessary when you have body fat to burn. Exogenous ketones will be used by the body first instead of using fuel from stored body fat.

While some people rely on macro calculators, I prefer to use my internal gauges to determine how much protein and fat I need. On days when I feel more physically hungry, I choose foods that are higher in fat and lower in carbs. When I eat more than 10 grams of total carbs per meal, I tend to feel sluggish. I also get hungry within two to three hours after eating, and my cravings for higher-carb foods are worse. Through trial and error, I have determined that keeping total carbs below 7 grams per meal works best for me. Protein, for me, works best at a range of 10 to 35 grams per meal. If I eat more than 35 grams, I feel sluggish within two hours. If I eat fewer than 10 grams, I crave protein. While fat per meal varies, I am generally satisfied at roughly 60 grams, and I make sure to keep fat grams higher than protein grams.

To determine whether a ketogenic meal has the right macronutrient ratios for your body, look for two telltale signs. The first is a lack of hunger. A meal that is very low in carbs, moderate in protein, and high in fat should keep you satiated for four to six hours or longer. If you find yourself hungry within a few hours of eating, then your meal probably needed more fat. The second sign is your energy level after eating. If I find myself feeling tired or sleepy within one to two hours after eating, then I know I need to evaluate what I ate. Feeling tired or sleepy after eating often means that my insulin is high. That meal may have had too many carbs (an extremely rare occurrence for me) or too much protein and not enough fat. When I have had "enough" fat and protein, my energy level remains stable after eating. On keto, the nefarious afternoon slump should be gone for good. If you're concerned about how a particular food or meal is impacting your blood glucose, using a monitor is often a helpful way to know for certain whether your blood glucose has been affected. Follow the guidance on pages 101 and 102 for testing your blood glucose before and after a meal. Over time, you will know whether you're eating the "right" foods by looking at your long-term results.

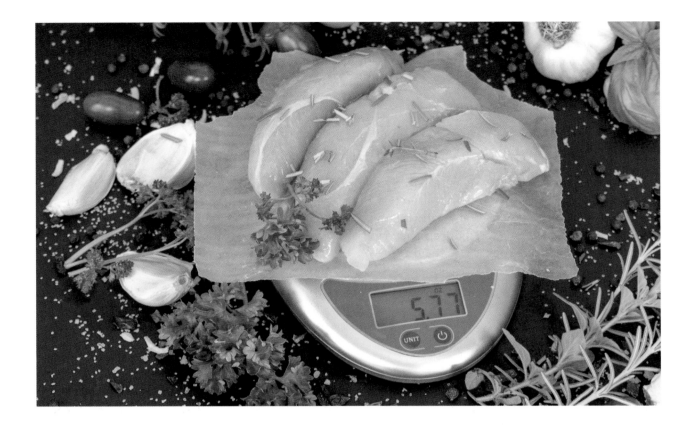

A Few Words About Hunger

Most of us with a history of obesity have been dogged by hunger our entire lives. We fear hunger because we know firsthand how miserable it can be. We've gone to bed hungry and woken hungry. We've battled hunger in every way possible. In the past, I tried so many tricks to stave off hunger, such as drinking a full glass of water at least thirty minutes before a meal, undergoing acupuncture, eating small, frequent meals, taking over-the-counter medications and prescription meds, and eating in front of a mirror. None of them worked. Even though I fought to control it, hunger always had control over me. I always considered it the worst part of dieting, but I also thought hunger was a necessary part of losing weight.

Keep in mind that the hunger you've fought your entire life is primarily physiological. Hunger is influenced by a lot of factors, many of which are not fully understood. Researchers believe that there is a complex interplay of hormones such as insulin, leptin, ghrelin, motilin, and thyroid hormones. The gut-brain axis is also not well understood but is believed to be an important player in the regulation of hunger. If you are obese or morbidly obese, it stands to reason that your body's hunger signals are dysfunctional. If your body, like mine, is carbohydrate intolerant, which interferes with insulin signaling, then it also seems reasonable that your hunger signaling is dysfunctional.

Hunger was nearly always the reason I could not sustain diets in the past. On keto, for the first time in my life, my hunger is finally tamed. Hunger used to be this wild, angry animal that dictated my actions every minute of the day. Suddenly the beast walked beside me, and I eventually learned to tame it as my body healed and the hormones that regulate hunger normalized. With your hunger tamed, you can use it as your onboard gauge. Hunger is how your body communicates with you about its energy needs, and it should take precedence over any macro calculator or chart. Once you begin to eat very-low-carb and high-fat, you will be able to trust your hunger signals to decide whether your meals are right for you. Eventually, you will be able to trust your hunger signals to decide when to eat.

One way to use hunger as a gauge, especially during the first few weeks of keto, is to use it to determine whether the foods you're eating are "right." Within the first week, most people are amazed at how their hunger levels have subsided. Some even worry that they aren't eating enough! If you're like me, your body is simply using its own fat stores, so it doesn't have to constantly ask for more fuel. If you're hungry—truly physically hungry—then you should eat, especially early on as your body is becoming fat-adapted. I always caution that if you're constantly hungry, then you're doing it wrong. You should not be physically hungry if you eat ketogenic meals that have the right macronutrient ratios for your body.

Another important component of identifying true physical hunger is minimizing processed foods. When we eat real foods from animals and plants and as close to the source as possible, we are more likely to avoid problematic food additives that exacerbate hunger and cause inflammation at the cellular level.

Notice that I talk about *physical* hunger. Most people find that the biggest challenge to managing hunger is differentiating true physical hunger from the desire to eat for other reasons. While much of hunger has a physiological basis, years of dysfunction can contribute to the development of unhealthy emotional attachments to food or at the very least to habits that have little to do with physical hunger. In the first few weeks on keto, you may find yourself eating breakfast at the same time you always have simply because that is your routine. You may find that you no longer need to snack, yet the smell of coffee in the breakroom at work might trigger you to reach for a snack as you grab a cup. You might also struggle with the timing of shared meals, especially if others are hungry and you are not. Before eating, you may need to ask yourself, "Is this hunger or habit?"

Cravings pose another barrier to recognizing true hunger, especially in the beginning. Sugar is highly addictive. Not many people transition from burning glucose to burning fat without at least a little struggle. Earlier I described the cravings that hit me in week two and nearly threw me off course. I managed those cravings with a low-carb, high-fat peanut butter cookie (see page 374 for the recipe), but I might have done just as well if I had fought those cravings with bacon. In fact, had I known then what I know now, I would have increased the amount of fat in my diet instead of making peanut butter cookies. True physical cravings and hunger are often best satisfied with fat. Fat is self-limiting because eating too much of it can make you feel nauseated or suffer diarrhea.

Stress eating is another challenge related to recognizing hunger. Once you learn to identify true physical hunger, you will be better able to recognize when you are wanting to eat to fill an emotional need, not a physical one. (See the section "Avoiding Emotional Eating" on pages 104 and 105 for more on combating stress eating.)

Learning to manage hunger is one of the single most important reasons I've been able to sustain keto long term. Ironically, one of the biggest criticisms I've heard from my own physicians is that this way of eating isn't sustainable. For me, no longer being hungry is the primary reason I have been able to follow a ketogenic plan since June 2013. When I am hungry, my body wants fat, and I eat high-fat foods until I am satisfied. When I am not hungry, I simply do not eat. Finally, I can rely on my own body to know the difference.

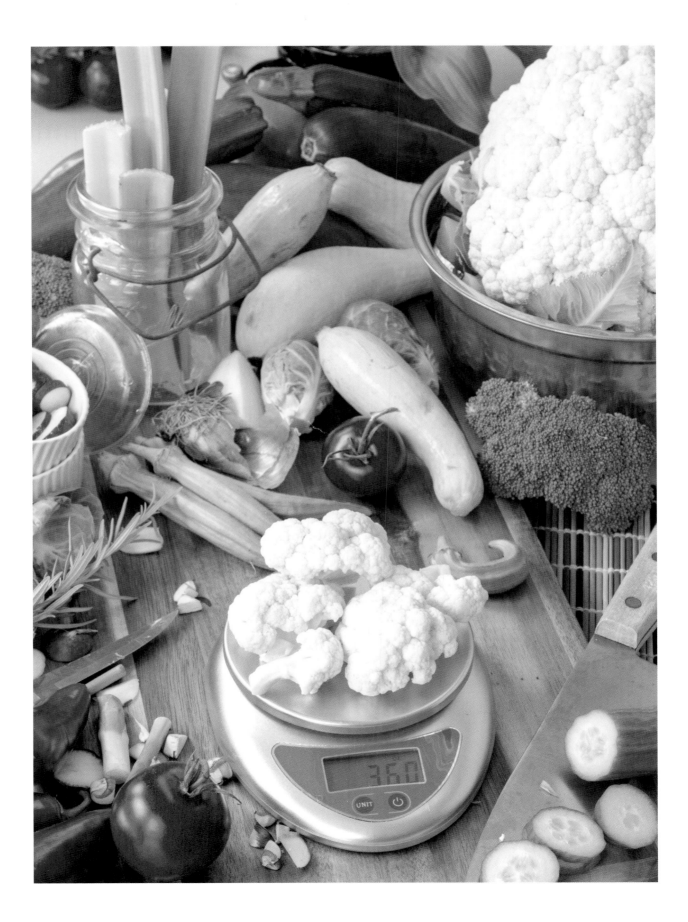

Chapter 2

The Food

Before keto, my kitchen was full of processed foods. My family ate from the freezer—breaded chicken tenders, frozen lasagna, and "diet" meals were standards for us. The fridge was stocked with low-fat milk for cereal and "healthy" juice for the kids. I kept canned veggies and fruits on hand as well as an endless supply of low-fat granola bars. The children snacked on crackers of all sorts, low-fat microwave popcorn, and packaged cookies. Muffins, brownies, and pancakes were frequently made from store-bought mixes. Ironically, many of my children's friends considered those treats "homemade" because I added eggs and oil and baked them myself.

Like many of yours probably do, my "recipes" began with a can of cream of something soup, a packet of seasonings, or a package of Cool Whip, powdered gelatin, or pudding mix. If I was "being good" and following a traditional calorie-restricted diet, I would buy the low-fat versions of those items. However, much of this stuff that we call food isn't really food, but foodlike products engineered by food scientists.

Because of our busy lifestyle, my family faced two primary challenges when switching to keto. The first was learning to eat real food—whole, unprocessed or minimally processed food that comes from plants and animals. A major part of this challenge was figuring out how to replace those convenient but highly processed packaged foods that had been staples for us. If we couldn't grab Pop-Tarts, granola bars, or low-fat (and sugar-filled) yogurt for breakfast, then what would we eat? Eggs are a great keto breakfast option, but our favorite egg casseroles had bread in them! Also, egg dishes aren't as quick as the grab-and-go items that we relied on.

I'll admit that I tried all the shortcuts that I believed were low-carb. I bought *cases* of Atkins bars, Quest bars, and premade sugar-free Jell-O, along with sugar-free Cool Whip, sugar-free pudding mixes, and whey protein powder drinks. I stocked up on sugar-free candies and "low-carb" wraps—which are not actually low-carb! When I ate those things, though, I stopped losing weight. Sometimes I even *gained* weight.

It took me months to figure it out. What I began to notice was that during the week, when I used those convenience products, my hunger was worse than it was when I took time to prepare my own meals from meats and vegetables on the weekends. Eventually, I realized that after eating those products, I had a heavy, tired feeling followed by hunger and then no progress on the scale. When I ate real food, that didn't happen. What I didn't yet understand was that the wheat, food starches, artificial sweeteners, and seed oils in those products were a problem for me. They spiked my blood glucose and/or raised my insulin and contributed to inflammation. When I avoided those things, I felt better. My hunger and cravings were more controlled, and I lost weight. It was no accident.

Now I understand that ingredients matter, and I do my best to follow what I call "clean" keto. For me, clean keto means not eating food that *has* ingredients, but eating food that *is* ingredients. I focus on vegetables in their purest forms, such as spinach leaves and whole heads of cauliflower. These are foods that I could (at least in theory) find in my garden. The same is true for animal foods. I generally avoid meat that is precooked or has added ingredients, such as a marinade. I can buy fresh meat and season and cook it myself. Ask yourself whether your great-grandparents would recognize something as food. A Pop-Tart? No way. A plate of bacon and eggs? Yes, please!

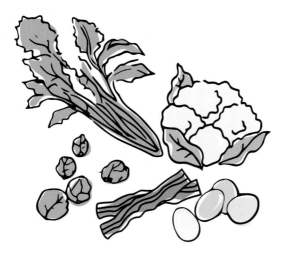

"Low-Carb" Doesn't Always Mean Low-Carb

Food manufacturers frequently add fiber to their "low-carb" products to lower the net carb count. The danger in this practice is that the fiber doesn't necessarily blunt the carb impact of those products; therefore, blood glucose can be impacted. Too often these packaged convenience foods derail people who are trying to follow a ketogenic diet.

Is it convenient? Not always. Are there short-cuts? I *have* found a few tips and tricks that make it easier. Meal planning and prepping one day a week has been my salvation. (See "Meal Planning 101" for much more on how to approach meal planning on a ketogenic life-style.) Many of us would love to replace our high-carb convenience foods with low-carb convenience foods, but doing so isn't going to resolve our health issues, particularly for those of us with severe metabolic dysfunction. Learning to eat real food is worth every second for the better health that is the result, and it really isn't that difficult to do.

The second challenge my family faced when switching to keto was learning to eat high-fat foods while restricting carbohydrates, especially carbs from wheat, sugar, and starch. Eating high-fat is not only contrary to traditional medical advice, but very different from what we were used to. When we began to discard carbs from our grocery cart and kitchen, we were left searching for replacements. Our internal GPS had to recalculate daily, it seemed. Instead of reaching for cereal or whole-wheat bagels with fat-free cream cheese, we needed to reach for bacon, sausage, eggs—anything that had fat and protein, but not bread, pasta, or rice. Breaded meats are not allowed on keto, but meat can be fried in healthy fats like butter, ghee, lard, or coconut oil. Of those fats, butter was the only one I bought before keto. I also learned that the vegetable and seed oils that were once staples in my kitchen are inflammatory, so I tossed those along with the flour and rice.

With the refrigerator, cabinets, and pantry devoid of foods that aren't appropriate for a ketogenic diet, where do you begin when it comes to stocking the "right" foods?

The easiest way to follow a ketogenic diet is to eat very simply. Meals comprised of meats and vegetables are generally safe. Focus on eating foods that *are* ingredients and avoiding foods *with* ingredients. For example, buy a pound of ground beef rather than frozen premade burgers that are more likely to have unnecessary added ingredients. Choose fresh or frozen chicken over frozen entrees that contain preservatives, food starches, and added sugars for flavor.

What Are "Healthy" Fats?

Healthy fats include saturated fats, which are less vulnerable to oxidative damage, tend to be solid at room temperature (think butter and coconut oil), and are generally best for cooking. Monounsaturated fats (avocado oil and olive oil) are liquid at room temperature, are relatively resistant to oxidation, and have antioxidants and polyphenols, which are important for good health. Polyunsaturated fats include omega-3 and omega-6 fats. Omega-3 fats are found in fish, seafood, and some plants. Omega-6 fats are found in industrially produced oils, including corn oil, peanut oil, and soybean oil. Polyunsaturated fats are more likely to oxidize and should be avoided in large amounts. Trans fats should be avoided entirely.

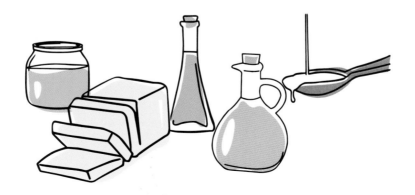

Meal Planning 101: The Basics

Some folks loathe the very idea of meal planning. Others break out in nervous twitches without a weekly or monthly meal plan. Either personality can follow a ketogenic lifestyle. Admittedly, though, it's far easier to do if you plan at least a little bit.

The easiest way to plan without planning, so to speak, is to keep your kitchen well stocked and to develop a repertoire of quick, freezer-friendly meals that you make frequently. In this section, I focus on the basic items that you can keep on hand to make keto cooking easier. I also encourage you to work on finding easy and enjoyable meals that you can throw together and that won't stress you out even if you don't have a lot of time to shop, prep, and cook (or you just really dislike cooking). Remember that meal planning can be as simple as considering your favorite dishes and thinking about the ingredients needed to make them. If you keep those items on hand consistently, then making meals becomes much easier.

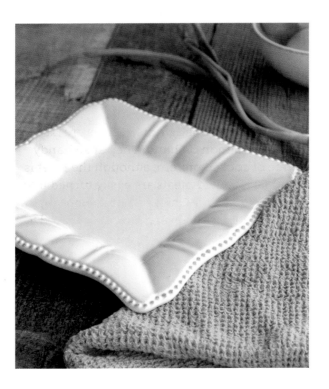

Stocking for Success

My first strategy for meal planning is to have food available. I've developed a list of low-carb staples that I always keep on hand. Even if I'm not completely out of an item, I buy more if it's on sale or if we don't have enough to get us through the week. I tend to grocery shop once a week and avoid running to the store on busy weekdays unless I absolutely have to.

Keeping meats stocked is easy with the help of a freezer. I tend to buy fatty meats when they are on sale. If I'm not going to use them before the sell-by date, I freeze them. *Tip:* Try to find out when your local grocers mark down meats; around here, they mark them down in the morning and then again in the afternoon. You can stock up on ground beef, steak, chicken wings, and whole chickens at great prices! By buying meats on sale and freezing them, you can easily pull something from the freezer for dinner without making a special trip to the store or breaking the budget.

Vegetables are a little more difficult to plan around, as they don't always stay fresh for a whole week. I tend to use the same vegetables frequently and choose those that have a longer shelf life, such as broccoli, cauliflower, and romaine lettuce. I also keep frozen vegetables on hand all the time, as well as one or two cans of veggies for when we are super busy. As mentioned earlier, sticking to just one vegetable side dish per meal will save you money, time, *and* carbs.

Because pantry items generally have the longest shelf life, those items are easy to keep stocked. I often buy them only once or twice a month—less frequently than meats, dairy, and vegetables.

My food shopping lists generally fall into four categories: meats, dairy, produce, and pantry. Here are the items that I always stock (or over-stock!) so that I am prepared to make a variety of satisfying low-carb dishes.

Meats

Meats are my primary source of protein. I try to select meats that have some fat, such as marbled beef or poultry with skin. The list that follows will give you an idea of which meats are the most keto-friendly. Use this list to identify your favorites and keep those on hand for meals. My fridge and freezer always contain at least a few meats that can be prepared quickly, including meats that I have already seasoned and cooked, such as taco meat, grilled or shredded chicken, and hamburger patties.

Ground beef is especially budget-friendly and can be used to make a variety of ketogenic meals, such as these recipes from this book:

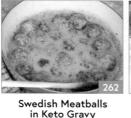
Swedish Meatballs in Keto Gravy — 262

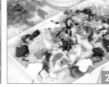
Open-Faced Taco for Two — 280

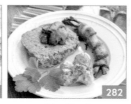
Meatloaf — 282

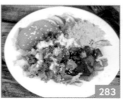
Big Mac Salad — 283

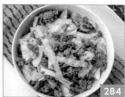
Kristie's Crack Slaw — 284

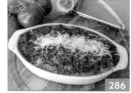
Noodle-less Lasagna — 286

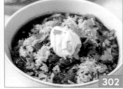
Taco Soup — 302

In a pinch, I fry up a batch of burgers (see my Basic Fatty Burgers recipe on page 276), and my family tops them with their personal favorites, such as cheese, bacon, mayonnaise, Sriracha sauce, and sliced avocado—all of which I generally keep stocked. Most often, I purchase 80 percent lean, or 80/20, ground beef. For meatloaf and meatballs, I tend to use 93 percent lean beef to avoid shrinkage. When buying whole cuts of beef, I look for fatty cuts like ribs or steaks with a lot of marbling.

I tend to purchase dark meat chicken or whole chickens that can be slow cooked without requiring much attention. (See page 316 for my Whole Roasted Chicken recipe.) My family does not eat a lot of seafood, but seafood is one of the fastest proteins to cook. Shrimp, when cleaned, can be sautéed in minutes. (My Sautéed Lemon Garlic Shrimp is delish; turn to page 336.) Most seafood keeps well in the freezer, too.

I also keep canned meats such as chicken, tuna, and salmon on hand. They are a handy source of cooked protein, although the meat is low in fat. Canned meats are easily turned into cold salads (see my Chicken Salad recipe on page 328, for example) and can also be used to make casseroles.

Beef

Beef bones (for broth)

Beef ribs

Beef roast

Ground beef

Hot dogs*

Liver

Steak (which can be shaved for Philly cheesesteaks)

Stew beef

Pork

Bacon

Ground pork

Pork chops

Pork ribs

Pork roast

Pork shoulder or pork butt

Pork steaks

Pork tenderloin

Sausage*

Poultry

Canned chicken

Chicken breasts

Chicken feet (for bone broth; see page 186)

Chicken leg quarters

Chicken thighs

Chicken wings

Turkey breast

Whole chicken

Whole turkey

Fish and seafood

Canned salmon

Canned tuna

Cod

Flounder

Salmon

Shrimp

Other

Deli meats*

Ground lamb

Pepperoni*

*These selections can contain undesirable ingredients. Search for grain-free products and choose those that are the lowest in carbohydrates. If they contain additives such as dextrose, make sure that those additives are listed near the end of the ingredient list. Avoid anything that contains high-fructose corn syrup.

Dairy

Dairy is a good source of fat and protein. When shopping for dairy, be sure to purchase full-fat varieties—the fewer ingredients, the better. For example, butter should contain only cream and salt or just cream. Real butter doesn't need "natural flavors." Always compare nutrition information and ingredients. Some brands of cream cheese have just 1 gram of carbs per serving, while others have 2 grams per serving. Please go out of your way to find the lower-carb brands. Also, heavy cream has 36 percent milk fat, while heavy whipping cream has 30 percent milk fat, making heavy cream the better choice for a keto diet. Heavy cream is also more stable when whipped because of its higher fat content. Avoid half-and-half, which has less than 18 percent milk fat; some brands have only 10.5 percent. Less milk fat means not only less fat, but also more carbohydrates in the form of lactose (a form of sugar).

With regard to cheese, use full-fat cheeses and avoid processed cheese products that contain undesirable oils. Cheese that comes in a box, can, or jar is generally a bad idea. American cheese is often highly processed; the only kind I buy is a brand that does not contain inflammatory oils and is made from dairy. When possible, my family enjoys cheeses made from raw milk.

Butter

Cream cheese

Crème fraîche

Heavy cream

Mascarpone

Sour cream

Full-fat cheeses, including:

Asiago

Blue cheese

Cheddar

Double cream Brie

Feta

Goat cheese

Gouda (regular or smoked)

Havarti

Mozzarella

Parmesan (fresh, not from a can!)

Port Salut

A Note About Dairy

Some folks find that dairy is problematic and must be avoided due to sensitivities to lactose, casein, or whey. At the very least, you may need to limit dairy to one meal per day or a few ounces per meal. If you feel bloated or if you aren't making as much progress as you'd like, dairy might be the culprit. The best way to determine whether you should avoid or limit dairy is go without it for a minimum of one week. It can take as long as five or six days to notice a difference. During that time, you can enjoy other sources of fat, such as coconut cream, coconut oil, avocado oil, ghee, olive oil, tallow, and bacon fat. If you go dairy-free and choose to reintroduce it later, start with dairy foods that are low in lactose, such as cheddar cheese, Parmesan cheese, and butter. If you do well with those, you might try adding in foods that are higher in lactose, such as heavy cream, cream cheese, and sour cream.

Produce

Produce is mainly carbohydrate, so I buy limited amounts. Fresh veggies and fruits don't stay fresh for long, so I tend to limit my purchases to those that I expect we will consume within the week. I generally keep spinach or leaf lettuce on hand for lunch salads or a quick side dish with dinner. Bell peppers, broccoli, cabbage, cauliflower, mushrooms, onions, and zucchini are also staples. Although I usually purchase fresh produce, I do keep canned green beans and collard greens on hand. For variety, we sometimes enjoy asparagus and Brussels sprouts, although I buy those only occasionally and when they are on sale.

Though technically a fruit, avocados contribute healthy fat to a meal, so those are also in frequent rotation. I buy tomatoes occasionally, but I limit those because of their higher carb content. The only sweet fruits I eat are the occasional berries. I limit those to less than ¼ cup per serving since the fructose (a form of sugar) in fruits can be problematic and can cause cravings.

Asparagus	Cucumbers	Romaine lettuce
Avocados	Green onions	Sauerkraut
Bell peppers	Jalapeño peppers	Spinach
Broccoli	Mushrooms	Tomatoes
Brussels sprouts	Olives	Zucchini
Cabbage	Onions	
Cauliflower	Pickles	

Pantry Items

Most folks find that the pantry clears out quickly when they stop buying boxed cereals, crackers, and other processed and carb-filled "treats." My pantry generally holds dried herbs, spices, and salt and shelf-stable sources of fat, such as ghee, avocado oil, and coconut oil. I also stock a variety of vinegars and condiments to flavor foods without adding carbohydrates. I keep peanut butter and nut butters on hand for my family, but I avoid them myself because of their higher carb counts. The same is true for nuts. While almonds and macadamia nuts are frequently included as part of a low-carb diet, portion control can be a concern. If you do consume nuts, be mindful of portions and eat them with a high-fat meal; avoid snacking mindlessly. Using condiment cups or plastic baggies to measure out portions can help.

Similar to the way I shop for dairy, I purchase pantry items as we begin to get low. It is not unusual for me to pick up an extra jar of ghee so that I always have some on hand and can avoid a trip to the store because we emptied a jar.

The following is a list of standard keto pantry items. Additional items are listed in the later section that discusses ingredients for Asian, Italian, and Mexican dishes.

Fats

Avocado oil

Bacon fat (rendered from cooking bacon; see page 188)

Coconut oil

Ghee

Olive oil

Sesame oil

Walnut oil

Vinegars and acids

Apple cider vinegar

Balsamic vinegar*

Coconut vinegar

Lemon juice

Lime juice

Rice wine vinegar*

White vinegar

Condiments

Buffalo sauce**

Coconut aminos*

Mayonnaise**

Mustard (Dijon, prepared yellow, and stone-ground)

Sriracha sauce**

Worcestershire sauce**

Nuts

Almonds

Macadamia nuts

Pecans

Walnuts

Canned goods

Green beans

Tomato sauce

Spices and seasonings

Bay leaves

Chili powder

Dill weed

Dried basil

Dried ground oregano and/or dried oregano leaves

Dried minced onions

Dried parsley

Dried rosemary leaves

Dried rubbed sage

Dried thyme

Garlic powder

Ginger powder

Ground cinnamon

Ground cumin

Italian seasoning

Jane's Krazy Mixed-Up Salt

Maple extract

Mustard powder

Onion powder

Paprika

Pumpkin pie spice

Vanilla extract

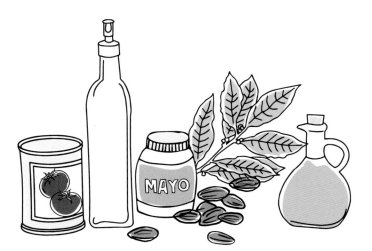

---

*The ingredients and carb counts in these items vary widely. Be sure to look for the brands that are lowest in carbs and do not contain added sugars.

**These products often contain undesirable oils or added sugars. Use them sparingly and buy brands with the best-quality ingredients you can find. Homemade mayonnaise is great. Making it yourself may take a little practice, but you may find that you prefer it to store-bought. See my recipe on page 192.

Meal Planning by Type of Cuisine

Another way to think about keeping your kitchen well stocked and planning your meals is to consider cooking by type of cuisine. My family typically enjoys the flavors found in Asian, Italian, and Mexican dishes. When they ask for a dish with an Italian flair, for example, I know that I have the staple ingredients on hand to create that flavor profile.

I've organized the basic ingredients for each of these three types of cuisine into handy lists to help you plan and shop. For example, to create an Asian-inspired dish, you want to have fresh garlic and ginger, along with coconut aminos or tamari (both of which are wheat-free substitutes for soy sauce). These lists are not exhaustive, but if you have these ingredients on hand, you can generally create the flavor profile you want.

Basic Asian ingredients

Asian-inspired dishes are ideal for those who avoid dairy. Unfortunately, eating keto at Asian restaurants in the United States can be difficult because rice and noodle dishes are ubiquitous and so many sweet sauces are used. I find very little that I can order. Fortunately, the same flavors are easy to produce in your own kitchen, without the carbs. Sautéed spinach, mushrooms, cabbage, and shirataki noodles made from glucomannan (such as the Miracle Noodles brand) make excellent substitutes for rice or noodles. You can also use asparagus and bean sprouts as a base for your dish.

Here are some Asian-inspired recipes that you will find in this book:

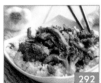
Asian-Style Beef and Broccoli

Moo Goo Gai Pan

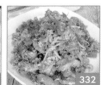
Skinny Chicken Fried "Rice"

Fats and oils

Ghee

Peanut oil*

Toasted sesame oil*

Meat and seafood

Beef

Chicken

Fish

Pork

Shrimp

Dairy substitutes

Coconut cream**

Coconut milk**

Produce and noodles

Asparagus

Bean sprouts

Cabbage

Miracle Noodles

Mushrooms

Spinach

Spices and aromatics

Chinese five-spice powder

Garlic

Ginger

Turmeric powder

Sauces and vinegars

Broth

Coconut aminos or tamari**

Fish sauce**

Rice vinegar**

Sriracha sauce**

---

*Use these as finishing oils and drizzle them over dishes rather than using them to cook foods.

**Be careful when purchasing these items. Look for brands with no added sugars. Coconut aminos and tamari are common substitutes for soy sauce, which is wheat based. Coconut aminos is a good option for those who avoid soy altogether; tamari is a wheat-free soy sauce (some brands contain small amounts of wheat).

Basic Italian ingredients

Italian foods are rich in flavor and can be part of a ketogenic lifestyle if you eliminate pasta and limit tomato products, which can contribute a lot of carbs. Lasagna made with alternative "noodles," Bolognese with added fat, and cream-based sauces are excellent choices. Antipasti platters are also keto-friendly. Avoid commercial Alfredo sauces because most are made with flour and/or food starches. Alfredo sauce is surprisingly quick, easy, and inexpensive to make at home and is an excellent way to add fat and flavor to a keto meal. See my recipe on page 204.

These are some of my favorite Italian-inspired recipes in this book:

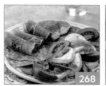
Antipasti Platter

Noodle-less Lasagna

Bolognese

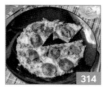
Skillet Pizza

Fats and oils

Bacon fat

Butter

Lard

Olive oil

Tallow

Meat and seafood

Chicken

Fish

Ground beef

Sausage

Shellfish

Dairy

Heavy cream

Mozzarella cheese

Parmesan cheese

Ricotta cheese*

Produce and noodles

Asparagus

Broccoli

Miracle Noodles

Mushrooms

Olives

Spinach

Tomatoes

Herbs, spices, and aromatics

Basil

Bay leaves

Garlic

Italian seasoning

Oregano

Parsley

Rosemary

Sage

Thyme

Sauces and vinegars

Balsamic vinegar

Pesto

Tomato sauce

White wine vinegar

---

*The fat and carbohydrate counts in ricotta cheese vary greatly from brand to brand. Often store brands have the fewest carbs. Be sure to read and compare labels.

Basic Mexican ingredients

What my family calls Mexican food really has more of a Tex-Mex or Southwestern flavor profile, but it is among their favorites. I can generally use whichever meats I have on hand, pair them with the spices and veggies listed below, and serve them with the sauces, cheeses, and other dairy I have available. These are the most frequently requested meals in my home. My only caution about Mexican food is that spices do have carbs. Chili powder and cumin, which are common ingredients in Southwestern dishes, are some of the higher-carb spices that I use. Calculating the nutrition information for recipes always reminds me to measure those spices carefully.

These are some of my favorite Mexican-inspired and Southwestern recipes in this book:

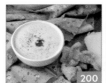
Chile con Queso 200

Southwestern Frittata 234

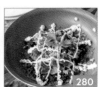
Open-Faced Taco for Two 280

Taco Bake 312

Shredded Mexican Chicken 329

Fats and oils

Bacon fat

Butter

Lard

Olive oil

Tallow

Meat and seafood

Beef

Chicken

Chorizo

Pork

Dairy

Cheddar cheese

Heavy cream

Monterey Jack cheese

Queso fresco

Sour cream

Produce

Avocados

Bell peppers

Jalapeño peppers

Limes

Onions

Tomatillos

Tomatoes

Herbs, spices, and aromatics

Chili powder

Cilantro (preferably fresh)

Cumin

Garlic

Onion powder

Sauces

Guacamole (see my recipe on page 205)

Salsa Fresca (see my recipe on page 206)

Adapting Your Meals to Keto

Even if you disdain meal planning, staying on plan is much easier when you have meals you enjoy that you can make easily. Now that you have a shopping list and an idea of the ingredients you need to create popular flavor profiles, take some time to think about what low-carb meals you might like.

To begin, consider the foods that you currently eat. Most of us are creatures of habit. We put our keys in the same place, sit in the same chairs, park our cars in the same spot at work, and keep to the same general routine. With few exceptions, our eating habits tend to follow patterns, too. Most of us appreciate variety, but if you wrote down your meals for the past three weeks, you would likely find a dozen or so common foods or dishes.

Look at your current eating habits and think about what needs to change in order for you to succeed on keto. First, jot down what you ate for breakfast for the last five days. Consider the times, the portions, and your level of hunger each morning. Then do the same for lunch, dinner, and any snacks you had.

Before keto, this is how my typical day looked:

Breakfast	At 7:00 a.m., a bagel with fat-free cream cheese or two waffles with low-fat peanut butter and reduced-sugar jam, with a diet soft drink, consumed while standing up in the kitchen or driving the kids to school.
Snack	Between 9:00 and 10:00 a.m., a low-fat granola bar and/or a package of peanut butter crackers, eaten at my desk at work, with a diet soft drink or coffee with Splenda and half-and-half.
Lunch	Between noon and 1:00 p.m., a chili cheeseburger, coleslaw, fries with ketchup, and a diet soft drink, or a large salad with grilled chicken, low-fat cheese, and fat-free dressing and a baked potato.
Snack	By 3:00 p.m., another low-fat granola bar and/or package of peanut butter crackers, along with a diet soft drink.
Dinner	Dinner with the family, usually at 6:00 p.m., included a lean meat like chicken breast, a starchy side like rice, pasta, or potatoes, and a vegetable side like green beans, peas, cooked carrots, or a salad, with water to drink.
Snack	Before bed, I had a snack so that I could take my pain medications. Typically, that snack was peanut butter crackers, low-fat crackers or granola bar, or cheese, with a diet soft drink or water.

Let's begin by considering which habits I could keep and what had to change in order to adopt a ketogenic plan.

Revamping breakfast

It is clear that I need breakfast options that are quick to make and can be eaten on the go. Bagels and frozen waffles have no place in a ketogenic lifestyle, so I began to brainstorm what I like to eat for breakfast that is also low-carb. That list includes omelets, quiche, sausage, and bacon. I began cooking several pounds of bacon and large batches of sausage patties every weekend so that my family could eat them on busy weekday mornings. For variety, I began to get creative with crustless quiches, often called frittatas. Starting with a base of eggs and seasonings, I added fats such as heavy cream, cream cheese, ghee, butter, shredded cheese, or bacon fat along with protein and low-carb veggies. The frittatas could be baked on Sunday evenings while we ate dinner. Once they had cooled, they could be sliced and eaten cold or reheated for quick breakfasts during the week.

Another option for the morning meal is to eat foods that are not considered traditional breakfast foods. My daughter dislikes most low-carb breakfasts and is especially reluctant to eat eggs. Her favorite breakfasts are warmed Kristie's Crack Slaw (page 284) and Bolognese (page 300). I've even seen her happily eat Taco Bake (page 312) or Skillet Pizza (page 314) before school. As long as breakfast includes a good source of fat and protein and limits carbs, breaking tradition is fine.

Think about *your* favorite breakfast foods. Look through the recipes in Chapter 7 for ideas that fit your tastes and lifestyle. Make a list of the low-carb, high-fat foods that you would enjoy eating in the morning. Decide whether you are okay with eating the same breakfast every day—some people like to eat the same morning meal throughout the week because it simplifies food prep and cleanup—or whether you need some variety from day to day, which will require a bit more time and effort in the kitchen.

Keto-fying lunch and dinner

When I look over my former lunch and dinner habits, I see some foods that I can enjoy in a ketogenic lifestyle. For example, a cheeseburger is still one of my favorite meals, but I eat it a little differently now. My keto cheeseburger typically includes bacon, lettuce, dill pickles, mayonnaise, and mustard. I order it without a bun. Ketchup is full of sugar, so I avoid it or make it myself (see page 190). I no longer order chili or coleslaw; restaurant chili often contains wheat fillers, sugars, food starches, beans, and too many carbs from tomato products, and most commercial coleslaw is made with inflammatory oils and added sugars. I avoid it in restaurants but make it often at home (see page 366). What I have discovered is that the best and most flavorful parts of this meal are the fatty meat, cheese, bacon, and mayonnaise. Buns are truly flavorless, and I do not miss them at all.

I also continue to eat salads for lunch, but I make sure to limit the carbohydrates from vegetables and add full-fat cheese and dressing along with a good source of protein. Dark-meat chicken, bacon, and boiled eggs are good high-fat options.

Dinner is easy to adapt, too. I plan dinners around the protein, just as I always have. The caveat is that instead of focusing on lean meats, I opt for fattier cuts, such as chicken wings and thighs rather than chicken breasts. A ketogenic dinner often works better with just one vegetable side that includes a source of fat rather than two sides, one vegetable and one starch. Salads with high-fat dressing and roasted or pan-fried vegetables cooked in fat or served with a high-fat sauce are good options. For me, the hardest part of adapting dinner was minimizing portions of vegetable sides so that I did not overeat carbs. Because high-fat dishes are very filling, I soon learned that it took far less food to satisfy my hunger. Another bonus of cooking just one side dish is less time spent in the kitchen cooking and cleaning up!

Sizing up snacks

Lastly, I had to change how I thought about snacking. The most dramatic change occurred in the first week: I no longer *needed* snacks. My hunger was drastically reduced because my blood glucose levels had stabilized. While I did stock peanut butter, almonds, and macadamia nuts in my desk and other usual hiding places, I quickly found that I did not require them.

If you want to keep a supply of keto-friendly snacks handy, though, especially when you're just starting out on keto, some good high-fat, low-carb options are pork rinds dipped in room-temperature butter, bacon, deli meats, cheeses, Cheddar Cheese Chips (page 256), salami, and Crispy Pepperoni Chips (page 257). You can also add fat to snacks, like pickles spread with cream cheese, beef jerky dipped in mayo, and hard-boiled eggs dipped in mayo or salad dressing. Some people snack on macadamia nuts or sliced avocado, but if you do, be sure to monitor portions, as these foods do have carbs.

What's on Your Plate?
An Inventory of Eating Habits (Sample)

Breakfast	At 7:00 a.m., a ~~bagel~~ with ~~fat-free~~ cream cheese or two waffles with ~~low-fat~~ peanut butter and ~~reduced-sugar~~ jam, with a diet soft drink, consumed while standing up in the kitchen or driving the kids to school.	Bacon, sausage, eggs, low-carb pancakes, frittatas, Dutch Baby.
Snack	Between 9:00 and 10:00 a.m., a ~~low-fat granola bar~~ and/or a ~~package of peanut butter crackers,~~ eaten at my desk at work, with a diet soft drink or coffee with ~~Splenda~~ and ~~half-and-half.~~	Snack only when hungry. Choose portioned nuts, pork rinds, cheese, pepperoni, or bacon. Use fatty sauces like mayonnaise, ranch dressing, or blue cheese dressing to increase fat.
Lunch	Between noon and 1:00 p.m., a ~~chili~~ cheeseburger, ~~coleslaw, fries~~ with ~~ketchup,~~ and a diet soft drink, or a large salad with grilled chicken, ~~low-fat~~ cheese, and ~~fat-free~~ dressing and a ~~baked potato.~~	Cheeseburger without a bun, with bacon, cheese, and mayo. Add homemade ranch dressing to salad with grilled chicken. Skillet Pizza, Swedish Meatballs.
Snack	By 3:00, another ~~low-fat granola bar~~ and/or package of ~~peanut butter crackers,~~ along with a diet soft drink.	
Dinner	Dinner with the family, usually at 6:00, included a ~~lean~~ meat like chicken breast, a ~~starchy side like rice, pasta, or potatoes,~~ and a vegetable side like green beans, ~~peas, cooked carrots,~~ or a salad, with water to drink.	Roasted chicken with green beans, Spinach Salad with Hot Bacon Fat Dressing, Meatloaf with Cauli Mash, Moo Goo Gai Pan, Chicken Philly Cheesesteak Casserole.
Snack	Before bed, I had a snack so that I could take my pain medications. Typically, that snack was ~~peanut butter crackers, low-fat crackers~~ or ~~granola bar,~~ or cheese, with a diet soft drink or water.	

Consider *your* current eating habits. What can you continue to eat as part of your new ketogenic lifestyle, and what will you need to do differently? Using a worksheet like the one on the previous page, record a few of your typical meals, then look through the list. Cross out the items that do not fit on a ketogenic diet. Highlight those that do. Those are the foods that you know you enjoy and can continue to enjoy. Next, turn to the keto food lists on pages 44 to 47 and highlight your favorites. You can also look through the recipes in this book for new dishes to try. Jot down the foods or recipe names that appeal to you. The highlighted foods and the foods you add to this worksheet will become the foods that you enjoy as you embark on your journey.

Meal planning starts with knowing what you like and making sure you have healthy foods on hand. If you aren't sure what to eat or you don't have keto-friendly foods to choose from, the journey is harder. Surround yourself with foods that will help you succeed.

Take the New Recipe Challenge

Now that you've identified some keto-friendly foods that you enjoy, commit to using those foods to create new meals. One of the smartest things I did early on in my journey was to commit to trying two new recipes per week. That decision had a huge impact on my success. In fact, I believe that single commitment was one of the main reasons I was able to switch from a high-carb, low-fat diet to a ketogenic lifestyle.

As I experimented with new recipes, I strategically created new habits in the kitchen. The ways in which I planned meals and combined foods changed. With each new dish that I made, I expanded my family's options. Those recipes became the building blocks for trying even more new recipes and combinations.

I found it helpful to use Pinterest to track the recipes I tried. First, I created boards for the recipes I wanted to make. After I made a recipe, I moved it to a new board and added comments about how we liked the recipe or how I might change it if I made it again. In that way, I developed a reliable list of tried-and-tested recipes.

Even if you don't use Pinterest, I encourage you to commit to trying a couple of new recipes each week. Doing so will help you add variety to this new lifestyle and become more confident in the kitchen if you don't have a lot of cooking experience. (If you already enjoy cooking, then this commitment will be easier for you.)

A word of caution: For any recipe that you find online, please calculate the macronutrients yourself. Often a recipe is promoted as low-carb or keto but is higher in carbs than you might think. That is especially true with low-carb breads and treats, which should be enjoyed only on rare occasions. When I calculate the nutritional information for my recipes, I use either the USDA Food Composition Database or the information provided by the manufacturer on the food product label. As an example, the following chart shows how I calculated the information for the Creamy Alfredo Sauce recipe on page 204:

Creamy Alfredo Sauce	Protein	Fat	Carbs	Fiber	Calories
½ cup (1 stick) salted butter	0g	96g	0g	0g	800
2 ounces cream cheese (¼ cup)	4g	20g	1.5g	0g	200
¾ cup heavy cream	0g	72g	2.4g	0g	720
1 teaspoon minced garlic	0g	0g	1g	0g	4
Dash of ground nutmeg	0g	0g	0g	0g	0
Freshly cracked black pepper	0g	0g	0g	0g	0
5 ounces Parmesan cheese	60g	30g	0g	0g	600
Totals	64g	218g	4.9g	0g	2,324
Per serving, based on 6 servings	10.7g	36.3g	0.8g	0g	387

The amount of each ingredient in the recipe is listed in the first column, followed by each macronutrient, plus fiber and calories. The numbers for each category are summed, and then each of those totals is divided by the number of servings the recipe makes—in this case, six servings.

As another example, the Whipped Coconut Cream with Macadamia Nuts recipe (page 380) illustrates an important point. The carbohydrates in coconut cream vary widely by brand. The brand that I used has only 3 grams of carbs per ¼-cup serving, whereas other brands can contain up to 6 grams per serving. Be sure to read labels and select the product with the lowest carb count so you do not go over your carb limit.

Whipped Coconut Cream with Macadamia Nuts	Protein	Fat	Carbs	Fiber	Calories
1 (13.5-ounce) can coconut cream	8g	77.4g	12.9g	0g	774
¼ teaspoon vanilla extract	0g	0g	0g	0g	0
3 drops liquid sweetener, or 1 tablespoon granulated sweetener	0g	0g	0g	0g	0
¼ teaspoon ground cinnamon	0g	0g	0g	0g	0
¼ teaspoon salt	0g	0g	0g	0g	0
3 ounces macadamia nuts	6g	63g	12g	7.8g	600
Totals	14g	140.4g	24.9g	7.8g	1374
Per serving, based on 4 servings	3.5g	35.1g	6.2g	2g	344

I suggest that you take the time to record the new meals you make, whether you and your family enjoyed them, and any changes you might make next time. If you like, you can use the My Keto Meals form, which you can download from my website, cookingketowithkristie.com. Filling out this form is entirely optional, but I used to use one just like it. Because my family's lifestyle is so busy, I found it helpful to jot down notes about which low-carb pancake recipe we enjoyed most, whether a recipe called for too much salt for our tastes, or whether I could think of ways to add more fat or protein to a meal or lower the carb count further.

Meal Planning 102: Advanced Topics

While some people refuse to meal plan or find it too restrictive, others want to plan to exact portions. These are the people who often color-code their freezer shelves! While my meal plans are not that precise, I do follow some general guidelines that keep my family eating well most of the time:

1. **Choose times for meal planning, shopping, and food preparation and/or batch cooking. Try to set aside two to three hours over the weekend or on a free weeknight.**

    Typically, I shop early on a weekend morning when the stores are quiet and do food prep on Sunday afternoon or evening. There are times when my planning is as simple as designating two meals to be cooked at once and expecting to eat out at least once and enjoy leftovers at least once. My planning also includes making sure that each member of the family has a few breakfast options for the week. The kids need lunches for school, and David and I often take lunches to work. I cook dinner two or three times during the week depending on our schedules.

2. **Consider your schedule for the week. Think about any changes or disruptions to your typical schedule that might affect the amount of time you have to prepare meals or enjoy meals with others.**

    Before I plan meals or shop for food, I check my family's schedules for the week. Typically, we all eat dinner together at around 6:00 p.m. when David gets home from work. I usually get home between 5:15 and 5:30, which leaves me little time to cook. Meals have to prepped ahead of time or made in a slow cooker or electric pressure cooker. If I have only thirty minutes to get food on the table, roasting a chicken is not an option. If any of us have evening activities, I factor those in as well. On nights when I'm picking up or dropping off kids, I have less time in the kitchen. I also make sure that whatever I've planned for dinner can be reheated for anyone who needs to eat later. On the nights when I'm away from home, I plan meals that the family can prepare without me or can reheat on their own. For example, sometimes I make a big batch of Bolognese in the morning before work. The children can heat it when they are ready to eat, and leftovers travel well in a Thermos for lunch the next day.

    Reviewing our schedules for the week ahead gives me an idea of how much time I have to cook each meal, whether I need to thaw meats or other foods from the freezer, and whether I need to plan meals that can be cooked extra quickly or reheated easily.

3. **Determine main dishes based on family requests, grocery store sales, or foods you already have on hand. A quick inventory of the fridge, freezer, or pantry will help you save time and money.**

   Before I plan meals, I look at which meats and vegetables are on sale at my favorite local grocers, and I try to plan meals around those discounted items. I also check the fridge and freezer to identify which protein(s) I already have on hand. For example, if chicken is on sale or if I have a package in my freezer, I think about favorite chicken dishes that can be prepared ahead of time, made in a slow cooker, or cooked quickly. Often, I ask my family if they have a taste for anything in particular. I try to honor any requests, because if they request something, they are more likely to enjoy it.

4. **Plan multiple meals around the same ingredients to save time and money and reduce food waste.**

   When I meal plan, I not only consider which foods are on sale, but often buy multiple packages of the same ingredient to use in more than one meal. For example, if spinach is on sale, I might buy several bags. One bag can be used to make Spinach Salad with Hot Bacon Fat Dressing (page 353), while another can be sautéed as a side dish for another meal.

Meal planning is easier when you start with what your family likes and then think through your weekly schedule, budget, and fridge/freezer/pantry inventory. Once you've taken those steps, you can begin to fill in your plan for the week.

Note: If you are the only member of your household following a ketogenic lifestyle, then you can simplify family meals to keep everyone happy. Before my family switched to keto, I continued making meals with one meat and two sides. The meat option was one we all could enjoy. One side was low-carb and high-fat, such as broccoli, cauliflower, or green beans, and the other was a starchier vegetable or other side that the rest of my family enjoyed, such as pasta, rice, or potatoes.

The following are some common keto ingredients. Whether you're looking at what's on sale or considering what is currently available in your kitchen, multiple meals with a variety of flavor profiles can usually be made from these same ingredients (check the index for additional recipes featuring these ingredients):

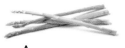

Asparagus

egg scrambles
frittatas
omelets
stir-fries
bacon-wrapped

pizza topping
roasted
sautéed
steamed

Bell peppers

 294
Savory Pepper Steak

 312
Taco Bake

 231
Western Quiche

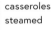 322
Chicken Philly Cheesesteak Casserole

egg scrambles
frittatas
omelets
pizza topping
soups
roasted
sautéed

Broccoli

 350
Homecoming Broccoli Salad

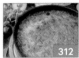 292
Asian-Style Beef and Broccoli

 351
Roasted Broccoli

casseroles
steamed

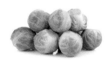

Brussels sprouts

 361
Creamed Brussels Sprouts

chopped and fried
roasted
steamed

Cabbage

 342
Cabbage Noodles

 284
Kristie's Crack Slaw

 366
Mom's Creamy Coleslaw

 363
Roasted Cabbage Steaks

stir-fries
fried

Cauliflower

 288
20-Minute Skillet Dinner

 368
Baked Cauliflower Mac and Cheese

 346
Cauliflower au Gratin

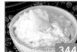 344
Creamy Cauli Mash

 354
Faux-tato Salad

soups
roasted
steamed
twice-baked

Cucumbers

 356
Cucumber, Tomato, and Feta Salad

 206
Simple Salsa Fresca

 273
Smoked Salmon Cucumber Bites

 365
Southern Table Pickles

dips
tzatziki

Eggs

 264
Classic Deviled Eggs

custards
egg drop soup
egg salad
frittatas
ice creams

omelets
scrambles
stir-fries
tossed salads
hard-boiled

Green beans

 348
Peppery Roasted Green Beans with Parmesan

 358
Slow-Simmered Country Green Beans

bacon-wrapped
grilled

Jalapeño peppers

 205
Guacamole

 260
Pork Rind Nachos

329
Shredded Mexican Chicken

206
Simple Salsa Fresca

egg scrambles
frittatas
stuffed

Radishes

 347
Herb-Roasted Radishes

 296
Mississippi Roast

boiled
fried
raw in salads

Spinach

 269
Baked Spinach Bites

 353
Spinach Salad with Hot Bacon Fat Dressing

egg scrambles
omelets
salads
creamed
sautéed

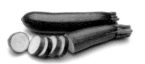

Zucchini

 286
Noodle-less Lasagna

 340
Zoodles

casseroles
soups
baked
boiled
sautéed

You can also use the index to identify recipes that can be made with beef, pork, poultry, or seafood.

	SUNDAY	MONDAY	TUESDAY	
BREAKFAST	Coffee with Baked Bacon (page 188)	Leftover pork tenderloin with scrambled eggs, butter, and cheese	Hard-boiled eggs with bacon and cream cheese or butter	
LUNCH	Simple Roasted Pork Tenderloin (page 310) and Creamed Brussels Sprouts (page 361)	Leftover chicken wings with blue cheese dressing	Leftover pork tenderloin and roasted broccoli loaded with sour cream, cheese, and bacon	
DINNER	Roasted Chicken Wings (page 259) with Blue Cheese Dressing (page 213)	Noodle-less Lasagna (page 286) with Roasted Broccoli (page 351)	Basic Fatty Burgers (page 276) with bacon and leftover creamed Brussels sprouts	
PREP AND COOKING TASKS	• *Bake bacon for the week* • *Roast pork tenderloin* • *Make Brussels sprouts* • *Roast chicken wings* • *Make dressing* • *Prep lasagna* • *Shred cheese for the week*	• *Bake lasagna* • *Roast broccoli* • *Boil eggs*	• *Cook burgers* • *Make and cook breakfast sausage*	

Sample meal plan 1

Here's an example of a weekly meal plan. I use a grid to write out my plan for the week and make sure I have enough ingredients on hand to make everything; therefore, once I begin cooking, I don't have to worry about running to the store for missing ingredients. (You can find a printable version of this grid to use for your four-week ketogenic journey on my website, cookingketowithkristie.com.)

Notice that I intentionally do most of the cooking on Sunday when I typically have more free time. I also make larger batches of certain foods on Sunday so that we have leftovers to eat throughout the week. I did not include Saturday because we are often away from home on weekends, or we enjoy dinner out. We also tend to eat leftovers to clean out the fridge for Sunday meal prepping.

In this example, some of the same foods are prepared in different ways. For example, the blue cheese dressing is served as a dipping sauce for chicken wings and later in the week as a topping for burgers. The dressing can also be used in egg salad or for deviled eggs (see page 264). In a pinch, you can dip pork rinds or bacon in the high-fat blue cheese dressing for a quick meal on the run. Taking the time to make one batch of dressing gives you options for multiple meals. Similarly, hard-boiled eggs are used in both the egg salad and the spinach salad. You boil eggs only once but eat them in three different meals.

Prepping future meals while cooking a meal helps me be more efficient. I typically start the week by baking at least 3 pounds of bacon. (If you haven't made bacon in the oven, it's easy.

WEDNESDAY	THURSDAY	FRIDAY
Sunny-side-up eggs with Breakfast Sausage (page 224)	Leftover pork tenderloin with scrambled eggs, butter, and cheese	Scrambled eggs with leftover breakfast sausage and cheese
Leftover burgers with bacon and blue cheese dressing	Egg salad with pork rinds	Leftover burgers with bacon and creamed Brussels sprouts
Leftover lasagna and creamed Brussels sprouts	Spinach Salad with Hot Bacon Fat Dressing (page 353) and leftover burgers	Leftover spinach salad and pork tenderloin
• *Make egg salad*	• *Make salad dressing*	

I use lower heat to avoid grease spatters. See page 188 for my method.) Lunch on Sunday is pork tenderloin with creamed Brussels sprouts. Pork tenderloin often comes in packages of two. My family will eat less than one tenderloin for Sunday lunch, and we will have another tenderloin left over for breakfast on Monday and Thursday and an easy dinner on Friday. The double batch of creamed Brussels sprouts made along with the pork will be perfect for three different meals later in the week. For Sunday dinner, I do something similar and make an extra-large batch of chicken wings. While I'm in the kitchen, I also put together a lasagna, which will just need to be baked on Monday evening. Finally, I use my food processor to shred a whole pound of cheese for us to use throughout the week.

On Monday morning, I scramble eggs in butter and top them with shredded cheese. The tenderloin can be warmed in the same skillet I used to cook the eggs. For lunch at work, I enjoy chicken wings with blue cheese dressing. After work, I put the lasagna in the oven and then chop and roast the broccoli. While we eat dinner, I boil a dozen eggs and let them cool.

On Tuesday morning, we grab hard-boiled eggs and bacon from the fridge. (If I have time, I might make egg salad for breakfast.) I add cream cheese or butter to the eggs and bacon to keep the fat content of the meal high. For lunch, I pack a slice or two of pork tenderloin and some leftover roasted broccoli from Monday's dinner, and top it with a little sour cream, cheese, and bacon—loaded broccoli! When I cook burgers for dinner Tuesday night, I will use at least 2 pounds of ground beef so that we have leftover burgers for lunches on Wednesday and Friday. When the skillet is already hot, it's just as easy to fry eight burgers as it is to fry four. I can also fix the breakfast sausage while the burgers cook. Multiple meals, one cleanup! These are also meals that my family can heat up if I'm not home to cook for them.

On Wednesday morning, I fry a pound of sausage (if I didn't cook it the night before) and make myself a sunny-side-up egg. The yolk will run into the sausage and make a creamy, high-fat breakfast. Lunch is one of the burgers cooked on Tuesday night with the blue cheese dressing and bacon made on Sunday. Notice that bacon is on the menu several times, but I took the time to cook it only once. Dinner requires no cooking on Wednesday since we are just heating up leftovers. With the extra time, I can make egg salad while I talk to the children about their day.

On Thursday, I enjoy more of the pork tenderloin for breakfast. Lunch is quick and easy: egg salad (made the night before) and pork rinds for extra fat and protein. For dinner, we eat the rest of the burgers with a spinach salad. The dressing takes less than fifteen minutes to prepare. The salad also has a sliced egg and some bacon in it, and both of those ingredients are already prepped. With the fatty dressing, the salad has perfect macros and makes a full meal even without the burger.

Finally, on Friday morning, I make breakfast fast and simple by scrambling eggs, heating some of the sausage cooked on Wednesday morning or Tuesday evening, and sprinkling it all with shredded cheese. For lunch, I finish off the creamed Brussels sprouts and have a burger with bacon. If all the bacon from Sunday has been eaten, I keep store-bought precooked bacon on hand and can have that instead. On Friday evening, we finish up the pork tenderloin and spinach salad.

Even if your family doesn't like the foods used in this sample meal plan, you can benefit from using the same approach:

1. Pick times for meal planning, shopping, and food preparation and/or batch cooking.

2. Consider your schedule for the week.

3. Determine main dishes from family requests, grocery store sales, or foods you already have on hand.

4. Plan multiple meals around the same ingredients to save time and money.

Turn the page for another sample meal plan that follows this same process. On the opposite page is a weekly food plan that you can use to plan your own meals for the week. If you would like to print out copies of this worksheet, you'll find a downloadable version on my website, cookingketowithkristie.com.

Weekly Meal Plan

Having a visual guide to what you plan to eat for the week helps you see how many servings of food you need, which affects how much food you buy and when you cook. A chart like this (also available for download from my website, cookingketowithkristie.com) lets you see the whole week at a glance.

	BREAKFAST	LUNCH	DINNER	PREP & COOKING TASKS
SUNDAY				
MONDAY				
TUESDAY				
WEDNESDAY				
THURSDAY				
FRIDAY				
SATURDAY				

	SUNDAY	MONDAY	TUESDAY	
BREAKFAST	Sweet Dutch Baby with Vanilla and Cinnamon (page 246) with Baked Bacon (page 188)	Broccoli, Ham, and Cheese Frittata (page 232)	Breakfast Pizza (page 238)	
LUNCH	Pizza	BLT Boats (page 258) with Ranch Dressing (page 209)	Leftover Taco Bake	
DINNER	Taco Bake (page 312) with sour cream, shredded cheese, guacamole (page 205), and Simple Salsa Fresca (page 206)	20-Minute Skillet Dinner (page 288)	Savory Dutch Baby with Bacon, Gruyère, Mushrooms, and Caramelized Onions (page 248)	
PREP AND COOKING TASKS	• *Bake bacon for the week* • *Make salsa fresca* • *Par-bake triple batch of Sullivans' KeDough Pizza Crusts (page 216)* • *Brown double batch of sausage* • *Shred cheese for the week* • *Make frittata* • *Cook Taco Bake*	• *Make dressing* • *Rice head of cauliflower* • *Cook 20-Minute Skillet Dinner*	• *Bake breakfast pizza* • *Bake Dutch baby*	

Sample meal plan 2

Here's another sample plan. Before I shop for ingredients, I check to see what's on sale, look at what I have on hand, and ask if the family has any special requests. Most often I shop early on Saturday morning and begin meal prep on Sunday because that is usually the least hectic day of our week, but meal prep could just as easily start on Saturday.

Meal prep starts with breakfast. Often, I cook for the meal we are eating as well as for a future meal, which minimizes the total time I spend cooking and cleaning. For example, if I already have a skillet full of a pound of sausage, cooking a second pound doesn't take much longer, and then I wash the skillet and stovetop only once. I like to shred cheese in large batches because I despise cleaning the food processor.

Even if it takes me thirty minutes to shred the cheese and portion it out into freezer-safe plastic bags, I would rather do that than wash the food processor five different times. The same is true for baking bacon and frying burgers. One cooking session and one cleanup yielding multiple meals makes life much easier.

On Sunday morning, I make a sweet Dutch baby as a weekend treat and bake at least 3 pounds of bacon. I also make the salsa fresca to serve with the Taco Bake for dinner. For lunch, I make a triple batch of The Sullivans' KeDough Pizza Crust, making 5-inch single-serving crusts. Four of those crusts will be used for Sunday's lunch, and I will have eight more to use later in the week or to freeze for when I need a Plan B. While the crusts are

WEDNESDAY	THURSDAY	FRIDAY
Leftover frittata	Breakfast Pizza (page 238)	Leftover frittata
Leftover Savory Dutch Baby and salad with ranch dressing	Leftover BLT Boats with ranch dressing	Pizza and salad with ranch dressing
Whole Roasted Chicken (page 316) with Homecoming Broccoli Salad (page 350)	Skinny Chicken Fried "Rice" (page 332)	Leftover 20-Minute Skillet Dinner
• *Roast chicken in slow cooker* • *Make broccoli salad*	• *Bake breakfast pizza* • *Make Skinny Chicken Fried "Rice"*	

par-baking, I brown a double batch of sausage. Some of the sausage will be used for pizza that day, and the rest will be used for breakfast or lunch pizzas later in the week. (I could also fry some of the sausage as patties for breakfast instead of crumbling it for breakfast pizza.) While I'm shredding cheese for pizza, I shred extra for later in the week. One pound each of cheddar, mozzarella, and Parmesan will be enough for seven days. Lunch prep ends by throwing together the frittata, which can sit in the fridge unbaked. I can bake it on Monday morning or on Sunday evening while we eat dinner. After it cools, I slice it into individual portions so that it can be reheated quickly on weekday mornings. For dinner, I finish making the Taco Bake and serve it with sliced

avocado, salsa fresca, shredded cheese, and sour cream.

Monday morning starts with a frittata that, if I baked it on Sunday night, requires only warming. Lunch is also quick, with BLT Boats made of bacon, sliced tomato, a few leaves of romaine, and homemade ranch dressing. For dinner, I'll rice a whole head of cauliflower and use half to make my 20-Minute Skillet Dinner. I'll use the other half for chicken fried "rice" on Thursday.

On Tuesday, I make a quick breakfast pizza with a cream cheese base, precooked bacon and sausage, a lightly scrambled egg, and some shredded cheese. Leftover Taco Bake with sour cream and cheese makes a great lunch. I'll add guacamole or diced avocado if we have some. For dinner, I make a Savory Dutch baby, which

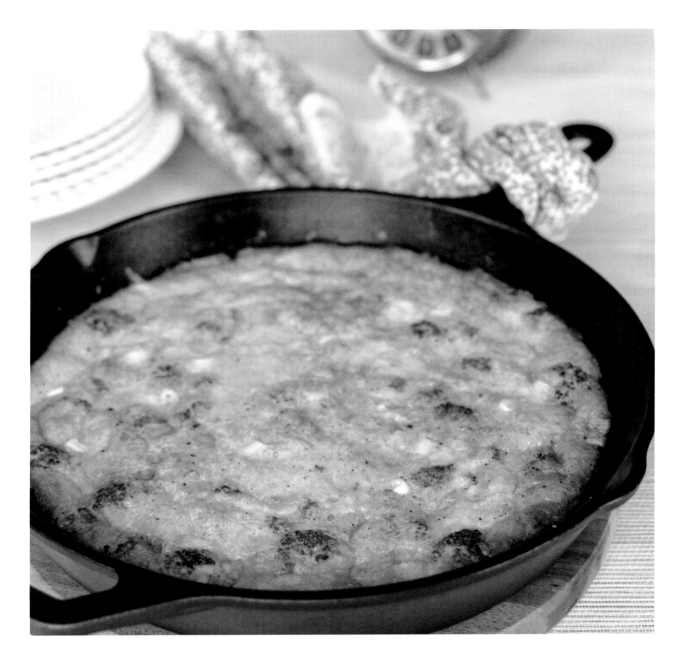

takes less than thirty minutes. I can add a salad if the family wants one.

On Wednesday morning, I enjoy more frittata for breakfast and leftover Dutch baby for lunch. Before leaving for work, I place a whole chicken in the slow cooker; it will be tender and juicy in time for dinner. All I have to do to get dinner on the table is make the broccoli salad. Having the cheese already shredded and the bacon already cooked means that dinner will be ready in less than twenty minutes.

On Thursday morning, I make another easy breakfast pizza and pack BLT boats for lunch. I use leftover roasted chicken and the cauliflower that I riced on Monday night to make chicken fried "rice" for dinner. Once again, dinner is done in less than half an hour!

On Friday, I finish the frittata and enjoy a quick pizza for lunch using leftover sausage, bacon, and pepperoni. For an easy evening meal, we can eat the rest of the 20-Minute Skillet Dinner.

Additional Time-Saving Tips

Because I can't always spend Saturday or Sunday planning, I try to take advantage of my time in the kitchen to do some simple prep work while I'm cooking other meals or when I have a little downtime. This saves time in the long run.

First, I've found that cooking the meat is often the part of a recipe that takes the longest. Cooking meat and then freezing it can help tremendously on days when time is stretched too thin. Instead of setting aside additional time, you can cook extra meat when you're already in the kitchen making a meal. For example, you can monitor two skillets at a time and use one to brown ground beef for taco salad and the other to cook hamburgers. After dinner, the burgers can be frozen individually or in packages of two or four or saved for a meal later in the week. Taco meat can be frozen in individual portions for lunches or in a larger batch for a family meal.

Similarly, roasting two whole chickens is just as easy as roasting one. One chicken can be eaten for a meal right away, while the meat from the second chicken can be used for chicken salad or frozen for later use. Sometimes I brown sausage as crumbles for quick omelets or pizzas. Other times I make sausage patties that can be rewarmed quickly for breakfast. Again, we can enjoy the sausage in a variety of ways without dirtying multiple pans or cleaning the cooktop more than once.

Foods that can be time-intensive to prepare are also good candidates for batch prepping. Meatballs are one example, and they freeze well, cooked or uncooked. I often freeze cooked meatballs in individual portions and pack them in lunch boxes. They are also great to eat on the run because they thaw quickly. Uncooked meatballs can be frozen on a rimmed baking sheet and then tossed into a freezer-safe plastic bag. They can go from the freezer to the oven for a fast meal with minimal cleanup. Uncooked jalapeño poppers can also be frozen on a rimmed baking sheet and then stored in a freezer-safe bag and baked when needed. Making two dozen poppers and freezing half is simpler than making one dozen poppers two separate times.

Lastly, I like to batch prep ingredients that I use frequently. For example, when I'm shredding cheese, I use a food processor or the shredding attachment for my stand mixer. The stand mixer method works well because I can position a freezer-safe plastic bag right under the grater to catch the cheese. I can easily shred 6 or 7 pounds, label it, freeze or refrigerate it, and clean the shredder in less than thirty minutes. Whenever we need cheese for a recipe or to top a dish, I can reach into the fridge or freezer and grab some preshredded mozzarella, Parmesan, cheddar, or Monterey Jack instead of having to stop and shred cheese and then clean up the mess.

Seasoning mixes can also be prepared ahead of time. Because my family eats so much ranch dressing, I keep a mason jar full of the dry seasoning mix used to make it (page 208). I use the seasoning mix not only for salad dressing but also to season meats, soups, and other dishes. The same is true for taco seasoning (page 207) and rib rubs (pages 298 and 306). Dinner comes together far more quickly when I'm not rummaging through the spice drawer and measuring out a half dozen spices. Instead, I reach for the labeled mason jar, use the amount of seasoning mix that I need, and keep on cooking.

None of these time-saving tips are difficult to implement. In fact, many of them have become second nature to me. It might take an additional minute to double the ingredients for a recipe, but it would take longer to make two separate batches. I also save a lot of time batch cooking meat when I cook and clean once but eat twice . . . or more.

When Meal Planning Fails: Turning to Plan B

My meal plans don't always go off perfectly. What happens when I've made eight servings of Sullivans' KeDough Pizza Crust and it's eaten within three days? Or when I've made a double batch of Healthy Hamburger Helper, but there isn't enough left over to feed the family a second meal? From time to time, someone in the family doesn't like a meal I've made or doesn't want leftovers. On other nights, a last-minute homework project or an unscheduled meeting keeps me from preparing the meal I'd planned. There are even times when I realize that I failed to pick up a key ingredient when doing my weekly shopping. My to-do list runneth over, and I fret over what I'll feed my family.

These are the times when I go to Plan B. Instead of fussing at myself for not planning better, I know that I can scrounge up something. With a well-stocked kitchen, I know that the freezer or pantry always holds promise. The following are some of my Plan B foods and easy meals.

From the freezer:

- **Hot dogs**—Though not ideal, hot dogs can be boiled on the stovetop or heated up in the microwave. We eat them with mayo, mustard, low-carb ketchup, cheese, and whatever easy sides are available, like coleslaw or creamed spinach.

- **Ground beef**—Raw ground beef can be pulled from the freezer and browned in a skillet for an open taco skillet. When there's lettuce in the fridge, we can have taco salad with shredded cheese and sour cream. If we're lucky, there's a fresh avocado, too. Ground beef can also be browned for Bolognese (page 300), which can be served on its own or over Zoodles (page 340), Cabbage Noodles (page 342), or glucomannan noodles (such as Miracle Noodles). I also defrost ground beef to make hamburgers, chili, or taco soup. Another tip is to freeze leftover cooked ground beef dishes. For example, if I have extra burgers, taco meat, meatloaf, or meatballs, I put them in labeled freezer-safe containers and use them for Plan B meals. They are excellent lunch options, too.

- **Thinly sliced beef**—If you have a bell pepper and an onion, you can fry up Philly cheesesteaks quickly. Top the mixture with shredded cheese and serve bunless cheesesteaks with mayonnaise and pickles on the side.

- **Cheese**—Frozen mozzarella can go straight from the freezer to a skillet to make a quick Skillet Pizza (page 314). I usually have pepperoni, bell pepper, black olives, and onion on hand for toppings. I can also open a can of tomato sauce to drizzle over the top.

- **Deli meat**—I generally have three or four packages of deli meat in the freezer, bought on sale. Most of it is used for lunches, but in a pinch, I can make roll-ups by combining cream cheese, my homemade ranch seasoning (page 208), and mayonnaise and spreading the mixture on slices of meat.

- **The Sullivans' KeDough Pizza Crusts (page 216)**—These can go from the freezer to a baking sheet, where I top them with whatever I have on hand, bake at 350°F, and serve. The children can also make pizzas without me, which is a bonus.

From the pantry:

- **Canned chicken, tuna, and salmon**—With mayo and dill pickles, you can make a quick salad with any of these options. Canned chicken can also be used in an easy broccoli casserole for a heartier meal.

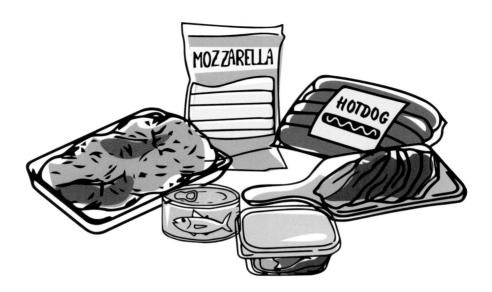

Plan B items like these may not make your list of favorite meals and may not be ideal in terms of ingredients, but you will be fed and remain on plan without a detour through the drive-through. Take the time to identify your new keto staples so that even at the last minute, you have a Plan B. It's always a good idea to keep a written list of Plan B staples that your family will enjoy.

Meal Planning Summary

Knowing what to eat and having foods that you enjoy on hand is paramount to your success. Take the time to identify your new favorite foods and meals. Also, take a little time to experiment with new recipes or new combinations of foods.

Meal planning can seem like a daunting task, but following a process makes it easier. Committing to meal planning often saves time, money, and sanity in the long run. When you can't meal plan or when plans go awry, having a well-stocked kitchen and a creative Plan B will keep you motoring toward your goals.

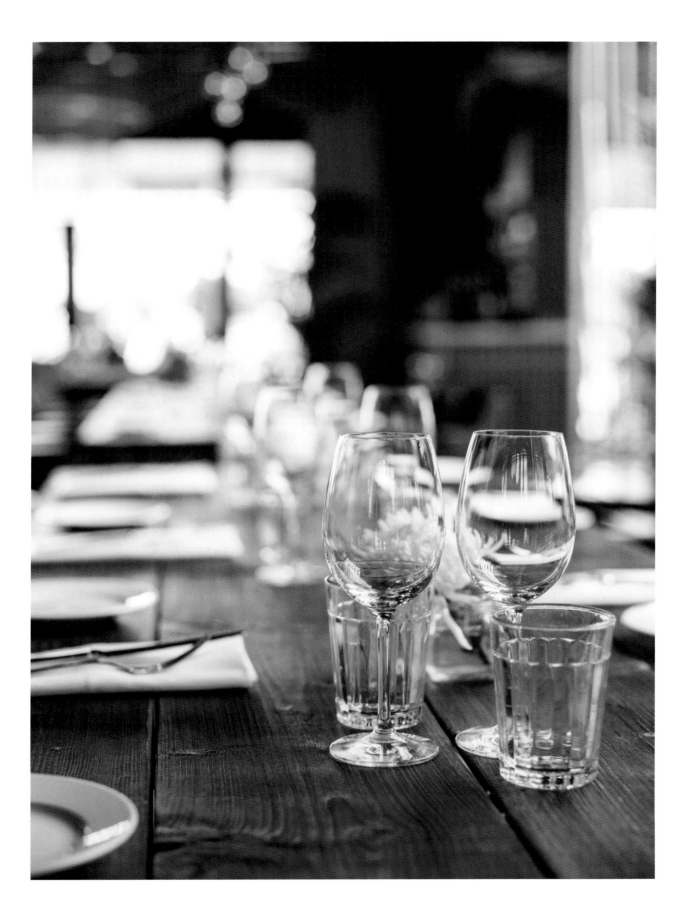

Chapter 3

Eating Keto
in the Real World

In the first month, following a ketogenic lifestyle is often easiest when you prepare your own food and eat your meals in the safety of your keto-fied kitchen. However, most of us are eventually faced with sharing meals with others who may not understand why we eat differently. In fact, because a high-fat ketogenic diet is the opposite of what most people consider healthy, how you eat may seem downright odd to those around you.

Whether you're celebrating with friends or family or simply eating at a restaurant for necessity, there are ways to navigate the common pitfalls associated with eating keto away from home so that you can stay on plan, make progress, and continue to get healthier. Now that you know how important good food choices are to your body, it's time to arm yourself with strategies for eating with others and for staying SAFE when eating out.

Staying on Plan in Social Settings

Eating with others is one of the top reasons people have difficulty adopting and sustaining a ketogenic lifestyle. First, food connects us. Whether it's lunch with a friend or a holiday celebration, food is involved in nearly every social interaction. We feel a tremendous need to assimilate. Also, we tend to enjoy "special" foods with friends and family. If we reject those foods, we might feel as if we are rejecting the people we care about. In addition, we tend to give each other indirect permission by sharing treats. One of my best friends always said, "When you eat dessert with a friend, the calories don't count!" She's right—the calories don't count, but the carbs do!

If you can learn to navigate eating in social settings, you will breeze through the journey.

Common Social Eating Struggles and How to Overcome Them

The following are some of the primary struggles people face when eating in social settings and some suggestions for managing them.

We don't want to be different

Relationships are often built on how we are similar to others. Whether we share mutual interests or common experiences, being similar matters. Often our food choices are about going along with the crowd. We don't want to be difficult by asking for different foods, bringing our own foods, or even needing alternative foods. The reality is that when food affects your health, you already *are* different. My daughter has two wonderful friends who have severe food allergies. Eating out with them or hosting them for meals can be a challenge, but never

once have I felt frustrated with them for having allergies. In fact, my entire family is careful to respect their needs. The last thing I want is for them to become sick because of the food I prepared for or shared with them.

When your body needs to follow a ketogenic diet, it is not a food preference. High-carb foods make me sick, as evidenced by the inflammation and obesity that I used to struggle with. Like it or not, I am different from someone who can eat higher-carb foods—and you might be different, too.

If pressed about why you're not eating "like everybody else," you can simply explain that high-carb foods make you feel bad. Then focus on shared interests other than food.

Sharing food creates an emotional bond ("Food is love")

Many of us have friends or family members who show love by preparing homemade meals or treats. (In fact, many of us may be guilty of using food to show affection ourselves.) Unfortunately, when that food contributes to our health issues, our loved ones may not understand that refusing the food they have prepared is not the same as rejecting *them*.

As difficult as it might be, we have to separate the food itself from the affection we are being offered. You do this by expressing sincere gratitude to the person who prepared it, explaining that while you cannot enjoy the food for health reasons, you genuinely appreciate the thoughtfulness. It might also help to suggest new ways to express their affection. One way is to tell them what foods or activities you enjoy now that you've adopted a ketogenic lifestyle. For example, if your aunt usually makes your favorite high-carb cookies, you could say something like, "I've always thought you were so special for making those cookies for me, and I looked forward to them every year.

Since I'm no longer eating sugar or flour, please don't make those. I would hate for them to go to waste. If you'd like to make something, I sure would enjoy *[insert a keto-friendly food such as chili, roasted pecans, or a favorite cheese]*." Alternatively, you could suggest doing an activity together or starting a new tradition that does not involve food.

My extended family has always enjoyed the foods that I've shared, and they still do. For a recent holiday gathering, I made several of my keto recipes, and each one was well liked. As long as the food is delicious, most people will be open to trying it. My family and friends don't think of the foods I share as "diet" foods or keto foods; they simply think of them as foods they will probably enjoy. If you don't tell people it's keto, they won't think twice about it. Try serving the Taco Bake on page 312, for example, and you'll see what I mean.

Celebrations are centered around food

I cannot think of a single holiday or celebration that does not traditionally involve food. Too often, the celebration *is* the food. We tend to celebrate with cake, and somehow partaking of a large sheet cake involves us in the party. While it seems odd to me now that I've been eating keto for so long, I have seen people struggle with what to do at a wedding or birthday party. A woman once said to me, "I can't refuse to eat wedding cake; it will hurt the bride's feelings!" This lady was neither the mother of the bride nor a member of the wedding party, so I asked, "How many people do you expect to be at the wedding?" She responded, "Oh, at least 100, maybe 200." I smiled as I asked, "And how many of those people are likely to notice that you aren't eating cake?" Most of us are far more self-conscious about what we are or aren't eating than anyone else will ever be. My own wedding reception was so busy and filled with emotion that I'm not sure I even ate cake, and I certainly could not tell you whether any of the guests refused cake. Even if someone had, I would not have been offended.

I had a similar conversation with another woman who was wringing her hands over her grandson's first birthday party. She told me, "You don't understand. It's my grandson's first birthday! I *have* to eat cake." She was right. I did not understand how keeping herself healthy by avoiding cake would diminish the celebration. Being part of a celebration is about being present. You can celebrate milestones or accomplishments by sharing time with others and recognizing that the joy is not in the food.

Holidays are often the hardest days to navigate. Holidays often come with a range of emotions, such as joy, stress, frustration, and nostalgia, and we are barraged with food connected to those emotions. In many families, tradition dictates that certain desserts or starchy sides simply *must* be served. Not only have those food traditions tasted good to us, but they connect us to our loved ones.

The first time my daughter helped me make my grandmother's pumpkin pie, she was only six years old. I was excited to share that experience with her since I was the only one in the family who had carried on the tradition. I remember snapping a photo and sharing it with other family members. We long for those connections. For the past five Thanksgivings, though, my family has not followed my grandmother's pumpkin pie recipe. Instead, I figured out a way to make that high-carb pie into a low-carb cheesecake that we can all enjoy while remaining healthy. Because I've shared the recipe, it has become a new family tradition not only at our house, but for thousands of others.

In addition to creating low-carb alternatives to some of our favorite holiday foods, my family has been intentional about creating new traditions that do not involve food. We look forward to these new traditions because they are all about spending time together and not about eating. In fact, many of our new traditions are even more enjoyable because they don't involve cooking and cleaning the kitchen. Here are just a few examples:

- **New Year's Day**—No black-eyed peas or corn-bread for us. We have a pajama movie day and take turns choosing our favorite movies to watch together. We tend to eat leftovers from the fridge or create simple meals that don't take us away from our movies, like antipasti platters.

- **Valentine's Day**—We make a meal together. The meal is ketogenic, but the focus is on the process. We use the good china, and the children set the dining room table. We take the time to dress up as if we were eating at a very nice restaurant.

- **Easter**—We avoid a lot of candy in the Easter baskets. Low-carb chocolates work well, but the children also get a book, new sunglasses, or other inexpensive toys or games. Often they get something related to summer, such as something to take to the pool or on vacation.

- **Fourth of July**—We go to a huge parade in my hometown and enjoy it with my childhood friends and their families. This is an easy holiday to stay on plan because it is often celebrated with cookouts, which are easy to make keto-friendly.

- **Halloween**—Trick-or-treating can be stressful! I don't like to give out candy, and I don't like my children getting candy. Fortunately, they are starting to age out of trick-or-treating. We've found inexpensive pencils, erasers, stickers, and so on that can be given to trick-or-treaters in lieu of sweets. We also carve pumpkins, and I make a big pot of low-carb chili that we look forward to.

- **Thanksgiving**—While I make several low-carb dishes for Thanksgiving meals with extended family, we have nonfood traditions, too. We typically begin decorating for Christmas over the Thanksgiving break. That tradition involves a six-hour drive round-trip to select a Christmas tree. The journey itself creates plenty of memories, such as the year when there were several inches of snow and Mom chose a tree that was so big it broke our tree stand.

- **Christmas**—In addition to the annual tree trek, we choose an evening or two to view Christmas lights. We simply drive around local neighborhoods, stopping at several of our favorites. Also, we go to a local performance of *The Nutcracker* that features many of the kids' friends. Over the years, it has been fun to hear the kids relate differently to the performance. Another nonfood tradition is the Elf on the Shelf. Even though my children have outgrown Santa, they still enjoy seeing what that elf gets into. Lastly, we have a tradition of gifting a puzzle to each set of grandparents. After opening presents, we often sit around working on the puzzle together with folks coming and going as we relax and chat and enjoy the company.

I encourage you to tackle holiday food traditions head on by letting others know in advance that you are no longer eating high-carb foods. Suggest new alternatives to high-carb favorites or simply explain that those kinds of foods make you feel unwell. You can still participate in the celebration without eating the food.

We fear that others are judging our decisions or feel as if we are judging theirs

First, rest assured that folks are not judging our decisions as frequently as we fear they are. Most people truly do not care what we eat unless it makes them feel bad about what they are eating. How many times have you sat with a group at a restaurant and heard the server ask if anyone will be enjoying dessert? Frequently everyone glances around the table to see if anyone else is going to order dessert. As soon as the first person says, "No dessert for me!" others begin shaking their heads. Likewise, if someone says, "Yes, please, can we see a dessert menu?" then everyone at the table has "permission" to order dessert.

When you follow a ketogenic diet, the dessert menu is literally off the table. Even restaurants that offer "low-carb" desserts tend to use higher-carb ingredients or sugar substitutes that are not keto-friendly. That might leave you as the lone diner choosing to abstain. Whether you intend it that way or not, your choice to decline might be seen as putting on airs, especially if you are avoiding dessert as part of a diet.

One way to address this is to order coffee or a glass of dry wine so that you are participating in the process but still remaining on plan. Another way to avoid seeming judgmental is to emphasize that sugar makes you feel bad. The choice isn't yours, but one that your body has made for you. Moreover, taking an interest in others' dessert choices is like giving them permission to enjoy dessert even though you know that it is not a healthy option for you.

Lastly, remember that of all the people with whom you share a meal, it is your opinion of yourself that matters most. Ask yourself what *you* will be happiest eating. A little discomfort in turning down food or choosing to eat differently is temporary, but feeling good builds confidence along with better health.

No one wants us to be deprived

Never, ever tell someone that you are on a diet. Never. Think about what it means to be on a diet. Traditionally, anyone who is dieting is miserably hungry and feels deprived. This is especially true on a low-fat, calorie-restricted diet. In social settings, folks want us to have fun! As we all know, deprivation is not fun.

When you say you are on a diet or trying to lose weight, you open the door to coaxing. "Oh, it's just one night! You can be good tomorrow!" Or "All things in moderation. You should enjoy yourself." Sadly, not everyone understands that truly enjoying yourself is about feeling good and being healthy. The happiness is not in those foods that make us sick.

When faced with limited food options

There will be settings where keto-friendly food options are limited. Whether it's a dinner party, a restaurant, or a work event, your best option may be to not eat. The wonderful thing about keto is that you can skip a meal. As strange as it may seem to you now, once you are fat-adapted, your hunger is diminished, so you can often skip a meal or go six or more hours between meals.

When I'm faced with zero good food options, I generally choose not to eat. If questioned, I try to be gracious and say either that I'm not hungry or that I plan to eat later. I avoid saying anything about the food not being good for me unless I'm pressed. Even then, I avoid being critical of the food that is available and focus on the fact that I avoid certain foods because I feel unwell when I eat them.

Five Tips for Navigating Social Situations

Eating in social settings is genuinely more difficult than eating at home in the safety of your own kitchen, where you control the ingredients; however, if you arm yourself with strategies ahead of time, you will be empowered to stay on plan. Regardless of where or with whom you're eating, follow these simple steps.

Step 1: Decide in advance of the event

Decide in advance what you will eat—before problem foods are tempting you and others are encouraging you to eat off plan. If you are unsure of what you will eat, you are far more likely to make poor choices.

Compare eating in social settings to shopping. If I go to the mall without a budget in mind, I am likely to buy on impulse and overspend; however, if I know my limits in advance, before I'm tempted by the 50 percent–off deals, then I'm more likely to stick to my budget and return home without regrets. Too often, when I make decisions in the moment, I react emotionally instead of objectively. Remind yourself of the progress you've made or want to make. Decide in advance that you won't invite cravings back in by indulging in high-carb foods.

Step 2: Never say diet!

Frame your food choices as healthy choices and not as a diet. When others believe that you are on a diet, they tend to focus on weight without regard for overall health. They also focus on the deprivation and misery that are so common on traditional diets. Someone on a diet is often told to eat "in moderation." When you're "on a diet," you are more likely to be met with comments such as, "Oh, just have a little bit! You can diet tomorrow," or assurances such as, "We'll go for a walk tomorrow and work it off." Others don't want you to feel deprived and may not understand the significance of weight as a marker of poor health.

Steer the conversation away from weight loss and focus on health instead. You might say, "I'm sure that's delicious, but I find that too much sugar (or bread or pasta) makes me feel bad. My body is just really sensitive to it. You enjoy it; I'll have some coffee." What you're communicating is that those choices make you feel bad. No one wants *you* to feel bad. You've turned your food choices into eating to avoid a sensitivity and not a diet to lose weight.

Step 3: Make it clear that your decision is *your* decision

Make food choices in ways that do not pass judgment on others. Whether they realize it or not, many people want you to eat high-carb foods, especially desserts or other treats, to absolve any guilt that they feel. If you've ever passed on dessert and then found that someone else at the table canceled his or her dessert order, then you understand.

Just as you do not want to be judged for your food choices, you want to foster positive relationships with others by not judging their food choices. In the suggested dialogue above, you aren't judging the other person's choice when you say, "*You* enjoy it." If, instead, you said, "I'm not going to eat that because it's unhealthy," you would be indirectly passing judgment on the person choosing to eat it.

Step 4: Shift the focus away from food

Once you have decided what you will and will not eat and have articulated that decision, divert the conversation away from food differences as quickly and naturally as you can. Comments about current events or the restaurant's decor, or even a sincere compliment to another person can get the conversation moving in a different direction. When in doubt, asking someone a specific question nearly always shifts the conversation. Children, pets, jobs, and hobbies are typically safe topics that folks enjoy discussing with others.

Step 5: Be the victor, not the victim

Enjoy your decision to stay on plan. Whether you settle on having a cup of coffee while others enjoy dessert or whether you order a bunless burger, keep any conversation about your food choices positive. The purpose of socializing is to have fun and enjoy the company of others. Even if you're thinking, "Dang, those onion rings look good!" don't say it aloud. Saying that you wish you could eat something opens the door to others encouraging you to eat it. Keep that door closed by being content with your choices outwardly, if not inwardly. When the moment passes, you won't regret what you didn't eat.

When you decide to be the victor, you refuse to think of food as something you're missing. Instead of approaching food from a perspective of deprivation or restriction, focus on what you *can* enjoy. I eat keto foods that I really like—chicken wings, bacon, butter, and cheeses. The fact that I've been eating those delicious, previously forbidden foods and became healthier while doing it makes it all the better. By focusing on what I "win" when I don't eat foods like bread and pasta, such as fitting into smaller jeans and being able to ride a bike again, I look forward to all the things keto gives me. Instead of focusing on what I miss eating, I focus on what I missed living when I ate those high-carb foods.

Perhaps most important, I make the choices. When people say to me, "Oh, you can't have that!" I have to stifle my inner three-year-old, who now wants exactly what she has been told she can't have. "I *can* have that, but I choose not to eat it," I reply. For my three-year-old who spent nearly all her life being monitored, criticized, and denied is no longer controlled by food and by others controlling her food. She controls her food, and when *she* chooses, she is powerful!

Some folks say, "Nothing tastes as good as skinny feels." I could never identify with that phrase because I never knew what it meant to be skinny. What I *can* identify with is how miserable it feels to be obese and in pain. When I look at bread, potatoes, pasta, or high-carb desserts, I see that miserable obese person I was for forty years, and the decision becomes far easier. I choose to be the victor, not the victim.

You can use those five steps to navigate most social settings. In case you're wondering how to implement them, I've included some sample lines that you can try when facing social challenges. These strategies have gotten me through every holiday, celebration, and social setting I've faced. At times I felt a little awkward, but I have never regretted choosing to stay on plan.

Each time you use these phrases, you should feel more empowered to speak up and choose wisely. When you make good choices, you feel good physically and mentally. Plus, you never know who else you might inspire. Someone who needs keto may be watching you and may need you to be an example they can follow.

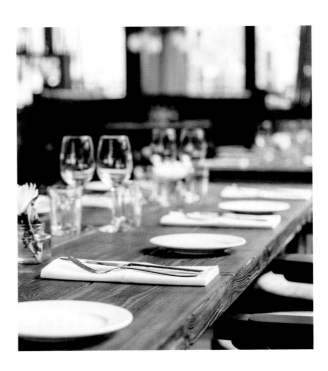

When you truly aren't hungry:

- "That looks great! I ate just a short while ago, but you enjoy."

- "Thanks so much, but I am stuffed from lunch [or dinner or breakfast]. I couldn't possibly eat another bite."

- "I'm sure that's delicious, but I'm looking forward to a big meal later today."

When you're dealing with food pushers or others who are challenging your ketogenic lifestyle and you want to emphasize that you truly feel better when you avoid sugar, grains, and starches:

- "The longer I go without eating sugar, the more I find that it makes me feel sick. Even one bite of something sugary, and it takes me a day or two to recover. I don't want to risk feeling bad because we are having so much fun!"

- "That has to be the most gorgeous cake I have ever seen in my life! Unfortunately, I can no longer eat flour and sugar. My doctor has been so pleased that my labs are better. I don't want to eat anything that might mess those up."

- "The last time I ate [insert food], I was miserable for three days! My body just does not tolerate it. I'll stick to eating [insert name of keto-friendly food, like steak or asparagus] and enjoying a glass of wine (or coffee)."

- "You know, I've been avoiding starches for several weeks now, and my digestion issues are so much better. I'm going to keep being careful with what I eat because I enjoy feeling good!"

When you're refusing food that has an emotional connection:

- "Aunt Sally, you know you make my favorite chicken pot pie! I have always loved sharing that with you, and I love that you made it just for me. Unfortunately, I've developed some food sensitivities, and I'm afraid I can't enjoy it anymore. I'd love to sit and chat with you for a while, though. I always enjoy when we have time together." Follow that comment by asking her about something important to her. Whether it's a new pet, a new car, or a pretty piece of jewelry she is wearing, deflect attention from the food to your sincere fondness for her.

- "I know that used to be our favorite food and we always ate it together, but I no longer eat foods high in sugar and starch. Let's grab a cup of coffee instead!" You could also suggest a nonfood activity, such as window shopping, taking a walk, or looking through old photos.

- "Grandmother always made the best coconut cakes. I loved that she made those for Christmas every year, and I loved that she always made an extra so everyone got an extra slice, but my favorite part was helping her make the cake. Do you remember the year she bought whole coconuts and we had to help crack them open? Granddad got a drill and we drained the coconut juice, and then she took a hammer to it! We ended up running to the store at the last minute to buy frozen shredded coconut!" Relating the recipe to another memory emphasizes that the true connection was made while making the cake, not eating it. You can enjoy the fond memories without eating the high-carb food.

Eventually you will come up with your own best responses for the situations you face and the people with whom you interact. Just remember to make your food decisions in advance, never say that you're on a diet, be careful not to judge or appear to judge the decisions of others, shift the focus away from food as quickly and as often as you can, and choose to be the victor, not the victim.

Eating at Restaurants

When I was adapting to a very-low-carb diet, I became comfortable preparing my own meals, but the first few times I went out to eat, I nearly panicked! Each time I worried that there would be nothing I could eat. I didn't want to be *that* person who asked too many questions or held up everyone else's orders because I was asking for something different. Over time, I learned a few tips and tricks that helped me order with far more confidence so that I could enjoy eating out again.

The easiest way to dine out successfully is learn as much as you can about the restaurant, the menu, and any specials in advance. When I review a menu, I follow a process that you can remember with the acronym SAFE:

- **S**can the menu.
- **A**sk questions.
- **F**ind options.
- **E**at until satisfied.

Scan the Menu

From appetizers to side items, I scan nearly every section of the menu. Sometimes appetizers are ideal portion sizes. Grilled meats, oysters Rockefeller, and platters of meats and cheeses are common on appetizer menus and can make a great meal or option to share. When I scan the salad listings, I look for a salad with plenty of fat and protein. Vegetables are primarily carbohydrates; therefore, a salad is not ideal unless it includes reasonable amounts of fat and protein. In a pinch, I order my salad with extra dressing, avocado, cheese, and/or bacon. Sandwiches, and especially burgers, can be good options if you order them without a bun or bread. Many restaurants will allow you to order a side of veggies with butter or a small salad with a high-fat dressing to go with it.

When I scan the menu, I look not just at potential entrees to order, but also to see which foods are on hand in the kitchen. For example, if I see that an entree comes with spinach but the entree I prefer is served with rice, then I know I can ask for spinach instead of rice with my entree. I've done the same thing with other low-carb vegetables, such as asparagus, green beans, and broccoli.

Ask Questions

As I scan the menu, I make a mental note of questions to ask if I plan to order a certain item. For example, I nearly always confirm that there is no sugar or flour in the sauces. When there is any doubt, I simply avoid the sauces. I also ask for substitutions that seem fair or appropriate, such as a vegetable instead of fries or a baked potato. While some people may be hesitant to ask for a sandwich without bread or a burger without a bun, I have never had a problem ordering food that way. I much prefer not wasting the bread and not having any of the cheese stick or any of the fatty goodness of the meat seep into the bun.

Find Options

As I scan the menu, I note the options that look best to me. I eliminate options by asking questions or by deciding just to avoid questionable items. By the time everyone is ready to order, I've usually identified at least two good low-carb selections.

Eat Until Satisfied

Restaurant portions never seemed large to me before I started following a ketogenic diet. Because I eat high-fat foods, I tend to fill up more quickly now. Instead of cleaning my plate, I often mentally draw a line across the plate and decide in advance to eat only half before taking a break. If I'm still hungry after I've eaten half, I continue eating, but if I'm starting to feel satisfied, I ask for a box and eat the leftovers as a second meal later. Learning to eat to satiety (I call it "eating to hunger"), even if it means leaving food on your plate, can help your long-term success.

General Tips for Eating Out

Here are some general tips for dining in restaurants:

- When possible, preview the menu ahead of time so that you have an idea of which options might be best. Most menus are available online, and many restaurants provide nutrition information, too.

- If you have a lot of questions or are uncomfortable asking questions in front of others, call the restaurant beforehand. If a restaurant is impatient with your questions over the phone, you might want to select a different restaurant.

- If you review the menu in advance and find no satisfactory options, eat before joining your group and have a cup of coffee or a glass of wine while the others eat.

- Ask if meat is breaded before it is fried. Look for roasted meats or seafood entrees without breading.

- Ask for melted butter to add fat to lean meats and seafood.

- If a dish is served with a sauce, ask about flour or thickeners that may be used in the sauce.

- Ask if there is sugar or corn syrup in the sauces or dressings. Avoid teriyaki, honey mustard, ketchup, Thousand Island, and BBQ sauce, which typically contain added sugars. If you want to avoid inflammatory oils, the best salad dressing is a simple olive oil and vinegar.

- Before ordering a dip or cheese sauce, check to see if it is thickened with flour.

- In general, choose butter or cream-based sauces over tomato sauces, which are higher in carbs; however, be sure to ask whether cream-based sauces have added flour or starches.

- Avoid pasta, even if the pasta is advertised as being gluten-free.

- Look for menu items that can be substituted for higher-carb sides, such as asparagus or steamed broccoli instead of rice.

On the following pages, I've provided sample menus from three different types of restaurants. For each menu, I've shared the SAFE process that I would use to identify keto-friendly meals.

American Restaurant Example

Ketogenic options are often plentiful at traditional American restaurants. Follow the general rules of eating out by remembering to stay SAFE.

Scan the menu

Among the starters, I would skip the egg rolls, jalapeño poppers, and corn dog nuggets because all have a batter or wheat-based wrap. The spinach artichoke dip and crawfish dip sound promising, so I would make a mental note to ask whether either has flour or a thickener in it. The dip would be easy to share with others at the table and should be high in fat if I need fat to add to an entree.

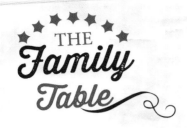

THE Family Table

Salads

House Salad
Organic green leaf lettuce, Applewood smoked bacon, cheddar cheese, cherry tomatoes, bell peppers, and Mama's homemade dill pickles

Caesar Salad
Romaine lettuce, toasted sourdough croutons, and Parmesan cheese topped with Caesar dressing

Family's Special
Crisp iceberg lettuce with black olives, red onions, pepperoncini, banana peppers, tomatoes, and freshly grated Romano cheese

Grilled Chicken Salad
Grilled chicken on a bed of green leaf lettuce, with roasted pecan chips, grilled red onions, bell peppers, cheddar cheese, and house-made sourdough croutons

Salad dressings: Thousand Island, Ranch, Caesar, French, Italian, or Family's Home-Style Garlic
Add grilled or fried chicken, grilled salmon, or a shrimp skewer to any salad for $2.00

Starters

Cheeseburger Egg Rolls
Crispy egg rolls stuffed with beef, lettuce, cheese, pickles, and mayonnaise

Jalapeño Poppers
Deep-fried jalapeños bursting with creamy cheese, bacon, and ham

Mini Corn Dog Nuggets
Fun-size big-kid bites of hot dog covered in a homemade cornmeal batter and deep-fried

Lighter Side Options

Citrus-Glazed Salmon
Salmon brushed with our perfect lime and orange glaze and oven-baked, served with an asparagus and mushroom medley

Lemon Pepper Whitefish
Mild whitefish seasoned with our lemon pepper butter and grilled to perfection, served on a bed of brown rice

Gorgonzola Spinach Artichoke Dip
Spicy cheese dip with spinach and artichokes, served with thick slices of toasted baguette

Crawfish Dip
Crawfish tails swimming in a thick three-cheese dip seasoned with Creole flavors, served with thick slices of toasted baguette

Served with your choice of seasonal veggies or sautéed spinach

Seared Sea Scallops
Lightly seasoned fresh scallops seared in a bacon-infused butter, garnished with bacon crumbles and served with quinoa

Lime Grilled Chicken
Grilled marinated chicken served with a citrus sauce over orzo pasta

Sides
Choose a loaded potato (butter, sour cream, cheese, bacon) for $0.75 extra

Baked potato*
Macaroni and cheese
Steamed broccoli
Seasonal vegetables

Sweet potato casserole
Country green beans
Sautéed mushrooms
Coleslaw

The salad menu looks safe if I can't find other options and if I ask for no croutons. Before ordering a salad, I would ask about the ingredients in the home-style garlic dressing. If the ingredients were not keto-friendly, I could substitute ranch or blue cheese dressing. (Both are likely to contain inflammatory oils, especially if they are not homemade.) I could ask whether olive oil and vinegar is available.

Under House Specialties, I spy a few good options, the most favorable being the roast beef, beef tips, and pork tenderloin. Other possibilities include the pork chop without the chutney. The Alfredo sauce is likely to have been made with flour, but a true Alfredo sauce is not. The fried chicken is coated in a breading that would be difficult to avoid, making it a bad option.

The Lighter Side options nearly always make me chuckle because they are low in fat, but too often sugar is added to enhance the flavor. Almost all of the dishes in this section of the menu have hidden carbs in the form of sweetened sauces or marinades. Citrus glazes are nearly always sweetened. All of these entrees are served with a low-fat grain. Nonetheless, the scallops and whitefish could be good ketogenic entrees when served with additional fat.

Among the side items, the keto-friendly choices would probably include green beans, steamed broccoli, mushrooms, and seasonal vegetables. The most exciting possibility is the loaded baked potato. While a potato is definitely not low-carb, the "loaded" toppings—butter, sour cream, cheese, and bacon—are a keto dream come true. Most restaurants will happily

Sandwiches & Burgers

Served with your choice of French fries, sweet potato fries, chips, potato salad, fruit cup, or house salad

Gourmet Angus Burger
½-pound Black Angus burger served with the Family Table's special sauce, perfectly seasoned crispy onions, your choice of cheese, tomato, lettuce, and Mama's homemade dill pickles

California Avocado Burger
½-pound Black Angus burger topped with sliced avocado, pepper Jack cheese, pico de gallo, and lettuce

Best Bacon Burger
½-pound Black Angus burger served with Applewood smoked bacon, cheddar cheese, lettuce, tomato, and Mama's homemade dill pickles

Western Burger
½-pound Black Angus burger served with our famous BBQ sauce, crispy fried onions, cheddar cheese, tomato, and lettuce

Family's Perfect Reuben
Sliced corned beef, sauerkraut, melted Swiss cheese, and the Family Table's homemade Thousand Island dressing, served on our freshly baked rye bread

Monte Cristo
Sourdough bread fried in butter and layered with smoked ham, juicy turkey, and cheddar cheese and topped with our bacon mayonnaise, served with lettuce, tomato, and dipping sauce

Free-Range Chicken Wrap
Breaded chicken tenders layered with Applewood smoked bacon, shredded smoked Gouda cheese, lettuce, tomato, and our bacon mayonnaise, neatly wrapped in a flour tortilla (grilled chicken available)

Philly Cheesesteak
Shaved Angus beef smothered in grilled peppers, onions, mushrooms, and a generous helping of cheese sauce

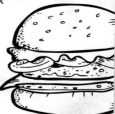

House Specialties

Spaghetti and Meatballs
A family favorite: two huge meatballs with Mama's spaghetti sauce, served over linguine

Slow-Roasted Roast Beef
Aged roast beef roasted for eight hours, topped with our mushroom and onion gravy

Char-Grilled Beef Tips
Perfectly charred beef tenderloin tips served with roasted peppers and onions

Family's Fried Chicken
Daddy's perfectly seasoned and battered chicken crispy fried in peanut oil

Creamy Chicken Fettuccine Alfredo
Chicken roasted in garlic sauce and topped with Alfredo, served over a bed of fettuccine

Grilled Pork Chops
Juicy bone-in pork chops topped with a slow-simmered apple chutney

Marinated Pork Tenderloin
Pork tenderloin marinated overnight and then roasted

---

serve you loaded broccoli instead of a loaded baked potato. You simply need to explain that you want the steamed broccoli and then you want the butter, sour cream, cheese, and bacon served on top of it. With the rich, fatty flavors of the loaded toppings, you will never miss a baked potato again. The coleslaw is likely to contain sugar, so I would avoid it.

A scan of the sandwich options reveals the possibility of ordering a bunless burger or a sandwich without the bread. Request a house salad with a keto-friendly dressing as the side. The Gourmet Angus Burger is probably not a great option because the special sauce is likely to be sweetened. Also, the fried onions may be breaded. The Avocado Burger and Best Bacon Burger look like very good options. The Western Burger would likely be okay without the BBQ sauce or fried onions. Nearly every BBQ sauce is full of sugar, so I avoid it when

eating out. Among the other sandwich options, I would avoid the Thousand Island dressing on the Reuben because those types of dressings are generally high in sugar. The Monte Cristo sounds good, although I would be concerned that the portion might be too small without the bread; however, the words "bacon mayonnaise" are promising. The bacon mayonnaise might also add tasty fat to steamed broccoli, green beans, or seasonal veggies. The Free-Range Chicken Wrap could be ordered without the wrap and with grilled chicken, but I might order a salad with grilled chicken instead. Lastly, a Philly Cheesesteak without the roll could be keto-friendly. On this menu, however, the mention of cheese sauce would give me pause. Cheese sauce is often made from cheese products that contain food starches and inflammatory oils, not from real cheese. I would request shredded cheese instead.

Ask questions

After scanning the menu, I would ask about ingredients in any sauces or dressings in the menu items I was likely to order and whether oil and vinegar was available as a salad dressing. Similarly, I would ask whether there is flour or thickeners in the dips listed in the appetizers section. Before ordering the roast beef, I would ask whether the gravy is made with flour or if I could have the roast without gravy. I would also ask about the ingredients in the pork tenderloin marinade, as it may have sugar in it. In addition, I would ask about substitutions. For example, if I wanted scallops, I might ask if the kitchen could omit the quinoa and have a side of steamed broccoli topped like a loaded baked potato. Alternatively, I could ask for two sides because I'm asking for the quinoa to be left off. Among the other side dish options, I would make sure that the green beans and mushrooms have no added sugar or starch, and I would confirm which seasonal vegetables are included.

Find options

The options that I find on this menu include the following:

- ***Crawfish Dip**—if there is no flour or thickener in the ingredients
- **House Salad**—add salmon, chicken, or shrimp and omit the croutons. Confirm that there is no sugar in the dill pickles. Ask for ranch or blue cheese dressing.
- **Caesar Salad**—add salmon, chicken, or shrimp and omit the croutons. Ask for ranch or blue cheese dressing.
- **Family's Special Salad**—add salmon, chicken, or shrimp and omit the croutons. Ask for ranch or blue cheese dressing.
- **Grilled Chicken Salad**—omit the croutons. Ask if the pecan chips are sweetened. Ask for ranch or blue cheese dressing.

- **Slow-Roasted Roast Beef**—without gravy, with a side of green beans and mushrooms, confirming no sugar in the green beans and no flour in the mushrooms. If the beef could be served without gravy, then I would not order it.
- ***Char-Grilled Beef Tips**—with loaded steamed broccoli and sautéed mushrooms, confirming no flour in the mushrooms
- **Grilled Pork Chops**—without apple chutney, with a side of either loaded steamed broccoli; sautéed mushrooms, confirming no flour; green beans, confirming no sugar; or seasonal veggies, confirming those are low-carb
- ***Marinated Pork Tenderloin**—confirming that there is no sugar in the marinade, with a side of either loaded steamed broccoli; sautéed mushrooms, confirming no flour; green beans, confirming no sugar; or seasonal veggies, confirming those are low-carb
- **Lemon Pepper Whitefish**—with no rice, with a side of either loaded steamed broccoli; sautéed mushrooms, confirming no flour; green beans, confirming no sugar; or seasonal veggies, confirming those are low-carb
- ***Seared Sea Scallops**—without quinoa, a side of either loaded steamed broccoli; sautéed mushrooms, confirming no flour; green beans, confirming no sugar; or seasonal veggies, confirming those are low-carb
- ***Avocado Burger**—without a bun, but with a side salad with ranch or blue cheese dressing. Ask for bacon mayonnaise on the side.
- ***Best Bacon Burger**—without a bun, but with a side salad with ranch or blue cheese dressing. Ask for bacon mayonnaise on the side.
- **Western Burger**—without a bun, without BBQ sauce, and without fried onions. Select a side salad with ranch or blue cheese dressing and ask for bacon mayonnaise on the side.

These are the items I would be most likely to order.

Mexican Restaurant Example

Ketogenic options are plentiful at many Mexican restaurants. Follow the general rules of eating out by remembering to stay SAFE.

Scan the menu

With the exception of guacamole, the appetizer section of a Mexican restaurant menu rarely has much to offer for those on a ketogenic diet. While there are often cheese (queso) sauces, those are typically made with a processed cheese product and include inflammatory oils and food starches and are higher in carbs than real cheese, so it's best to avoid them. Some Mexican restaurants offer chicharrones (fried pork rinds). These are perfect for dipping in guacamole or salsa in lieu of chips.

Often the House Specialties or Favorites section offers some good choices. If nothing else, the entree descriptions can tell you which ingredients the restaurant should have on hand and which substitutions you might request. On this menu, the Carne Asada is a good option. Before ordering, confirm that it does not come with rice or beans. If it does, request that those be left off your plate. The Molcajete, Chile Colorado, Chile Verde, and Carnitas could be excellent choices. Again, confirm that you don't want beans, rice, or tortillas. While the Huevos Rancheros is not a good option, the Chorizo con Huevos includes a fatty Mexican sausage and is a better alternative.

Fajitas are generally my pick at a Mexican restaurant. When possible, I select carnitas

CASA DE SULLIVAN

Starters

Nachos
Beans & tortilla chips topped with cheese, choice of meat, pico de gallo, guacamole, & sour cream

Guacamole
Served with tortilla chips

Chile con Queso
Melted cheese dip served with tortilla chips

Fajitas and Favorites

Fajitas
A half portion of our delicious fajita steak or chicken, served sizzling hot over sautéed onions & green peppers. Served with refried or rancho (cholesterol-free) beans, Mexican rice, corn or flour tortillas, lettuce, pico de gallo, cheddar cheese, sour cream, & guacamole.

Fajitas Quesadillas
Crispy flour tortillas filled with cheddar & Monterey Jack cheeses, pico de gallo, & our delicious fajita steak or chicken. Served with sour cream, guacamole, & your choice of refried or rancho (cholesterol-free) beans & Mexican rice.

Fajita Burrito
Giant 10-inch flour tortilla filled with your choice of delicious fajita steak or chicken, with Mexican rice, grilled onions, & green & red peppers. Your choice of refried or rancho (cholesterol-free) beans. Garnished with pico de gallo, sour cream, & guacamole.

Special la Casa
Tender sliced beef & chicken with cactus, onions, tomatoes, black beans, & two flour tortillas.

Taco Salad Jalisco
(Taco Salad Traditional) Served on a hot plate with cheese melted over your choice of ground beef, chicken, or picadillo & topped with lettuce, cheese, & tomatoes.

Fajita Chimichanga
Deep-fried flour tortilla filled with your choice of grilled chicken or steak, onions, & green peppers. Served with rice, beans, sour cream, guacamole, lettuce, tomatoes, & cheese.

Barbacoa
Shredded spicy slow-braised beef with onions & peppers. Served with rice & corn or flour tortillas. Garnished with lettuce & pico de gallo.

Mole Poblano
Shredded chicken breast with special dark sauce, rice, & guacamole salad. Served with two flour tortillas.

House Specialties

The Famous Macho
Giant 10-inch flour tortilla filled with Mexican rice, black beans, refried or rancho (cholesterol-free) beans, & your choice of ground beef, chicken, or picadillo. Topped with burrito sauce & cheddar cheese. Covered with lettuce, tomatoes, crema Mexicana, & Cotija cheese.

Carne Asada (Gluten-Free)
6-ounce portion of seasoned skirt steak char-broiled to perfection. Garnished with whole green onions, fried jalapeños, & freshly made guacamole.

Carne Asada Burrito
Burrito stuffed with tender skirt steak, refried beans, & Mexican rice, topped with Molcajete sauce, Cotija cheese, & green onions. Served with pico de gallo & fried jalapeños.

Molcajete
Chicken & steak strips sautéed in a mild sauce with mushrooms & onions, topped with melted Monterey Jack cheese. Garnished with pico de gallo & a jalapeño pepper.

Chile Colorado
Tender cuts of beef slow-simmered in a mild red chile sauce with onions & tomatoes.

Chile Verde
Chunks of slow-baked pork blended with a mild green tomatillo sauce, green peppers, onions, & spices.

Pollo a la Crema
Boneless breast of chicken sautéed with onions in a rich cream sauce. Garnished with Cotija cheese.

Carnitas
Tender chunks of stewed pork grilled with onions, green & red peppers, & spices. Served with sour cream, rice, & beans (no guacamole). Choice of flour or corn tortillas.

Huevos Rancheros
Three eggs over easy, topped with salsa ranchera & Monterey Jack cheese. Served with Mexican rice, refried or rancho (cholesterol-free) beans, & corn or flour tortillas. Garnished with lettuce & pico de gallo.

Chorizo con Huevos
Mexican sausage blended with a mix of tomatoes, onions, cilantro, & eggs. Served with Mexican rice, refried or rancho (cholesterol-free) beans, & tortillas.

A La Carta
- Quesadilla (chicken or cheese)
- Taquitos
- Flautitas
- Chiles Rellenos
- Tortas
- Chalupas
- Enchiladas (beef, chicken, shrimp, or cheese)
- Tostadas

and/or chorizo, which are higher in fat. Even if chorizo isn't on the menu, some restaurants will allow you to order it in place of shrimp or beef. I often ask for extra guacamole and sour cream instead of rice, beans, and tortillas. The Taco Salad might be a good option if it doesn't include rice or beans. Barbacoa, Mole Poblano, and Special La Casa all appear to be excellent options without beans or tortillas. Before ordering, I would confirm that the sauces do not contain flour.

The A La Carta menu items are not keto-friendly because each is wrapped in a wheat or corn-based product or served on a shell or wrap. Chiles Rellenos are one possible exception. Traditional Chiles Rellenos are made by roasting poblano peppers, dipping them in an egg wash, and then frying them. The poblanos can be stuffed with cheese or meat and are covered in cheese sauce. Unfortunately, many restaurants use flour in the batter and use a processed cheese product to make the cheese sauce. Also, note that a standard-sized poblano pepper averages 9 grams of carbs!

Ask questions

After scanning the menu, I would probably settle on something obviously keto-friendly, like the fajitas. I would ask for extra guacamole and sour cream instead of rice, beans, and tortillas. If I wanted to try something else, I would ask about the sauces on the other entrees before ordering. Specifically, I would ask whether any flour or thickeners are added.

Find options

The options that I find on this menu include:

- **Carne Asada**—without beans, rice, or tortillas
- **Molcajete**—without beans, rice, or tortillas
- **Chile Colorado**
- **Chile Verde**
- **Pollo a la Crema**—ask about flour in the crema
- **Carnitas**—no rice, beans, or tortillas, with a request for guacamole

- **Fajitas**—with carnitas and/or chorizo instead of shrimp or steak, because carnitas and chorizo are higher in fat than shrimp and steak and often are more tender and flavorful. Request extra guacamole and sour cream instead of rice, beans, and tortillas.
- **Taco Salad Jalisco**—confirming that the salad does not contain rice or beans and ask for shredded cheese instead of queso sauce
- **Barbacoa**—without rice or tortillas, but with added sour cream and guacamole
- **Mole Poblano**—without rice or tortillas
- **Special la Casa**—without tortillas

Here are some general tips for dining in Mexican restaurants:

- Refuse any tortilla chips brought to the table, but keep the salsa if you like.
- Avoid cheese sauces, as most are made with a processed cheese product and have inflammatory oils. When in doubt, ask whether cheese sauces are thickened with flour or starches. Choose grated cheese or queso fresco as a safer option.
- Order your entree without rice or beans. Be clear that you don't want tortillas, either.
- Ask if you can have guacamole, fresh avocado, or extra sour cream instead of rice, beans, and tortillas.
- Choose fattier meats such as carnitas (pork) or chorizo (Mexican sausage). Chicken or steak is fine but will be leaner.
- Avoid salads that have beans and rice in the base.
- Avoid too many peppers and onions in entrees such as fajitas. You can easily avoid eating those in most dishes.
- Avoid dishes that are wrapped in flour or corn tortillas. These include flautitas, quesadillas, taquitos, tortas, chalupas, sopas, enchiladas, and tostadas. You can choose to eat only the filling, but often there is very little filling, or the filling includes beans and/or rice, which are difficult to pick out.

Italian Restaurant Example

Ketogenic options can be plentiful at a good Italian restaurant. Follow the general rules of eating out by remembering to stay SAFE.

Scan the menu

Sometimes appetizers work well as entrees or as dishes to share with others at the table. An antipasti platter is usually large and offers a variety of fatty meats, mozzarella, and olives. Often these platters include assorted vegetables, such as artichoke hearts and roasted red peppers, that are slightly higher in carbs but can easily be avoided. The entire platter is often drizzled with olive oil, which makes it an even better ketogenic option. Avoid appetizers that are primarily bread, such as bruschetta, or are breaded and fried, such as calamari or mozzarella sticks.

Although I've rarely found fried squid that wasn't breaded, I could ask the server to be sure.

If nothing else, the menu offers some good salad options. Caprese salad has fat and protein from the mozzarella and olive oil. If I added a fatty protein like salmon along with some extra olive oil, I would have a filling high-fat entree. The Greek salad without red onions and/or red bell pepper would also work well with the addition of a protein. The feta cheese and olives add fat. A Caesar salad without croutons is generally high in fat, but it would also need a protein added. My main concern about salads is that the dressings are often made with poor-quality seed oils that contribute to inflammation. I could ask for olive oil and vinegar as a dressing instead.

While pizza is generally not an option on a ketogenic plan, from time to time you might find a restaurant that will make you a crustless pizza. The toppings are simply tossed

---

KRISTIE'S Cucina

Starters

FRIED CALAMARI
Fresh squid, house-made tomato gravy

ANTIPASTI PLATTER
Prosciutto di Parma, soppressata, capicola, imported provolone, homemade mozzarella, marinated vegetables

BRUSCHETTA
Grilled Tuscan bread topped with chopped vine-ripened tomatoes, garlic, basil, imported feta cheese, balsamic reduction sauce, olive oil

House Specialties
Choice of pasta: linguine, penne, rigatoni

FRUTTI DI MARE WITH TOMATO GRAVY OR ALFREDO
Shrimp, scallops, mussels, clams, calamari, spicy tomato broth, spaghetti, crusty bread (may substitute house-made Alfredo for spicy tomato broth)

CHICKEN PICCATA
Chicken, white wine lemon butter sauce, capers

CHICKEN CACCIATORE
Chicken, tomato gravy, mushrooms, peppers

VEAL SALTIMBOCCA
Veal, prosciutto, white wine lemon butter sauce

SALMONE AL GRIGLIA
Salmon, spinach, lemon garlic butter

CHICKEN MARSALA
Chicken, mushrooms, marsala cream sauce

Salads

HOUSE SALAD
Organic greens, crumbled gorgonzola, green olives, house dressing

CAPRESE SALAD
Roma tomatoes, fresh mozzarella, fresh basil, balsamic vinegar, olive oil

CAESAR SALAD
Romaine lettuce, garlic croutons, freshly shaved Parmesan, house-made Caesar dressing

GREEK SALAD
Romaine lettuce, feta cheese, Kalamata olives, cucumbers, red onions, red bell peppers, Greek vinaigrette

Pasta
Gluten-free pasta available upon request

ITALIAN GRANDMOTHER'S CLASSIC LASAGNA
Meat ragu, fresh pasta, mozzarella, Parmesan, ricotta, tomato gravy

EGGPLANT ROLLATINI
Eggplant, mozzarella, Parmesan, ricotta, tomato gravy

CHICKEN PARMIGIANA
Chicken, tomato gravy, mozzarella, Parmesan

MANICOTTI
Shells stuffed with meat ragu and ricotta, tomato gravy

Wood-Fired Pizza

MARGHERITA
Fresh tomatoes, basil, mozzarella

QUATTRO FORMAGGI
Mozzarella, fontina, ricotta, Parmesan

SICILIAN
Pepperoni, Italian sausage, tomato sauce, basil, mozzarella

FLORENTINE
Spinach, ricotta, herbs, Parmesan

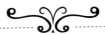

into a deep-dish pizza pan or oven-safe bowl, topped with cheese, and baked until hot and bubbly. If you don't ask, then it definitely won't be an option! I look at the pizza section of the menu to better understand which ingredients the restaurant has on hand. For example, I see that spinach is on the Florentine pizza, so I know that they have spinach. Spinach is also part of the salmon entree, so I could ask whether a pasta dish might be served over spinach instead of pasta.

Among the pasta dishes, lasagna and manicotti are not good options, as they are primarily pasta, which is difficult to eat around. Eggplant and chicken Parmigiana are generally dredged in flour and fried. I could ask how the dishes are prepared, but it is likely that they are high in carbs. Notice that there is a gluten-free pasta option. Unfortunately, just because a food is gluten-free does not mean that it is low-carb. Often higher-carb substitute flours are used, which make gluten-free pasta much higher in total carbohydrates than regular pasta made from wheat flour.

The House Specialties section offers some promising selections. The Frutti de Mare sounds good except for the crusty bread and the fact that it is served over pasta. I could ask for it to be served over spinach instead. The Alfredo entree would be higher in fat, but Alfredo sauce is often thickened with flour. The Chicken Piccata, Chicken Cacciatore, Veal Saltimbocca, and Chicken Marsala sound delicious (my mouth waters at the thought of lemon butter sauce or prosciutto, a fatty Italian ham), but nearly every Italian restaurant makes traditional versions of these dishes, which means that the meats are dredged in flour before being fried. You could ask if grilled meat could be substituted. Salmon is high in omega-3 fats. As long as the lemon garlic butter contains no flour or starchy thickener, the grilled salmon would be a good low-carb option. If the sauce is thickened with flour, you could ask for the salmon with plain butter instead.

Ask questions

After scanning the menu, I would ask whether the Alfredo sauce has flour or a thickener in it. I might also ask if some of the house specialties could be made with meats that are not dredged in flour. I would also ask if sugar is added to the marinara. If I wanted a salad, I would ask about sugar in the dressings.

Find options

The options that I find on this menu include the following:

- **Antipasti Platter**—to enjoy as an entree or share with friends
- **Caprese Salad**—with salmon or chicken and extra olive oil
- **Caesar Salad**—with salmon or chicken and extra olive oil
- **Greek Salad**—with salmon or chicken and extra feta and olive oil, no red onions
- **Sicilian Pizza**—crustless, with ricotta and extra cheese
- **Frutti di Mare**—served over spinach with just a little tomato gravy or with Alfredo sauce if it is not made with a starchy thickener
- **Salmone al Griglia**—with spinach and lemon garlic butter if it contains no thickener

Here are some general tips for dining in Italian restaurants:

- Refuse the bread basket. Never let it hit the table. If dining with carbivores, pass the bread as far away from you as possible.
- Ask whether salad dressings contain sugar or corn syrup. Many Italian restaurants offer olive oil and vinegar, which is a good option.
- Avoid eating a lot of marinara, since tomatoes are generally high in carbs and low in fat.
- Avoid pasta, even if it is advertised as gluten-free.
- Look for menu items that can be requested instead of pasta, such as spinach, roasted cauliflower, or steamed broccoli.

Practice using SAFE on the menus you find online. You can use a form like the one shown below or simply keep notes in a notebook. I also encourage you to keep track of your favorite keto-friendly restaurant meals; I've included a sample on the opposite page. Blank versions of both of these worksheets are available for download from my website, cookingketowith-kristie.com.

Staying SAFE When Eating Out (Sample)

Follow the general rules of eating out by remembering to stay SAFE:

Scan the menu.

Ask questions about ingredients and substitutions.

Find options.

Eat until satisfied.

Restaurant name: *Kristie's Cucina*

Scan the menu:
Write down any potential keto-friendly options. Focus on finding plain meats that are roasted or grilled. If you must choose a salad, look for salads that have fat and protein. Search for side items such as spinach, asparagus, or steamed broccoli that could be substituted for pasta, potatoes, grains, or other starches.

Antipasti platter, Caprese salad, Greek salad without onion and with added fatty protein, Caesar salad without croutons and with added protein
Frutti di Mare (seafood) with spinach instead of pasta
Grilled salmon with lemon garlic butter and a side of spinach

Ask questions:
Write your questions here. Call the restaurant in advance or ask before ordering if you are uncertain about ingredients or how a dish might be prepared.

1. Does the Alfredo sauce have flour or thickener in it?

2. May I have spinach as a side or in place of pasta?

3. Do you have olive oil and vinegar as a salad dressing option?

4. Are the meats in the chicken piccata, chicken cacciatore, Veal saltimbocca, and chicken marsala breaded?

5. Can the pizza be made crustless, with the toppings and cheese baked in an oven-safe bowl or skillet?

The options that I find on this menu include:
List the choices most likely to be keto-friendly here.

Antipasti Platter, Frutti di Mare served over spinach, salmon with spinach and lemon garlic butter with a Caesar or Greek salad without croutons

KETO LIVING *Day by Day*

My Favorite Keto-Friendly Restaurant Meals (Sample)

Name of restaurant: The Homesteader

What I ordered: Steak with side salad, no croutons, blue cheese dressing

Approximate carb count: 5 grams of total carbs

Hunger level 3 hours after eating this meal: Not hungry for 5-plus hours

Describe whether the restaurant or meal was keto-friendly.
No butter, only margarine. Ordered no croutons, but were still on salad.

Name of restaurant: Luigi's Trattoria

What I ordered: Shrimp scampi over spinach with fresh Parmesan

Approximate carb count: 3 grams of total carbs

Hunger level 3 hours after eating this meal: not hungry

Describe whether the restaurant or meal was keto-friendly.
Had real butter and fresh Parmesan. Had salmon, scallops, and steak options. Also offered broccoli and asparagus as side dishes.

Name of restaurant: Mama's Buffet

What I ordered: Grilled chicken and salad (chosen from buffet)

Approximate carb count: 6 grams of total carbs

Hunger level 3 hours after eating this meal: Hungry at 4 hours.
Needed more fat with meal.

Describe whether the restaurant or meal was keto-friendly.
Not a lot of good keto options. Could have had steamed broccoli and added shredded cheese and butter.

PART II:
A Four-Week Guide to *Beginning Keto*

I spent much of my life wondering what was wrong with me. As an obese kid, I daydreamed about a magical oil that I could put in my bathwater. The oil would dissolve the fat on my body without harming my skin. In the fantasy, the oil would make my arms and legs perfectly proportioned, but I'd have to submerge myself entirely to get the full benefit of this special oil. I wondered if my bathtub was big enough. I was eight years old.

Even before puberty, I knew I was different. I was *always* hungry and hopelessly fat. I hated that word; I feared it. That word had been tossed at me in utter disgust more than once by adults, peers, and even younger children. I couldn't even say it.

Growing up, I entertained myself by reading, eating, and daydreaming, and through my reading I knew there was something wrong with me. The characters in the books I read were never overweight. Sometimes there was a chubby sidekick, but that person was never the focus of the story. The fat kid was usually smart. Look at Velma from Scooby Doo! Velma is the smart one, while Daphne is a taller, thinner redhead who has a boyfriend. The gang always treats Daphne better than they treat the shorter, chubbier Velma. No matter the story, the heroines are always pretty. They always have nice clothes and boyfriends. I had neither.

While I will admit to serious crushes on a few TV favorites, daydreams about boys didn't come until late in high school. Weight loss, however—and the Holy Grail solution I dreamed about—was a recurring fantasy.

As I grew into adulthood, various gimmicks gave me hope—the cabbage soup diet, acupuncture, and restricting calories. Eventually I was prescribed weight-loss drugs. When gastric bypass surgery failed me—I lost 125 pounds in the first year and a half but then gained over 80 pounds back—I took it as the ultimate failure. Surgery had been my "last chance," and I couldn't even make that work; I was hopeless. I began to wonder whether science would ever figure out what was irrevocably broken in me. I held on to the hope that my miracle oil would be discovered. I never dreamed that the answer had already been found decades earlier.

When I eventually read Gary Taubes' book *Why We Get Fat,* it taught me that my lifelong struggle with weight wasn't a personal failure. This book gives examples of how carbs, protein, and fat behave in the body when the body doesn't process carbohydrates efficiently. It explains the roles of insulin and other hormones. I had never read anything like it before. For the first time ever, I read a book in which I was the main character. It was *my* story in print! My body was a classic example of metabolic dysfunction. It was clear that my hormones were out of whack, and I was eating the entirely wrong mix of carbs, fat, and protein.

By the time I got to the end of that book, I might have taken to hunting unicorns if Taubes had said it would make me lose weight. In spite of the fact that his book is explicit about weight being a symptom, not the disease, let's be honest . . . I still wanted to "treat" the symptom, which meant that I was only interested in losing weight.

Thankfully, Taubes wasn't selling meal plans, supplements, exogenous ketones, or any other "shortcuts" to weight loss. His book includes a thin little appendix of how to follow a very-low-carb diet—no sugar, no starch. It was written by Dr. Eric Westman, a doctor at Duke and a man I would eventually meet and get to know. I read his diet plan, and, seeing as how there were no unicorns to chase, I figured I'd give it a try just to see if these guys were on to something. After all, the plan didn't involve cabbage soup or needles. Duke University was just up the road from my home in North Carolina, and its medical school is highly respected. Taubes had spoken to me and seemingly *about* me throughout his book. I wanted to see if this story could give me the happy ending I yearned for.

And it did. After four decades of dreaming and struggling, I found my miracle oil. My miracle *oils,* really.

My miracle is in the form of butter, ghee, bacon fat, and mayonnaise and in the yumminess of fried chicken wings and roasted pork bellies. It may not have made me as perfectly proportioned as I'd like to be, but this story, with all of its plot twists, is finally headed toward a much happier conclusion!

Will the plan that I followed work for you? The only way to know for sure is to give it a try. This part of the book is designed to help you follow a ketogenic diet for four weeks. Each week begins with an introduction that outlines the focus for the week and encourages you to plan ahead for success. If you choose to plan your meals each week, you'll find tools for meal planning, shopping for ingredients, and meal preparation in Part I. In addition, I've provided daily tips and strategies that give you a glimpse into what helped me transition to a ketogenic lifestyle and some inspiration to help you stay on track.

In some ways, following this plan is taking the road less traveled. Although the plan focuses on real, whole foods, many families do not eat this way. No longer relying on processed and packaged foods can be a challenge, but it is not impossible, and the health benefits make it all worthwhile.

I spent much of the first part of the book telling you about my journey to better health; now let's get you started on *your* journey!

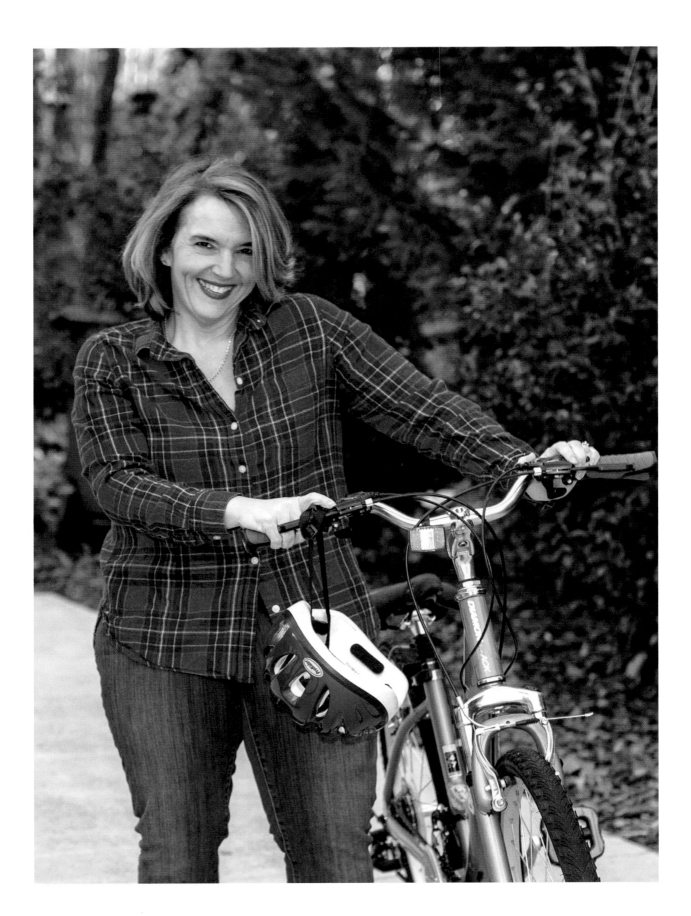

Chapter 4
Planning Your *Journey*

You've heard my story, and you've seen my "before" and "after" photos. What you can't see is everything that happened in between. To help you along your journey, I've spent considerable time identifying the things that helped me succeed. How was I able to stick to a ketogenic way of eating long-term when many others struggle?

In this chapter, you will be challenged to think differently. You will begin by exploring why you want to adopt a ketogenic lifestyle. Determining what matters most to you will be a starting point for the choices you make to stay on plan. Next, you will be challenged to ignore the scale as your primary measure of progress. There are more than a dozen other equally important physical and psychological markers that will help you to determine whether you're heading in the right direction. Lastly, I've included my top ten navigation tips and the four tenets that should guide you along your journey as last-minute reminders to ensure your success.

Know Your Why!

As I shared earlier in this book, when it came to my weight, my list of failures was long. All the times I tried to lose weight but never succeeded for long hung around my neck like leaden necklaces. I wanted to accomplish my goal, but nothing ever seemed to work. I struggled. Losing weight seemed impossible, but at the same time, the pain and limitations I was living with made me miserable.

When I decided that I was going to lose weight or die trying, I wrote down all the reasons I *had* to succeed this time. I scribbled reminders of what made me feel so despondent that I did not want to keep on living as an obese wife and mother.

Here is what I wrote:

- *Your children deserve more. They need a mom who can do things with them.*

- *Your husband deserves a wife he can be proud to be seen with. He needs a wife who can support his career and not drag him down because of all the things she cannot do. He needs a partner he doesn't have to physically help.*

- *Remember the wedding. (Turn back to page 12 for this story.) Remember the women older than you in the beautiful dresses. Remember how huge and unfeminine you felt; you felt ugly and clumsy. Remember the dresses you didn't have the confidence to wear.*

- *Your weight holds you back in your job. You sweat when you present. You can't easily find professional clothes. You get tired easily.*

- *Choose you. Choose you over food. Just for today.*

Why are *you* considering a ketogenic lifestyle? Spend a few minutes jotting down your thoughts about why this way of eating might be a good option for you. Use the following questions to guide your thinking:

- Does your health negatively impact your day-to-day life? If so, how?

- How does your health affect your relationships with others? Do you feel that your close friends and family are impacted by your health?

- Why is it important to you to follow a ketogenic lifestyle? What do you hope to accomplish?

- What do you want to be different about your health or your eating habits?

The following sample shows how I tackled these questions at the beginning of my ketogenic journey. If you'd like to print out a copy of this worksheet to fill out for yourself, you can find it on my website, cookingketowithkristie.com.

Whenever I struggled with cravings or in social settings, whenever I stared down Halloween candy or Girl Scout cookies, I looked to my list for support. Reminding myself that my children deserved more made it easy to stay on plan because that statement was so true. Visions of myself wearing sexy dresses motivated me to keep trying even when the number on the scale was not moving as quickly as I wanted it to. I knew my why. Referring to my list kept me centered when hormones, stress, and doubt threatened to push me off track.

You may never need a list of what matters most to you, but if you reach a crisis point in the early days of keto like I did, then you will be grateful that you took the time to write down your thoughts about why you want to undertake this journey.

Know Your Why!

Why are you considering a ketogenic lifestyle? Spend a few minutes jotting down your thoughts about why this way of eating might be a good option for you. Use the questions below to help guide your thoughts. Some of these questions may not be relevant to you. Respond only to those that are.

Does your health negatively impact your day-to-day life? If so, how?

Yes. At work I use a desk that raises up because sitting for a long time hurts my back. I can't easily go upstairs, and I can't walk very far. I need help putting on pantyhose for work or church, which is difficult when I travel alone to professional conferences. I can't participate in any physical activities with my children. After work, my back hurts so much that I often just go to bed. It is often difficult to find clothing that fits, especially professional attire.

How does your health affect your relationships with others? Do you feel that your close friends and family are impacted by your health?

My health affects my children because I cannot do things with them. At night my back hurts too much to walk upstairs to tuck them in. I don't take them to do activities. I avoid social situations because I don't feel well or I don't want to embarrass my husband. Sometimes I avoid seeing friends because of my weight. A lot of our family time is limited to the things that I can do.

Why is it important to you to follow a ketogenic lifestyle? What do you hope to accomplish?

I want to lose weight. I want to be able to do things with my children. I want to wear pretty clothes like other women do. I want my husband to be proud of me. I want to feel normal instead of always feeling like the fat girl. I want to be able to shop in any clothing store, not just in plus-sized stores. I want to be able to walk in the mall and go on hikes with my family without pain. I want to be able to fit into movie theater seats and airplane seats without being embarrassed. I don't want to have to worry about whether I will fit in a booth at a restaurant.

What do you want to be different about your health or your eating habits?

I want to be in control of my food, and I want to not be hungry. I want to feel good instead of having daily pain and inflammation.

Mile Markers of Progress

The best part of the ketogenic journey is feeling better. After you reduce inflammation and stabilize your blood glucose, you will simply feel good. Using ketones for fuel gives you energy you may not know you had. You will enjoy that your clothes become looser and you can wear smaller sizes. In addition to looking and feeling better physically, there are multiple psychological benefits. As your body shrinks, your confidence is likely to grow. Each day, as you practice new habits and build on your successes, you will be proud of yourself. You are capable and strong. Over time, you are likely to notice that your attitude toward food changes, and you will begin to see yourself differently, just as others may see you differently. These successes extend far beyond the scale.

As you make your way along this journey, I encourage you to monitor your non-scale progress. I think of these successes as mile markers along the ketogenic highway, marking the progress you're making toward your destination of better health. In this section, I outline some physical markers of success that include weight loss, but also include markers that are often far more important. After that, I offer a long list of psychological markers of success. Please use these markers as you record your daily and weekly progress in the four-week plan that follows.

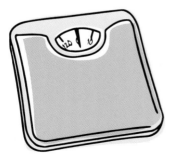

Physical Mile Markers of Progress

What do we traditionally do on day one of a diet? We jump on the scale! Okay, many of us don't actually *jump* on; we *step* on, usually with trepidation. The scale tells us things about ourselves that we don't want to know. We believe we can cover it up with loose clothing or Spanx, so we avoid reality by avoiding the scale. Truthfully, when I was obese, I thought that not weighing myself was okay. When I did, I was mortified at the thought of someone else finding out my weight. I didn't even want my husband to know my weight. The same was true for my clothing size. Cutting the tags out of garments was typical for me. When I tried on or brought home clothes, I often hid the sizes from others by strategically covering the tags with my hands. Somehow, by not having numbers to quantify my weight, I believed I was making myself look smaller.

In reality, my size was my size. Regardless of the number on the scale or the size of clothing I wore, my children could not stretch their little arms around me for a full hug. I could not chase after them. The airplane seatbelt stretched as far as it could to clasp around my girth, and I was breathless and sweaty after even a short walk from the parking lot to my office. Those were the markers that mattered most.

This time, start your new diet—your new *lifestyle*—differently. Begin by collecting some physical markers that will give you a reality check and provide an excellent baseline. As you prepare to embark on your journey, consider these measures as your starting location, and use them to orient you as you make progress toward your destination.

The scale

Whether I suggest it or not, most of you are going to weigh yourselves before you begin a ketogenic lifestyle and frequently throughout your weight-loss journey. If you do, please keep the following points in mind:

- Weigh yourself at the same time each day.
- Weigh yourself without clothes, or wear the same type (and weight) of clothing each time.
- Follow the product guidelines, such as by placing the scale on a level surface.

Perhaps most important, remember that the scale is only one marker, and it cannot give you an absolute number. It is not uncommon for body weight to fluctuate within a 5-pound range even within the same day depending on what you've eaten, your water intake, whether you've been to the bathroom, and so on. A more accurate measure is how your weight is trending over time.

For example, let's look at a week's worth of daily weighing:

- On Monday, you weigh 223 pounds.
- On Tuesday, you weigh 224.
- By Wednesday, the scale records 222 pounds.
- On Thursday, you weigh 225.
- On Friday, you weigh 222.
- By Saturday, you hit a new low of 221 pounds.
- On Sunday, you weigh 223.

Were you really gaining and losing weight each day? Probably not. Over the span of a week, you weighed between 225 and 221 pounds. What do you actually weigh? Something within that range.

If you determine that your weight range is 225 to 221, then as long as you stay within that range, your weight is fairly stable. You want to aim for dips below the bottom of your range, or 221 in this example. Over time, the dips will become more frequent, and the higher end of the range will come down. Your new range for week two might be 223 to 218. By week three, you might be celebrating a range of 221 to 216, and so on. Each week, you will likely see accumulating weight loss, and thus your range, and your absolute weight, will gradually decrease.

You should not be concerned with just one temporary fluctuation above the high end of your range. However, if you see more than one spike above that top number, with other days staying at the higher end of the range, then you might have legitimately gained weight. Using the same example, your weight range might go from 228 to 223 instead of 225 to 221. In that case, you need to look at your eating habits and your lifestyle and make some adjustments.

Another concern about using the scale as your primary measure of progress is "Only syndrome." Although there are other markers of success, sometimes people get stuck on the number on the scale and complain, "I only lost 1 pound this week!" or "I only lost 4 pounds this month!" Only? There are times when I would have been thrilled to have lost any weight at all, but I, too, have been afflicted with Only syndrome.

When you first begin a ketogenic lifestyle, weight loss will likely be pretty rapid. There might be times, however, when you lose just 1 pound in a week. There will also likely be times when your weight does not change, but you lose inches. Your body may need time to adapt to significant weight loss; your weight might stay the same for a while even as your body continues to heal.

For most people, dealing with Only syndrome is a matter of perspective. You have to remind yourself that any weight lost is a success. Also, any weight lost is not weight *gained*, which is what happened to me when I was not following a ketogenic plan. Moreover, regardless of the scale, I will always follow a ketogenic diet. This is simply the way that I eat now because I have found it to be the best plan for my body. My task is to stay focused on eating healthy each day, one day at a time. The scale will take care of itself.

Finally, a significant problem with using the scale as a measure of "success" is that many people obsess over it and weigh far too frequently. Too often the number on the scale influences our mood for the day: we are encouraged when the number is lower and discouraged when it isn't. Below is an example from someone following a ketogenic diet that I saw in a Facebook group. She wrote:

So today is day 3 of my new WOE [way of eating]. I had weighed a couple of days before starting and was shocked yesterday when the scale said I was down 6 pounds! I knew that seeing numbers will be my motivation, but today I weighed and was up 0.8! So how often do you all weigh? I need the encouragement of the numbers moving but don't want the discouragement of following the plan and seeing a gain.

This woman is three days into the plan and obviously is weighing herself every day. Her comment shows her elation at "losing" 6 pounds and then her discouragement at having "gained" 0.8 pound. Notice the use of the decimal? She is treating the scale as if it could give her an absolute number. Also, she is only beginning, yet she has very high expectations. Only a loss will make her happy. The most troubling part of her comment is her emotional connection to the weight reported by the scale. Yesterday she was excited, motivated, and encouraged, but today she describes herself as discouraged. After forty-eight hours, using absolute numbers, she still would have "lost" 5.2 pounds, yet she is discouraged by the scale going up less than 1 full pound.

Please learn from this example. We all want to wake up tomorrow having reached our goal weight, but no plan works like that. Accept from the beginning that your weight will fluctuate daily. Sometimes it will fluctuate in the way that you want, and some days it may go up. What matters most is that the cumulative impact—that your weight *trends downward.* If you are weighing yourself more than once per day, please reconsider that practice. Also, if the number on the scale influences your mood,

especially it if impacts your mood negatively and leaves you feeling discouraged, then you might want to take a break from the scale. Have a friend or family member hide the scale and weigh yourself only once a week or even a month. Spend time thinking about and using other mile markers of progress instead.

Body measurements

One of my biggest regrets (along with not taking "before" photos, discussed next) is not taking "before" body measurements. Because I had no idea whether this crazy diet might work, I neglected to measure my thighs, hips, waist, bust, and upper arms. You will want to take the time to do this for yourself.

Keep in mind that it can be difficult to take measurements exactly the same way each time, so don't be overly concerned if you get varying results, especially if you measure frequently. Use the following chart as a guide for taking measurements and as a place to record your numbers. (You can download a copy of this chart from my website.) This chart is designed to be used weekly, but you might prefer to use it no more than once per month. Choose what works best for you.

Guide to taking body measurements

Try to place the tape measure in the same area each week. Here are a few tips to get the most accurate circumference:

- **Upper Arm:** Measure just over your bicep, which is roughly 4 inches above your elbow, at the widest part of your upper arm.

- **Chest:** Measure just under your arms and across your chest at the widest part (across the nipples). Women might also measure just under the breasts where a bra band fits.

- **Waist:** Measure at the smallest part of your natural waist—typically, just above the belly button.

- **Hips:** Measure at the widest part of your hips, including the widest part of your butt.

- **Thigh:** Measure the fullest part of your thigh.

Pull the measuring tape firmly, but do not squish any body parts when measuring. If the tape is pulling hard enough to squish your skin, then you are pulling too snugly.

Keep the measuring tape flat against your skin as you wrap it around the area you are measuring.

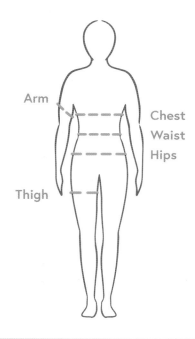

Starting Measurements

Weight	
Left arm	
Right arm	
Chest	
Waist	
Hips	
Left thigh	
Right thigh	

Measurements at End of Week 1

	Measurement	Difference
Weight		
Left arm		
Right arm		
Chest		
Waist		
Hips		
Left thigh		
Right thigh		

Measurements at End of Week 2

	Measurement	Difference
Weight		
Left arm		
Right arm		
Chest		
Waist		
Hips		
Left thigh		
Right thigh		

Measurements at End of Week 3

	Measurement	Difference
Weight		
Left arm		
Right arm		
Chest		
Waist		
Hips		
Left thigh		
Right thigh		

Measurements at End of Week 4

	Measurement	Difference
Weight		
Left arm		
Right arm		
Chest		
Waist		
Hips		
Left thigh		
Right thigh		

Before and after photos

Take "before" photos. I know you probably don't want to, but please hear me out.

When I was obese, I always ran from the camera because I hated seeing pictures of myself. Instead of being in photos, I was the photographer. While I have fantastic pictures of my children that I will always cherish, I have very few photos of us together. I regret that for several reasons, one of which is that I have very few "good" before photos as a record of my weight loss.

You can take your before photos with friends or family members or take them alone, but take them. After you begin your keto journey, I encourage you to pick one day of the month and take a photo on that same day every month. Many people select the first day of the month, but it can be any day; just be consistent. When the scale fails you, and it will, you will be amazed when you compare photos. Even a photo of only your face can reveal changes in your body. Remarkably, most people find that they look younger even when the "after" photo is taken years later. The following pictures of David and me are evidence of that. These photos were taken ten years apart, but we look younger in the more recent photo!

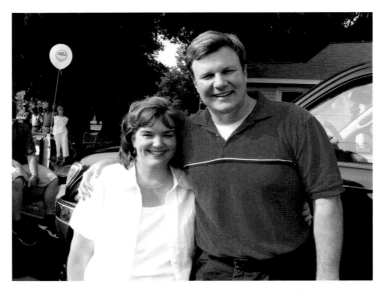

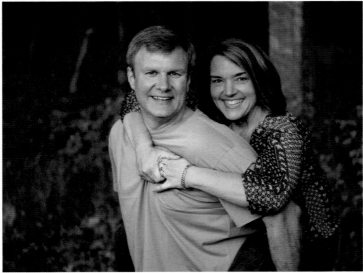

How your clothing fits

Clothing is my favorite way to monitor progress. Clothes do not lie—especially jeans, fitted dresses, and workout attire. Find at least two sets of clothing. First, find a pair of pants and/or a top that is too tight to wear comfortably. Take a picture of yourself wearing those garments or simply note how they feel on your body. At the same time each week, try on those same clothes. Within a week or two, you will likely feel a difference in how they fit.

Second, buy a new piece of clothing as a short-term goal. It can be a skirt, a pair of pants, a top, or a dress. You might even select a workout ensemble. Whatever it is, buy it one size smaller than you currently wear. By the end of your twenty-eight days, you just might find that it fits! Even though you might be disappointed in the number on the scale, you might see changes in the way your clothing fits that are reassuring indicators of success.

Moving from plus sizes into regular sizes

No longer needing plus-sized clothing was a huge marker of success for me. It took me nearly six months of following a ketogenic diet before I could shop in the misses' section. And when I did, I felt lost! As happy as I was to no longer need plus sizes, I was terrified to enter the dressing room. As I continued to lose weight, I spent months not knowing what size I needed. It wasn't unusual for me to try on at least three sizes. Growing up, I was so obese that I couldn't wear store-bought clothing. Now I can walk into any women's clothing store to shop, and I do not even buy the largest size on the rack. When you pass this mile marker, you will remember it. You will remember the stores where you shopped and the first clothes that you bought.

Blood glucose and ketone testing

On a ketogenic diet, blood glucose stays stable and is likely to remain in or fall into a normal range.

If you have type 2 diabetes, monitoring your blood glucose is one of the most important measures you can take. You might be surprised at how quickly blood glucose can normalize and how soon you may be able to discontinue medications after adopting a ketogenic lifestyle. If you are taking medications, please work with your physician to adjust them as needed.

Even if you do not have diabetes, testing your blood glucose can yield useful information. To test at home, you will need a blood glucose monitor and test strips, which are available over the counter. You can use a protocol similar to the Oral Glucose Tolerance Test administered at a medical facility by testing prior to eating (fasting), one hour after eating (postprandial), and two hours after eating. Ideally, your blood glucose will remain relatively stable at each postprandial check. If it rises more than fifteen points, then what you ate is considered to have spiked your blood glucose.

Typically, too many carbohydrates in a meal are the culprit, especially if the number rises to its highest point one hour after eating. A single ingredient such as coffee, pecans, or pork can also cause spikes. What causes spikes for one person may not cause spikes for another; blood glucose response is highly individual. Blood glucose testing is a good way to determine which low-carb sweeteners are safe for you; a spike after consuming a particular sweetener indicates that it is not a good option for your body. Just because a food or sweetener has no impact on *my* blood glucose does not mean that it is safe for you or anyone else.

At two hours postprandial, your blood glucose should remain close to the number you got when you tested before eating. If the number is higher, then this slower rise in blood glucose could signal too much protein in your meal.

I test my blood glucose from time to time just to see how a meal or sweetener affects me. When my blood glucose rises after a meal, I know that something I ate or the composition of the meal was not ideal for me. I make changes by avoiding those ingredients or adding more fat and lowering carbs and/or protein in future meals.

Stress, illness, and other factors can impact blood glucose readings, especially fasting ones, so keep that in mind if you choose to test your blood glucose.

Some people who follow a ketogenic lifestyle also test for ketones. You can test your blood, urine, or breath. While testing blood ketones yields the most reliable results, it is often unnecessary. High levels of ketones do not equate to weight loss or better health. If you consistently starve your body of glucose, then your body will have no choice but to burn fat (ketones). Too often, measuring ketones leads to unnecessary expense and frustration. Unless your doctor encourages you to track ketones as part of a medical protocol, you may be better served spending your money on bacon and butter.

Fitting differently in seats

Pretty soon you are likely to find that you need to adjust the driver's seat in your car. You will no longer need a seatbelt extender on an airplane, and the thought of sitting in a restaurant booth won't scare you. Staring at a booth or a theater seat and wondering whether it is wide enough to accommodate your body is terrifying. Others are watching, and you worry what people think about having to sit next to you. All that changes as you stay on plan and your body starts to shrink. Celebrate it! This mile marker says "Welcome" because you literally and figuratively fit beside everyone else.

Recognizing physical hunger

Are you hungry? Cues such as a rumbling stomach, headache, light-headedness, and slight weakness are powerful markers for deciding when to eat. Once you can identify true physical hunger, you are well on your way to success. Hunger is an excellent gauge along your journey. When I ate high-carb and low-fat, I could not trust my hunger signals because ghrelin, leptin, and insulin, the hormones that contribute to hunger, were all out of whack. But after spending some time listening to my body and giving it high fat, moderate protein, and low carbohydrates, I began to notice that my hunger had lessened. I missed meals by accident! Ghrelin, leptin, and insulin began to work more normally. My body was finally able to use stored fat for fuel, and I experienced fewer of the signs of physiological hunger.

Note: If you are diabetic or on medication to control blood glucose, your hunger signals may feel different. Please work with a medical professional to manage your medications.

Psychological Mile Markers of Progress

The mental changes that come with feeling healthier are often overlooked, even though these are the changes that truly make keto a lifestyle. While I can't possibly mention them all here, mile markers like these will soon become your milestones. When eating is controlled and hunger no longer dictates your days, amazing things begin to happen to your mood, your attitude, and your ability to manage your time. When you feel like moving, activities that used to be a chore become so much easier. Some even become enjoyable!

Eating to hunger

Reduced physical hunger is a physiological mile marker, but the ability to eat to hunger is a significant psychological mile marker. Like Pavlov's dogs, many of us are used to eating by the clock or eating when others eat. Regardless of our last meal, the clock striking noon can send us scrambling to the cupboards. Not only are we accustomed to eating at certain times, but many of the times we eat are dictated by work hours or family responsibilities. Even if we aren't hungry at our designated lunch hour, seeing people eating around us or smelling food nearby can trigger our wanting to eat. Sometimes we fear that we will get hungry before we have another opportunity to eat, so we eat during the lunch hour whether we are truly hungry or not. (We also eat because of boredom, stress, or emotions; see "Avoiding Emotional Eating" on the next page.)

Learning to ask yourself, "Am I really hungry?" when you're standing in the kitchen is so important. That's step one. Step two is answering that question honestly, and step three is choosing to eat only if you are truly hungry. Eating to hunger is a challenge for many, even after they have lost some weight and followed a ketogenic lifestyle for some time. Your body often needs less food than your brain thinks it does. Feed your body the fuel it needs, and keep your brain occupied with more important thoughts.

As you become fat-adapted and your body has access to its fat stores, you will find that you need to eat less frequently and that you require less fuel. When your meals are well balanced with high fat, moderate protein, and low carbohydrates, then going six to eight hours between meals is not uncommon. In fact, your meals should keep you satiated for four to six hours on average. Many people find that they eat only two meals per day when following a ketogenic plan. While you don't want to force yourself to forgo a meal, having the self-awareness to eat only when hungry, and not out of habit or because of the time, is another mile marker of progress.

Having the determination to avoid high-carb foods

You cannot be successful on a ketogenic plan if you continue eating high-carb foods. Keto simply does not work if you do not stay on plan. Each day, one of your most important goals is to avoid high-carb foods, which means that dogged determination is an important marker of success.

Unless you live alone in a cave, you will see others eating your old carby favorites. Someone will offer you a sweet treat. You will smell bread baking, and there will be popcorn at the movies. Decide each morning before your feet hit the floor. Are you going to stay on plan today? Deciding in advance makes your day far easier. When you're ambushed by bagels in the breakroom, your resolve will enable you to breeze right past them.

Each time you encounter a high-carb temptation and you choose to stay on plan, you will be empowered. Each small success reminds you that you *can* be successful. Your confidence will grow as your health improves and you see results. Without the powerful marker of staying on plan, progress simply isn't possible. Take the time to acknowledge that you have been tenacious and resolute.

Monitoring portions

When hunger signaling is dysfunctional, we tend to overeat. Many people are surprised by the size of a single serving when they use a scale to weigh food. The primary foods for which you need to control portions are carbohydrates, namely vegetables and limited fruits, since you will be eating very few packaged foods. Portion control is the most important way to avoid carb creep. In general, you don't need to worry about protein portions as long as you make sure to eat more grams of fat than grams of protein.

Manage your portions by using a food scale for accuracy. If you don't have a scale, use the photos on pages 29 to 33 as visual guides. Over time, you are less likely to need to measure your food since you will have a better sense of what a serving size looks like.

As discussed earlier, there will be days when you simply want more protein and fat, and you should eat to satiety. Managing portions is really about counting carbohydrates and eating until you are just satisfied and not overly full. When you begin to consciously monitor your carbohydrate portions, you're definitely passing another mile marker of progress!

Avoiding emotional eating

Nearly all my life, I ate when I was happy, sad, excited, anxious, angry, elated, or nervous. Our culture celebrates every holiday with food. When someone dies, you take food to the family. A new baby? Take the new parents a casserole or bring the new mother her favorite food. We have soothed and been soothed by foods since infancy. Often, our first instinct is to soothe a crying baby with a bottle.

Emotional eating is one of the hardest habits to break because it hits us when we are most vulnerable. Our brains believe that this extraordinary emotion *deserves* food. The reality is that what we truly deserve is to be healthy. We may long for the crunch of chips after someone has wronged us, but eating those chips will not soothe us for long. Instead, the influx of carbs may make us feel sick or tired and heavy. Later, we feel guilt or remorse.

Eating when stressed feeds a negative cycle. We feel bad, so we eat, which ultimately makes us feel worse. We feel bad about feeling bad. We feel guilty for making poor choices. Often, instead of correcting, we keep making bad choices because we're overwhelmingly frustrated. The cycle continues with thoughts such as, "I've already blown it, so I'll just eat what I want and start again tomorrow." Too often tomorrow never comes because we've awakened the cycle of cravings, making it harder to stay on plan.

Break the cycle by not starting the cycle in the first place. Find a better way to cope. When you manage the impulse to eat your emotions, you win. You succeed in objectifying food. Food is not a comfort, but being able to control food is comforting. When faced with emotional eating, I tell myself, "I've never regretted something that I did not eat."

After nearly five years on keto, I'm not immune to stress eating. It is still a huge issue for me. In my first year, I made myself sick stress eating sunflower seeds! Pork rinds can also be a problem for me when I'm stressed. I used to justify it by saying, "But what I'm eating is low-carb and high-fat!" Yes, but no. That doesn't make stress eating okay, because I am not eating out of physical hunger.

Over time, I've developed better coping skills. Here are a few strategies to try:

- **Get out of the kitchen.** Remove food items from your reach. Hide under the bed if you have to, but position yourself where there is no food.

- **Phone a friend or loved one.** You can't eat while you're talking, and your mother will always be happy to hear your voice.

- **Take a bath or shower.** Somehow the water running over me soothes me. It seems to knock out the anxiety and doubt just a little. I imagine those feelings washing down the drain.

- **If you're a person of faith, pray.** God always laughs at my fears and reminds me how silly they are. I find prayer humbling and reassuring.

- **Watch a funny movie or video.** Seeing other people laugh or laughing at a comedy can help change your own mood.

- **Go for a walk.** Walking is my favorite stress reliever and means to avoid stress eating. Even a quick lap or two around the house or ten minutes around the neighborhood has a significant impact on my mood. If you need an excuse to walk, run an errand and park as far away from the building as you can.

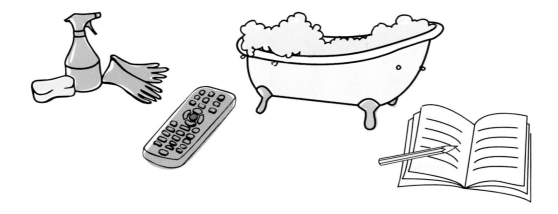

- **Write it out.** Writing about stressors or emotions is sometimes comforting. If you're feeling overwhelmed, making a list of what you need to accomplish now and what can wait until later can be helpful. Actually doing something from that list is a huge stress reliever for me.

- **Take action.** Do something that needs to be done, even if it's just cleaning out a drawer or sweeping the floor. Send the email or text that you've been meaning to return. Being busy often helps by giving you a sense of accomplishment and control.

When you find yourself heading toward a moment of emotional eating and you are able to stop yourself, celebrate that mile marker of progress. Recognize that you are acting differently and that you will get different results.

Doing the work of keeping carbs below your threshold

My personal threshold for carbs is roughly 7 grams per meal. Most meals I keep to around 4 to 5 grams of carbs, but I allow myself to go slightly higher on occasion. Even holiday meals are rarely above 10 grams of total carbs for me. In the beginning, staying below your carb threshold per meal is what will help you be most successful, so the ability to put forth this effort this is an important mile marker of progress.

As you learn the carb counts in various foods and watch your portion sizes to minimize carbs, give yourself credit for that hard work. Instead of mindlessly eating convenience foods, you are consciously creating meals that will give your body the better health it deserves. Eventually, staying below your carb threshold will become second nature. For the first four weeks, though, be sure to count this as a success that is helping you build future success.

Avoiding snacking and learning to leave food on your plate

Many of us snack out of habit or when stressed. When you find yourself no longer snacking between meals, it's a sign of two very good things. First, you are eating well-formulated ketogenic meals that sustain you for at least four hours. Second, you are learning to eat to hunger, which is one of the single most important markers of success.

Similarly, when you learn to eat to hunger, you will find that you eat smaller portions and you are more likely to leave food on your plate, especially when eating out. Often I mentally halve my plate and ask for a box as soon as I get close to eating half. By the time the check is paid, my tummy is fully satisfied, and I'm happy to have leftovers for another meal.

Staying on plan when eating out

When you can pass the bread basket without even peeking in, you've reached an important milestone. You've made the decision to eat foods that fit your plan. Eating out is riddled with challenges. You may have to be brave enough to ask questions about how food is served or what ingredients are used. You might have to ask for substitutions or request that the server not bring you certain foods. You might also have to plead for an alternative side item that isn't normally paired with your entree. Speaking up can be hard. When you've done it, you should be proud. You're eating differently and creating new habits. Each time you do these things, it gets easier and you get healthier.

Eating at restaurants with friends can be especially challenging. The strategies mentioned earlier, such as deciding in advance to stay on plan, planning ahead, and asking questions, are still important even when others are watching. When you stick to your plan in spite of the carbivores around you doing otherwise, you set an example that this plan is important to you. Seeing you enjoying your "diet" food just might convince someone else to give it a try. Pages 79 to 89 provide tips on eating out, including how to order.

Staying on plan in social settings

Our society is fixated on serving food at nearly every celebration and gathering. Wherever two or more people are gathered, there shall be food! Unfortunately, those foods that we use to celebrate are often high in carbs and therefore are not ideal choices for a ketogenic plan. However, many of the recipes in this book are perfect for parties and celebrations, which is one reason why I've included a chapter called "Small Bites," beginning on page 254.

On your ketogenic journey, you will learn to enjoy socializing with friends and family while food becomes less important. Once you survive those first gatherings while remaining on plan, you will know that your mindset has changed. I find myself talking more with others instead of hovering by the buffet table or lurking in the kitchen. My family has also become more intentional about creating new traditions that do not revolve around food. (See pages 73 and 74 for more on creating non-food traditions.) I have a lot of fun sharing the keto-friendly foods that I eat on holidays, too. Rarely do I share a ketogenic dish and not get rave reviews. In fact, most of the time I end up sharing the recipe!

Give yourself credit for passing this milestone by staying on plan, creating new ways to celebrate, and sharing your new favorite foods.

Using Mile Markers of Progress Along Your Journey

As you journey through this four-week guide, I encourage you to keep track of your successes. At the beginning of each week, I've provided a chart for you to record your non-scale victories. (You can find a downloadable version on my website, cookingketowithkristie.com.) This chart is a place to note the physical and mental changes that you notice as well as to record your daily macros if you choose to track them. Even if you don't track protein and fat, counting carbs can be helpful. You can use the mile markers of progress described on the previous pages as a guide, but you will likely discover many more of your own. To give you an idea of how to complete this weekly summary, I've provided an example below that includes some non-scale victories that many people enjoy within the first four weeks.

Notice that I have deliberately omitted a place to record your weight on this chart. You can add that information if you like, but please take the time to celebrate the other mile markers that signal your progress on your ketogenic journey.

Mile Marker Summary (Sample)

	MACROS FOR ALL MEALS AND SNACKS			MILE MARKERS OF SUCCESS
	Daily Total Carbs	Daily Total Protein	Daily Total Fat	
MONDAY	18	60	98	I had to move my seat forward in the car! There is definitely more room between me and the steering wheel.
	Daily Total Carbs	Daily Total Protein	Daily Total Fat	
TUESDAY	14	75	98	I did not eat lunch because I wasn't hungry. Instead, I ate a big keto dinner that I had prepped on Sunday.
	Daily Total Carbs	Daily Total Protein	Daily Total Fat	
WEDNESDAY	20	67	125	My pants are too big! I've been wearing a belt, but I'll definitely need to shop for clothes soon.
	Daily Total Carbs	Daily Total Protein	Daily Total Fat	
THURSDAY	12	48	102	My favorite donuts were sitting on a table in the breakroom, so I just avoided it all day. When I was tempted, I did a quick online search for a smaller pair of pants!
	Daily Total Carbs	Daily Total Protein	Daily Total Fat	
FRIDAY	16	55	96	I went to lunch with friends. I ordered a burger without a bun and added bacon instead of fries. Everyone said my plate of food looked the best.
	Daily Total Carbs	Daily Total Protein	Daily Total Fat	
SATURDAY	15	58	90	I went to a birthday party and stayed on plan! While everyone else ate cake, I enjoyed a cup of coffee.
	Daily Total Carbs	Daily Total Protein	Daily Total Fat	
SUNDAY	17	61	88	I went shopping, and the walking did not make me feel out of breath.

My Top Ten Navigation Tips for Your Ketogenic Journey

If you haven't read any of Part I, then read these pages before beginning the four-week program that follows. These are my top ten tips for making a ketogenic lifestyle work. When you finish reading these tips, read them again. After you've read them a second time, begin implementing them one by one. They are listed in order of importance.

1. Count *all* carbs.

Keto doesn't have to be complicated. Despite the detailed information in this book, you don't need to wait for perfection. Don't drive yourself insane calculating macros or weighing and measuring your food. If the food you're eating has a label, then use the nutrition information on the label. For accurate carb counts of other foods, use the USDA Food Composition Databases (https://ndb.nal.usda.gov/ndb/search/list). Know the carb count of *every* food you put in your mouth *before* you put it in your mouth.

When I first started keto, I didn't know a macro from a micro, but I knew that I had to count carbs. The physicians I follow who recommend a ketogenic diet generally advise patients to count total carbs, not net carbs, which means not subtracting fiber. Some forms of soluble fiber, especially those found in packaged foods, can impact blood glucose; therefore, counting total carbs is a more conservative but safer approach.

For the first four months, I counted only total carbs, and I lost more than 40 pounds and discontinued all my medications in that time. While "low-carb" can be interpreted in different ways, remember that a ketogenic diet requires that 5 percent or less of your calories come from carbs.

2. Commit for two full weeks.

I hope you will follow my full four-week plan, but if four weeks sounds like a long time, start by deciding that you're going to follow a ketogenic plan 100 percent for two weeks. Just two short weeks, one day at a time—no sugar, no starch, no grains. Keto can be unforgiving for those of us with metabolic dysfunction; even one little Hershey's Kiss can throw your body off and keep you from seeing the results you want. Moreover, during those two weeks, you will be able to push through cravings and start enjoying the benefits. Once you successfully make it through two weeks, eating this way gets easier. Decide "Come heck or high water, I'm following this plan for two solid weeks." Then do it.

3. Find your favorite keto foods to eat.

Use the food lists, sample meal plans, and recipes in this book to identify your favorite keto-friendly foods and find some new ones. My favorites include chicken wings (page 259), creamed spinach, and homemade ranch dressing (page 209). When I'm tired of those things, I've got Meatloaf (page 282), Savory Pepper Steak (page 294), Taco Soup (page 302), and coffee with heavy cream. As you develop your keto menu, pick mostly from the lists of keto-friendly foods found on pages 43 to 47.

4. Limit total carbs per meal.

The "magic" that makes a ketogenic plan work is linked to keeping blood glucose stable. Eating higher-carb meals raises blood glucose, which is why you have to remain vigilant about counting carbohydrates. The body responds to each single meal. While some people talk about grams of carbs per day, keep in mind that eating your entire daily allotment of carbs in one meal can be counterproductive if that higher-carb meal raises your blood glucose. While you may find that you can tolerate up to 15 grams of total carbs per meal, many people cannot. Cravings are worse for me when I exceed 7 grams of total carbs in one meal. Through trial and error or by testing your blood glucose (see pages 101 and 102), you can find your own carb threshold.

5. Eat to hunger.

A ketogenic diet does not starve your body. On keto, you eat high-fat foods, such as bacon and chicken with crispy skin, that keep your blood glucose stable and keep you feeling full longer. As I explained to my husband, "If you're hungry on keto, you're doing it wrong." When you *are* hungry, eat. There are days when I am truly hungry, and on those days, eight strips of bacon and three eggs are not "too much" for me. On other days, two strips of bacon and a cup of coffee are sufficient. Fat tends to be self-limiting and can make you feel sick if you overeat it. You will learn quickly when you've overeaten fat. Stop eating when your hunger is satisfied; don't gorge. Moreover, do not eat again until you are physically hungry.

6. Learn to listen to your body.

Know whether you're eating what's "right" by listening to your body. An ideal ketogenic meal meets these requirements:

- You leave the table feeling satisfied—not stuffed, but comfortable.

- You feel energized, not tired or sluggish, one to two hours after eating. If you do feel tired or sluggish, then your meal was not ideal; these feelings may be linked to having eaten too much protein or carbohydrate or may be related to a food sensitivity. Make note of what you ate so that you won't make the same mistake again. (See pages 24 to 28 for tips on creating a balanced keto plate.)

- You do not feel true physical hunger for at least four hours after the meal. It takes a body that long to metabolize a meal when the balance of macronutrients is right.

7. Learn your hunger cues.

Hunger is not about feeling anxious, frustrated, angry, or happy. Hunger is not an emotion. True physical hunger is not triggered by a commercial on television or by someone eating near you. Physical hunger is disruptive. It stops you from what you're doing and says, "I need a little fuel here!" If you're busy and you get distracted by hunger, you're truly hungry. When you're hungry, eat. If you're not physically hungry, drink some water, phone a friend, run an errand, clean, or go for a walk. Learning to recognize true physical hunger is a key to success.

8. Don't try to take shortcuts.

There is no substitute for real food. Whether you're tempted by the convenience of "low-carb" products that are not really low in carbs, or you're tempted by supplements that promise a quicker path to ketosis, or you're simply toying with the idea of a three-day gimmicky "diet," "detox," or "fast," don't. Learning to eat real food and changing your habits for the rest of your life is going to make you healthier in two weeks, two months, two years, and two decades. Easy shortcuts won't get you further along in your journey for any length of time.

9. Pay attention to ingredients.

If a food is marked "low-carb," "sugar-free," or even "keto," it probably isn't a good option. Looking for convenience, I made this mistake often early on. Many of the sweeteners used by food producers will impede your progress. For example, diet soft drinks can cause stalls in weight loss, and many people find that drinking them increases hunger. If you pay attention to ingredients and steer clear of those that will keep you from succeeding, you are more likely to see better results.

10. Create new eating habits.

You will not succeed by doing the same things you've always done. You have to think differently about food and meals. What you eat, when you eat, and why you eat are going to be different on a ketogenic plan. For example, in the morning, I often eat nontraditional breakfast foods, such as a bacon cheeseburger or a Skillet Pizza (page 314). For quick lunches, I sometimes eat sandwich fillings that are high in fat and protein without the bread. Even if you don't like to cook, you can still create low-carb meals that you enjoy instead of giving in and eating your old high-carb ordering habits. If you don't *do* something different, you will never *be* different.

Traversing the Keto Flu

There may be an adaptation period as your body switches from primarily burning glucose to burning fat. While "keto flu," as it is commonly known, doesn't affect everyone, common complaints include fatigue or feelings of weakness, dizziness, headaches, extreme cravings, nausea, irritability, and difficulty sleeping. As one friend described her symptoms to me, she asked, "How can this be healthy?!"

The good news is that the keto flu is a signal that your body is transitioning to burning fat. As it does, it may need some additional support. Here are some tips:

First, a ketogenic diet has a diuretic effect, so you can expect your body to release fluids. Be prepared for increased urination and thirst. Water is the best option when you're thirsty. I keep water close by at all times, including by my bed at night. Be careful not to force fluids beyond thirst, however, as this can flush the body of necessary electrolytes.

Second, balance electrolytes by drinking salty bone broth, adding sea salt to foods, or even sipping pickle juice, which is full of sodium. On a ketogenic diet, your body will need salt. Don't underestimate the power of bone broth. Not only does it provide sodium, but it is rich in vitamins and minerals as well.

Third, fight cravings with fat! Cook veggies in bacon fat. Slather your plate with more butter than you think is polite and dip everything into it. Fat will keep your body satiated and help you avoid hunger and cravings. Some people swear by pickle juice as a way to fight cravings, too; if you're struggling, then it's certainly worth a try.

Lastly, remember to stay the course. The keto flu lasts a few days at most. Once you push through to ketosis, the journey becomes much easier. You will be amazed at your energy level, mental clarity, and lack of hunger.

The Four Tenets of Keto

Following a ketogenic lifestyle and staying on plan can be difficult long term. Four basic tenets will help you make the transition last a lifetime and ensure your success:

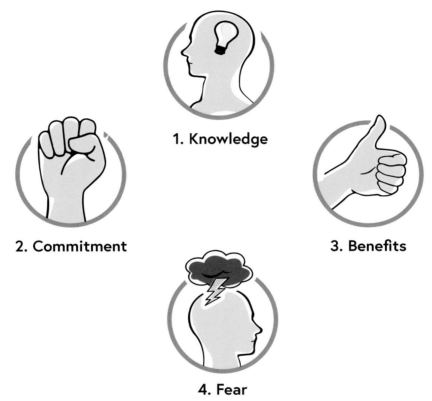

1. Knowledge

2. Commitment

3. Benefits

4. Fear

Knowledge

Knowledge is power. When you know something another person doesn't know, you have power over that person. The reason we pay attorneys, electricians, and plumbers so well is that they have knowledge and skills that we don't have, so they have the power to charge us for that knowledge.

Don't follow this plan just because you want to lose weight like someone else did. Take the time to know why eating this way matters. Remember, you lower blood glucose, reduce insulin, burn fat, and control hunger by eating low carbohydrates and high fat. Understand that the three macronutrients—fat, protein, and carbohydrate—impact the body differently. Know what happens when you eat foods that are high in each of those macronutrients. When you have a basic understanding of how each macronutrient is metabolized, you can objectify your decisions about food. Understanding the science helps you override emotional attachments to food and learn to see foods for the value of their macronutrients.

When my grandmother passed away years ago, I inherited many of her things—furniture, glassware, dishes, and so on. Even though it doesn't match our tastes or lifestyle, I want to keep all of it. I have an emotional attachment to her things that goes beyond the reasonable objections expressed by my husband. He can rationally see that we don't have room to store the furniture. We can't use the furniture because it is uncomfortable, impractical, or too fragile for daily use. While I know logically that we should not keep the furniture in storage, I still struggle with the thought of not keeping it.

Making food choices can be somewhat similar. When we logically choose foods based on how they nourish our bodies and impact blood glucose, we begin to see those foods not as "my favorite yeast roll" or "Grandma's tastiest cake," but as "foods that harm my body" or "foods that make me sick." Armed with knowledge, we can look beyond taste and emotional attachments to objectively consider what happens when we eat more carbohydrates than fat or protein. Knowing that high-carb foods cause physiological responses that result in sickness (high blood glucose, inflammation, overweight) makes it easier to choose not to eat them. Just as we might struggle to give away Grandpa's old recliner, we also struggle to pass up a food that we "love" or that is linked to a family tradition. But when we objectify it and see food as fat, protein, and carbohydrate, it's easier to make better choices. No matter how many rooms or cabinets I fill with those antique possessions of theirs, I will miss those departed family members. They are not found in those possessions any more than comfort, joy, or happiness are found in the foods that make us sick.

Commitment

Even with a clear understanding of food as macronutrients and the metabolic impact of each, food choices can be hard unless you have commitment. Commitment is integral to almost every setting. Without it, we rarely achieve our goals. Commitment is a decision. Every day an athlete decides whether he or she will practice, work out, or eat in ways that help him or her compete. Even when tired or sick or pressed for time, the athlete makes decisions about whether to commit to what he or she knows to be best for performance. Married couples, parents, academics, professionals, and even pet owners are similar. When we commit, we do things we don't always want to do to work toward bigger goals.

When we commit to a ketogenic diet, we commit to eating in ways that keep us healthier. Regardless of what others are eating, regardless of not having enough hours in the day, regardless of having to learn new ways of selecting and preparing food, we commit. Every day.

The wonderful thing about keto is that the commitment is primarily limited to our food choices. We don't have to exercise; activity is an important part of overall health, but it isn't required to be successful on keto. Keto requires only that we control our food choices and rewards us with the realization that food no longer controls us.

When starting keto, it might help to commit to a short time frame. I decided that I would try this "diet" for two weeks. That was it. Just two weeks. I never promised to give up bread or doughnuts or chocolate pie for the rest of my life, but I did promise that I would give this new plan a two-week run. If Gary Taubes (see page 13) knew his stuff, I thought, two weeks should tell me whether this plan might work for me. I could do anything for two weeks.

Benefits

The commitment to keto gets easier each day when we learn to look for and see the benefits. Most folks look first to the scale as a measure of progress, but you also see other benefits. Reduced hunger was one of the first benefits I enjoyed during my two-week commitment to keto. On day three, I called my best friend and nearly shouted into the phone, "I forgot to each lunch!" She understood the significance of that moment. By week two, my clothes were looser, so I knew I was losing inches even though I wasn't measuring myself at the time. My pain lessened, and eventually I began to take fewer medications. My mobility improved, and I began to marvel at the things I could do.

A significant benefit for me was being able to participate in activities with my children. I have photos of myself flying kites with the kids. I was running to get the kite lifted off the ground. Me! Running! While having fun! If eating a yeast roll or a bagel meant that I couldn't play with my kids, then that certainly reinforced my resolve. How could I ever choose carbs over the joy I discovered from feeling good and enjoying active time with my children? I focused on the rewards.

As if the rewards of buying smaller clothes, having reduced hunger, being active with my family, and increasing confidence weren't enough, there was another significant benefit that I had never known with any other diet: I loved the delicious food! Who could not love eating butter? I was eating steak, bacon, full-fat cheese, and other foods that I had been told to avoid all my low-fat life, yet here I was wearing the smallest clothes I'd ever worn.

In every other diet, I had been hungry and felt deprived. The list of "allowed" foods was grim. Few people ever truly enjoy the food on a low-fat diet. For example, a baked potato without butter, cheese, or sour cream is just paste. What tastes good is the fat. Take that same butter, cheese, sour cream, and bacon and load it onto some roasted broccoli. Those are the kinds of foods that I eat now, whenever I want! All that fat and my health improved each day.

As you begin your ketogenic journey, look for benefits to help you focus on why this lifestyle change is worth it. As you leave behind old habits, think about what feels better about this way of eating.

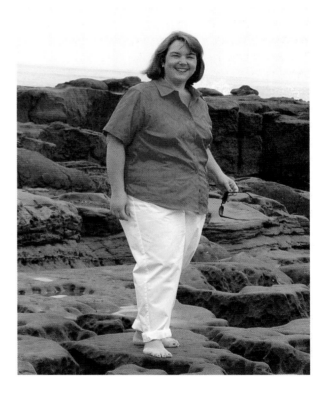

Fear

After you've harnessed the power of knowing about keto, made the commitment to give it an earnest try, and focused on the rewards, don't forget your fear. Fear can be a powerful motivator. In those first few weeks, I was very much afraid that this "diet" wouldn't work. I feared that I was forever stuck being obese and in significant pain. My life was framed by all that I had to say no to. Much of what I couldn't do involved activities with and for my children. Feeling as if you can't be the parent you want to be can be a strong incentive to change. Each time I chose to stay on plan, I knew that I wasn't choosing just for me and my health, but for Grace and Jonathan, too. I was opting to be the mother my children deserved and to be the wife my husband wanted on his arm. The fear of failing them motivated me to make the effort to stay on plan.

People have told me that they've watched a loved one lose their sight or a limb to diabetes, and the fear of facing that same fate themselves motivated them to control their blood glucose to prevent or reverse diabetes. I was fearful of becoming disabled because of back pain. When you understand that high-carb foods result in a life you don't want, then you can better understand that your daily choices do matter to your long-term success.

I run from my fear of obesity by eating foods I love—like bacon! That bacon empowers me in ways that a doughnut can never do. The doughnut belonged to the mom who had to lie down each night after work because her pain was severe. The yeast bread was eaten by the wife who could only shop in plus-sized stores. The stack of pancakes was served to the woman who would not pose for family photos. I have been that woman, and while I love her for making the decision to try a ketogenic diet and for doing the hard work, I do not want to take back her struggles. She deserves for me to stay on plan. She worked hard to acquire the knowledge, make the commitment, and look for the benefits. She lived through the things I now fear most. I love her, but I will not *be* her again. I will stay on plan for her, for my children, for my husband, and for me.

Use these four basic tenets to follow the ketogenic diet with me for four weeks. Don't worry, I will be there with you every day of those twenty-eight days, and you will eat some delicious food. You will need to make the commitment to see it through every day, 100 percent. Along the way, I will remind you to look for the benefits, and before long, you will be able to harness your fear to move forward in your journey.

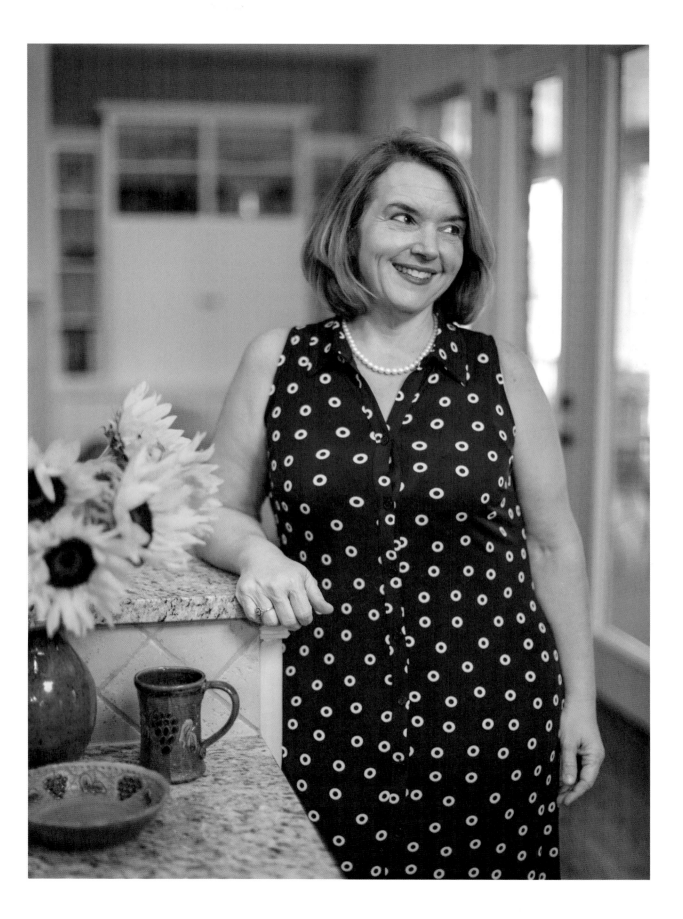

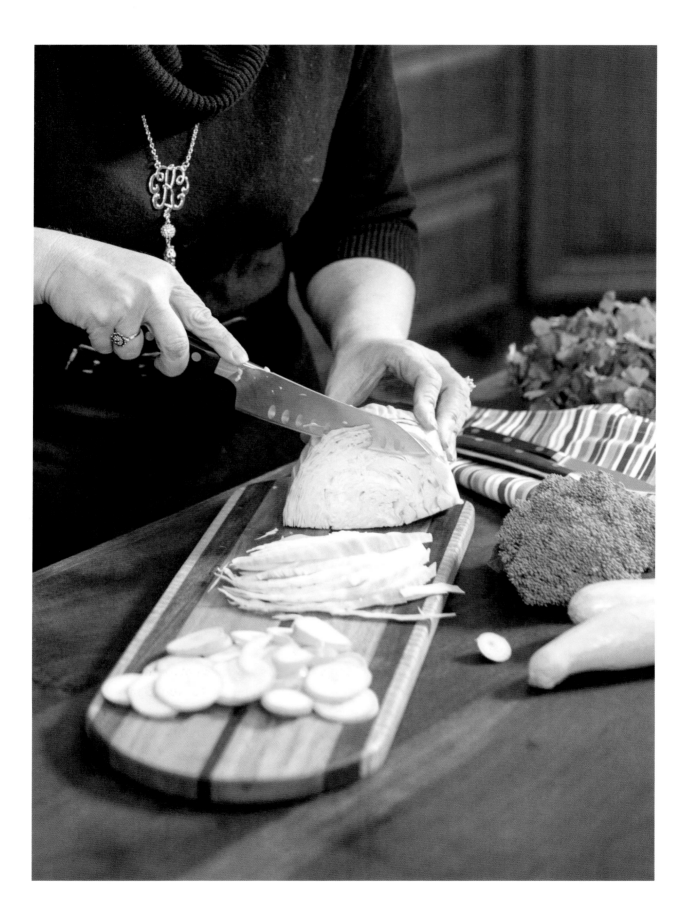

Chapter 5
Your First Four Weeks *on Keto*

For twenty-eight days, we will journey together as you adapt to a ketogenic lifestyle. For each of the four weeks, I've identified common challenges and provided information to help you succeed, including a checklist of action items that you can use to prepare for those seven days. Each week, you should begin with a weekly food plan as well as a fresh Mile Marker Summary. The food plan helps ensure that you have appropriate, and delicious, foods so that you aren't hungry or unprepared. (For more on meal planning, see pages 42 to 69.) The Mile Marker Summary is a place to record what you eat as well as to monitor your progress. This summary encourages you to make notes about how you feel after you eat and to monitor your hunger before and after each meal. (An explanation of how to use the summary is on page 107, and various mile markers of progress are described on pages 96 to 106.) You are likely to be surprised at how quickly you notice positive changes!

I've treated each day of the week like a devotional, providing you with a story that illustrates a message that I think is particularly relevant for that point in your ketogenic journey, along with some inspiration for you to take with you as you face the day. At the end of each day, I've added a "Just for Today" affirmation that I hope will motivate you to make good choices and, most importantly, to choose *you*. I used many of these same affirmations to help me when I struggled to stay on plan. Carry them with you, tape them to the fridge, or simply read them when you need them.

Week 1

Welcome to the first week of your journey! I'm really excited that you've decided to join in this big adventure. All that planning will come in handy this week as you take the driver's seat and begin to navigate the lifestyle changes that will help you follow a ketogenic plan long term.

Week 1 will not always be easy. There will be times when you may not know which path leads in the right direction. There may be flashing signs tempting you to stop or veer off course. Don't worry, I'll be here encouraging you every day, pointing out the directional signs that you need to follow. There may be times when you need to yield, slow down, recalculate your route, or refocus on your destination—we all need to do that from time to time. What is important right now is that you have decided to take the journey!

Following a ketogenic path is not a journey you will ever complete, only a journey that you start. You begin each day by deciding what you *will* eat and what you *will not* eat. You can't speed up the journey, so you will learn to focus on navigating each day, one day at a time. Eventually, you will learn to simply enjoy your travels as navigating becomes second nature, and you can relax and focus on the people and activities that matter most to you. Your primary goal for this week is to begin the journey and start down the path.

Here are your points of focus for Week 1:

1. Use what you learned about creating a ketogenic plate to put together tasty meals that keep you on plan. (See pages 24 to 28.)

2. Pay attention to how hunger feels. Hunger is not about boredom, stress, fear, or excitement. Identifying and managing physical hunger will keep you moving forward. A complete discussion of hunger is on pages 36 and 37.

3. Manage cravings by using the power of balancing macronutrients and being intentional about what, when, and with whom you eat.

4. Control your food decisions even when faced with questions or advice from others who mean well but may doubt what you're doing.

5. Harness your fear to make important lifestyle changes that ensure your ongoing success. (See page 114 for more on harnessing fear.)

The first key to success for Week 1 is consistency. You must stay *100 percent on plan* every single day as your body adjusts to burning fat instead of glucose for fuel. If you don't stay on plan, then you will never know whether this way of eating works for you.

Another key to success is to focus on food! Learn about the macronutrients in the foods you are eating so that your blood glucose remains balanced and eating this way becomes natural.

Week 1 Checklist

☐ Complete your shopping and meal prep for Week 1 and decide on your weekly food plan. Pick out five easy breakfasts, five simple lunches, and five delicious dinners. Determine which meals can be made or prepped ahead of time and do the prep work by purchasing all the ingredients at least one day in advance of Day 1. See the sample meal plans on pages 60 to 66 for inspiration.

☐ Make or buy bone broth (see pages 186 and 187) in case you experience the keto flu (see page 110).

☐ Complete the "Know Your Why!" worksheet (see pages 94 and 95).

☐ Review the section "My Top Ten Navigation Tips for Your Ketogenic Journey" on pages 108 to 110.

☐ Take photos, try on clothing, jot down your measurements (see pages 98 and 99), and so on so that you have a baseline from which to track your progress.

☐ Throughout the week, use the Week 1 Mile Marker Summary to record your progress. Pages 96 to 107 discuss how to monitor your progress and provide some examples of mile markers of progress. This summary may be useful to you in later weeks as a baseline to see how much your eating, your habits, and your mindset have changed. You might also want to record your daily total macronutrients so that you can start to understand what works well for your body. While keeping carbs low, focus on how your hunger levels change as you eat varying amounts of fat and protein. See page 107 for a sample to help you get started.

Daily Food Journal

Use a journal like this to record what you ate, what time you ate, how hungry you were when you ate, and how satisfied you felt after eating. Remember to eat only when hungry. For good ketogenic ratios, make sure that each meal has fat grams equal to or higher than protein grams, with carbohydrate grams lower than protein and fat. To print out copies of this chart, go to my website, cookingketowithkristie.com.

First Meal

Time: ....   Hunger level: 1   2   3   4   5   6   7   8   9   10

What I ate: ....

....

Carbs: .... Protein: .... Fat: ....   Satisfaction after meal: 1   2   3   4   5   6   7   8   9   10

Second Meal

Time: ....   Hunger level: 1   2   3   4   5   6   7   8   9   10

What I ate: ....

....

Carbs: .... Protein: .... Fat: ....   Satisfaction after meal: 1   2   3   4   5   6   7   8   9   10

Third Meal

Time: ....   Hunger level: 1   2   3   4   5   6   7   8   9   10

What I ate: ....

....

Carbs: .... Protein: .... Fat: ....   Satisfaction after meal: 1   2   3   4   5   6   7   8   9   10

First Snack

Time: ....   Hunger level: 1   2   3   4   5   6   7   8   9   10

What I ate: ....

....

Carbs: .... Protein: .... Fat: ....   Satisfaction after meal: 1   2   3   4   5   6   7   8   9   10

Second Snack

Time: ....   Hunger level: 1   2   3   4   5   6   7   8   9   10

What I ate: ....

....

Carbs: .... Protein: .... Fat: ....   Satisfaction after meal: 1   2   3   4   5   6   7   8   9   10

Mile Marker Summary, Week 1

Use this summary to record your progress throughout the week. You might also want to record your daily total intake of carbs, protein, and fat so you can begin to understand what works best for you. For a printable version of this worksheet, go to my website, cookingketowithkristie.com.

MONDAY

MACROS FOR ALL MEALS AND SNACKS			MILE MARKERS OF SUCCESS
Daily Total Carbs	Daily Total Protein	Daily Total Fat	

TUESDAY

MACROS FOR ALL MEALS AND SNACKS			MILE MARKERS OF SUCCESS
Daily Total Carbs	Daily Total Protein	Daily Total Fat	

WEDNESDAY

MACROS FOR ALL MEALS AND SNACKS			MILE MARKERS OF SUCCESS
Daily Total Carbs	Daily Total Protein	Daily Total Fat	

THURSDAY

MACROS FOR ALL MEALS AND SNACKS			MILE MARKERS OF SUCCESS
Daily Total Carbs	Daily Total Protein	Daily Total Fat	

FRIDAY

MACROS FOR ALL MEALS AND SNACKS			MILE MARKERS OF SUCCESS
Daily Total Carbs	Daily Total Protein	Daily Total Fat	

SATURDAY

MACROS FOR ALL MEALS AND SNACKS			MILE MARKERS OF SUCCESS
Daily Total Carbs	Daily Total Protein	Daily Total Fat	

SUNDAY

MACROS FOR ALL MEALS AND SNACKS			MILE MARKERS OF SUCCESS
Daily Total Carbs	Daily Total Protein	Daily Total Fat	

Day 1: Learning to Drive

My first day following a ketogenic plan was not all that memorable. All I knew was that I should count carbs. I hadn't taken the time to plan my meals, and I worried about keeping my portions small because I still thought of keto as a diet, and diets left me feeling hungry all the time. For *your* first day on this journey, keep it simple. Eat when you're hungry, but only when you're hungry. Don't worry about how many slices of bacon you eat or whether it takes two servings of breakfast to feel satiated. Pay attention to portions only to limit the number of grams of carbohydrate you consume; do not restrict fat or protein.

When I was learning how to drive, I fell in love with a car that had a manual transmission. My dad promised that if I learned how to drive a manual transmission, he would buy the car for me. With that kind of motivation, I was determined to succeed! We spent hours talking through the process and practicing. There were plenty of lurches and stalls as I tried to figure out how to release the clutch and accelerate smoothly. I knew that there was a friction point and that as I raised my left foot off the clutch, I had to press my right foot down on the gas pedal. In those first few weeks, all I focused on was releasing the clutch slowly and accelerating so that the car moved forward smoothly and didn't roll back, lurch forward, or choke. My dad could explain it to me while we sat in the driveway, but it wasn't until I was stopped at a stop sign on a hill that I *experienced* exactly how it felt to disengage the clutch while increasing the flow of gas. Knowing how the car felt at that moment was the key to accelerating successfully.

Similarly, knowing how your body feels with regard to hunger is the key to knowing how much to eat and when. Keeping carbs low, protein moderate, and fat high will help you feel those signals of true hunger. If your blood glucose runs high and your insulin signals aren't functioning properly, you often remain in a constant state of hunger. The goal for today is to keep your blood glucose stable by avoiding sugars and starches (carbohydrates) while fueling your body with fat and protein. Only your body can tell you how much you should eat, but it can only do so when your signals are functioning properly.

You may get some false signals today as your body craves sugar. Meals may seem "incomplete" because you are not experiencing those blood glucose spikes afterward. That feeling will go away over the next week if you consistently keep carbohydrates low and eat enough fat and protein. Instead of giving in to cravings, focus on how you feel before and after meals. Concentrate on your energy level. In my first week on keto, I noticed that I did not feel heavy or tired after meals, but lighter, with more consistent energy throughout the day. By choosing to eat only low-carb, high-fat meals, you will learn how your body responds to a ketogenic way of eating.

JUST FOR TODAY I choose me by eating high-fat, low-carb foods that keep my blood glucose stable and help me learn what true hunger feels like.

Day 2: Following the Signs

When I was about six years old, I was chased by a pack of dogs. One of the leaders of the pack was Whiskers, who belonged to my grandmother. He was a Chow and fiercely protective of us grandchildren. We adored him. He allowed us to snuggle, harass, and antagonize him at will. Yet one day, as I was walking to my grandmother's house to get my bike, he seemed to turn on me. My grandmother had a long driveway that curved slightly around the house. The side yard was obscured by a hedge. As I rounded the curve and was able to see just around the hedge, there were the dogs. They were in a circle, and Whiskers and another large neighborhood dog were squaring off in the center. Their postures indicated an impending fight. While I never fully understood what the pack was doing, I followed my instincts and ran. The dogs gave chase. I ran as hard as my chubby little legs allowed, hollering all the way. To get to safety, I had to cross a busy highway. Thankfully, a neighbor heard my cries for help, and a passing motorist who recognized my plight was able to safely stop traffic. The neighbor called her dog, and the entire pack followed him to her house while I bounded across the road to my mother. I shook for hours afterward. I never became irrationally fearful of dogs, but I did develop a healthy fear of them.

A healthy fear is a fear that causes us to take action or reminds us to be cautious. Unwittingly, a dear friend created a healthy fear in me when I first started keto when she told me, "Even one little Hershey's Kiss can throw you off plan!" That friend didn't know it, but her words struck terror in my heart. It was such a defining moment that I remember standing in my kitchen as we chatted on the phone. My size-22 jeans were tight, and I had just opened the refrigerator door. When she said that, I promptly closed the fridge and sat down to finish our conversation.

More than anything else, those words stayed with me in the first few months of following a very-low-carb lifestyle. Because I understood what sugar did to my body, I understood why it was so important to avoid it. When I was hungry or faced temptation, I remembered my friend's words and then chose fat and protein over carbohydrates. I had a healthy fear of being thrown off plan.

As you go through Day 2, remember that your body is changing in ways that you cannot yet see. Continue to pay attention to hunger. If you notice that you are urinating frequently, feel thirsty, or have headaches, you may need more sodium and more water. Dehydration is not uncommon in the first week or two as your body adapts. If you have any symptoms of the keto flu, follow the tips outlined on page 110.

Use the food lists on pages 43 to 47 to choose foods that are very low in carbs. When in doubt, eat high-fat selections like butter, heavy cream, olive oil, mayonnaise, and full-fat dressings. Some excellent foods to keep at the ready are bacon, full-fat cheeses, and macadamia nuts (measure serving sizes). Eating enough fat will help you avoid hunger and lessen your chances of going off plan. When you know *what* to eat, you can focus on *when* to eat.

 JUST FOR TODAY I will use my healthy fear to avoid sugar and starches. My healthy fear will make me cautious about the foods I choose so that I will not fail.

Day 3: Maybe Tomorrow

"I can't imagine saying that I will never eat donuts again!" That's what my skinny friend said to me about my new diet. She either has a healthy metabolism or has underlying health conditions that are not physically obvious, because she eats all the sugar and processed junk that make me sick. Still, I need to confess something: I have never promised that I will never eat donuts again. What I say is, "Just for today, I am not going to gobble down donuts. Tomorrow or next week, I might eat a dozen, but today, I'm going to choose me. I'm going to see if this crazy diet works—just for today!" You see, I knew the plan wouldn't work if I didn't follow it. If I ate a donut, then I wouldn't be on plan. How would I know if it worked? I had to give it a chance, even for just one more day.

When I started keto, I promised myself that I would follow the plan to the letter for two solid weeks, because I desperately needed to see if it would work. At the end of those two weeks, I would assess whether this plan was right for me. I never told myself that life with bread was over. I never swore that I would never eat donuts again. Nope. I left my options open. For two weeks, I would not eat sugar or starch. Two weeks. After that, all bets were off.

Somehow, I knew that if I didn't give it 100 percent, I could not blame the diet. I was tired of failing. My body was getting bigger, and I needed to buy larger clothes. My prescriptions were increasing, and so was the back pain that often radiated down my legs. Standing to cook meals and walking even small distances was getting harder. Losing weight could make it all better, and my husband and children deserved at least two weeks of me giving it my best.

Eating keto has a cumulative effect. The formula is:

$$\begin{array}{r} \text{today} \\ \text{yesterday} \\ \text{the day before yesterday} \\ +\ \underline{\text{the day before that}} \\ \text{better health} \end{array}$$

This equation adds up to lower blood glucose, reduced inflammation, and weight lost, which feels good all over.

Whenever I'm faced with cravings or temptations, I remind myself that I may choose to eat off plan tomorrow, but not today. Today I'm going to push through. I don't want to go back to where I started, so I will get to the end of today just to see what's on the other side.

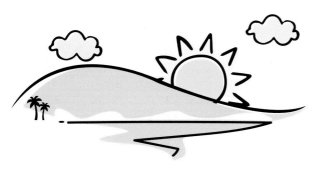

JUST FOR TODAY I choose to do this for just one more day because I want to see what tomorrow looks like when I stay on plan. I know what will happen if I give up.

Day 4: You *Can* Have That!

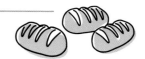

"You can't have that!" The words stung, and the young child who lives inside me immediately shouted, "Oh, yes, I can!" It was the first week of my new diet, and my family and I had gone to dinner with David's parents at a steakhouse that is famous for its yeast rolls. The waiter presented us with a big basket of warm, buttery rolls just as we were seated. Those big, fluffy rolls were on the table even before we had squeezed into the booth! Not only did my five dining companions eagerly devour the rolls, but they were very vocal about how *delicious* the rolls were, smeared with cane syrup–sweetened fake butter spread. Then they requested a second basket. My mother-in-law asked for more of the fake butter spread, too. She looked at me and asked, "Don't you want some?" and then remembered, "Oh, you can't have that!"

I looked at those rolls and saw Trouble. At the time, my rudimentary understanding of why keto works was that eating carbs (sugar) raises blood glucose. To deal with that glucose, the body releases insulin. That release of insulin isn't necessarily a problem in metabolically healthy individuals, but my morbid obesity was an outward sign of inner metabolic dysfunction. In that first week, I also understood that insulin is a hoarder hormone; it helps store fat in cells. While sitting in that booth and looking at those rolls, I had an image of insulin being like thousands of mean little soldiers running through my bloodstream, locking fat into my cells. No wonder we're hungry again so soon after eating; there's no energy to be used because it's locked away as fat! Obesity can be described as a condition of starvation because energy cannot be accessed. If blood glucose is kept stable, though, insulin levels should fall, and stored energy (or fat) can be used.

I knew that even one bite of a yeast roll would release a cascade of hormones, including insulin. I visualized the insulin meanies shoving fat into my cells, and I felt my upper arms getting bigger. While others saw an unlimited supply of a delicious food, I saw poison. In those high-carb rolls, I saw the morbid obesity that I was desperately trying to fight off. It was only the first week of my keto journey, but I could already tell that it was working. When I ate very few carbohydrates, my hunger disappeared. I replied, "Oh, I *can* eat those. I just don't want them."

At the time, I didn't understand the power of my reply, but it saved my life in two ways. After a lifetime of hunger and deprivation, I knew that I could eat anything I wanted. By saying "I *can* eat those," I was giving myself the power of control. No one else was restricting me. The child inside me was not being chastised for sneaking food from the refrigerator or eating a second helping of dessert. My inner adult was in charge, and she was empowered to make the decision. She looked at those poison rolls that would only contribute to her morbid obesity and decided, "I just don't want them"—and that is the second powerful mind shift I verbalized that night. I didn't want them even when others were raving about how delicious they were. In those rolls I saw obesity, plus-sized clothing, sweating after little exertion, back pain, and diabetes. Since that day, I have been able to reject high-carb foods simply because I see them differently. Instead of seeing foods that taste good, I see foods that make me sick. Disease and obesity do *not* taste good.

That night, I ordered a steak, a salad with full-fat dressing, and steamed buttered broccoli, and I could not finish everything on my plate. While others complained of being overly full and sleepy, my energy level stayed high for the rest of the evening. I was proud of my choices.

It was over four years and 100 pounds ago that I stared down those poison rolls. I am still empowered to eat anything I choose, and I continue to choose low-carb, high-fat foods that keep me healthy.

JUST FOR TODAY

I can choose to eat anything I want, and I choose not to eat the high-carb foods that make me sick.

Day 5: When the Bread Basket Comes

What if someone said to you, "How do you go into a store and not shoplift? I mean, there are so many things I see that I want—pretty dresses, warm sweaters, and so many great shoes! How can you not stick just one item in your purse?"

Can you imagine? Most of us would never dream of shoplifting, especially when the object is something we can afford or don't even need. We wouldn't consider stealing because we set boundaries for what we will and will not do. When I walk into a store, I don't even have to think about whether or not I will steal. I simply won't. I decided not to steal decades ago. It's a decision from which I have not wavered and cannot imagine ever wavering, except perhaps in extreme circumstances.

The same is true for me with regard to food. When the bread basket comes, I don't have to think about whether I will have a roll. I know that I won't because I have set boundaries for myself. I know my whys—the reasons why staying on plan matters to me (see pages 94 and 95). Because I have made the decision in advance, there is no struggle. I will not eat the bread. Instead, I will have a delicious fatty steak with steamed broccoli loaded with butter, cheese, bacon, and sour cream, and I will focus on enjoying time spent talking with my companions over dinner.

Yet folks often ask me, "How do you go to a party and not eat cake? How do you refuse the bread basket at a restaurant when those rolls look so good? How can I keep myself from eating the Valentine candy my friend gave me?" Resisting these kinds of temptations is far easier when you set boundaries for yourself. I don't take things that don't belong to me, and I don't eat high-carb foods, either.

Imagine what would happen if you didn't set boundaries in advance. Imagine sitting at the table when the bread basket comes, and everyone else picking out rolls and smearing them with butter. You sit there wondering if maybe you should, too. You remember the taste and texture of rolls like these, and then you have a choice to make. At that moment, deciding whether to eat a roll is difficult. Refusing the roll feels like deprivation. You think about how unfair it is that everyone else is enjoying a roll. Others may feel bad for you because they sense your wavering. They might try to make you feel better by encouraging you to "Have just a bite," or by saying, "One roll won't hurt you." You might hear rationalizations like "You can always start over tomorrow."

Most of us have started over way too many times. The one bite that turns into a hundred bites *does* hurt. "One roll" has never ended well for me. Set your boundaries before you are staring down the bread basket or tub of popcorn or Valentine treat. You decided when you started this twenty-eight-day guide that you were going to give keto your best shot. If you don't stay on plan for at least two solid weeks, then you will never know whether a ketogenic diet really works for you. Just two weeks, and if it doesn't work out, you can come back and eat an entire basket of bread all by yourself. Remind yourself, "Just for now—for two weeks—I will stay on plan."

See pages 76 to 78 for more strategies and tips for handling social situations. I've provided examples of what you can say and do to make eating in social settings much easier.

JUST FOR TODAY If I am tempted by what others are eating, I will remember why staying on plan matters to me and why I must set boundaries with others. No matter how hard it might be to pass up food in the moment, I have never regretted something that I didn't eat.

Day 6: Enjoy the Silence

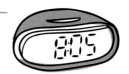

About six months after my husband and I started a low-carb, high-fat diet, I awoke to absolute quiet. It was 3 a.m., and the only thing I could hear was a clock ticking. David was lying beside me, but there was no noise! The man who could wake a hibernating bear with his snoring wasn't even breathing heavily. That's when it occurred to me: "Is he breathing?" I leaned closer to him but still didn't hear anything. I didn't want to wake him, but worry began to rise up into fear, so I leaned even closer. I felt his arm. It wasn't cold, but it wasn't as warm as my worry wanted it to be. I decided to put my hand near his face to see if warm air was coming from his nose or mouth. In the dark, as I propped myself up on my right elbow, I reached across his body with my left hand, lost my balance, and accidentally popped him right in the face! He sat straight up in bed.

Now, when you wake your husband with a pop to the face at 3 a.m., he typically wants an explanation, so I exclaimed, "You're alive!" He knew that already, so I had to explain that I had awoken to complete silence and had begun to panic. We'd fallen into a pattern of me desperately trying to get to sleep before he did because his snoring had gotten so bad. Even when I did manage to fall asleep first, it wasn't unusual for his seismographic snorts and gasps to rouse me. His snoring was worse when he slept on his back, so most nights I tried to nudge him onto his side by pulling the covers or gently tugging or pushing him. On other nights, sleep deprivation left me less "understanding," and I would utter a grumpy, "You're snoring!" We even discussed sleeping in different beds at one point. After losing about 40 pounds, he was no longer snoring, and neither of us had even realized it until I awoke to silence.

When we reached our mid-forties—we were both obese at the time—we considered our snoring, high blood pressure, aches and pains, poor lipid panels, and tiring easily to be "normal" parts of aging. We joked that getting old wasn't fun, but it was better than the alternative. What we didn't attribute to aging we attributed to genetics. My father-in-law had high blood pressure, so we figured it was inevitable for David to have it, too. But with a low-carb, high-fat diet, David's blood pressure is now at the low end of the normal range after years of being high enough to require medication.

We began keto to lose weight, but along the way, we gained a unique perspective about weight and health. As our bodies changed, our lives changed. We came to realize that eating low-carb and high-fat was giving us far more than just slimmer bodies. Obesity was just a symptom. When we addressed the underlying issues—inflammation, insulin resistance, and metabolic dysfunction—our bodies healed and the pounds melted away. Our hunger decreased, and we didn't feel as if we were starving all the time. Our morning aches and pains abated. Our lifestyles opened up to bike rides, hikes, and kayaking and longer periods of working in the yard. We marvel at the better health we enjoy simply because we no longer eat sugar, starch, or grains. We are eating the most delicious foods we've ever enjoyed— butter, cheese, and fatty meats. Our vegetables are roasted in fat or smothered in rich sauces. Although our portions are half the size they used to be, our bellies are not grumbling. And most of the time, we sleep quietly in our bed without fearing the silence.

JUST FOR TODAY

I choose to be healthy. If I don't *do* something different, my life will never *be* different.

Day 7: Your Team Plate

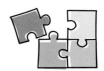

Have you ever put together a team to accomplish something? Suppose you need a team to build a new playground in your community. First, you need a planner—someone to keep the slide from being built to end under the monkey bars and to make sure that seating is situated in the shade. Next, you need workers—folks who are strong and dependable and know their way around power tools. Third, you need people who can spread the word and build community support. Networkers get donations and garner support for the team's efforts. Lastly, you need energy and fun. A team needs members who will keep the Bluetooth speaker streaming with music. A team may need additional strengths depending on the task at hand, but those are the four general areas that can get a project completed.

Use those same components of building a team to build your ketogenic plate. You have the role of planner. You determine the project scope, budget, and schedule. You have three different team members to work with: protein, fat, and carbohydrate.

Protein is a hard worker—dependable, strong, and knowledgeable. Too much protein will slowly raise blood glucose, so you don't want to eat too much in any meal; however, you do want to have at least some protein with every meal. (See pages 24 to 28 for a discussion of building a ketogenic plate.)

The second team member—the networker—is fat. Fat, including both dietary fat (the fat you eat) and stored fat, should be your primary source of fuel. Of the three team members, fat is the *least* likely to raise blood glucose. Can you eat too much fat? Yes, but if you overeat fat, you may experience nausea or intestinal distress, and you aren't likely to want to do it very often.

The third and final team member is carbohydrate. Carbs can be fun teammates who bring texture and tunes, but they often play the music way too loud! You want to employ carbs in small amounts because they can rile the neighbors (raise blood glucose) and derail your goals.

The team you create on your plate is what matters most to your long-term success. Your body processes each meal individually. If you put together a good team, then you can easily go four to six hours or longer without hunger. If you are hungry sooner than that, look at whether the team you assembled for your last meal had the right mix of members. Do you feel tired or sleepy? Then you've eaten too much protein or too many carbs. Do you still feel hungry after the meal? Then you didn't eat enough fat or protein. In subsequent meals, you need to adjust the makeup of your team.

It takes time and patience to figure out what sort of team—or what ratio of protein to fat to carbohydrate—works best for you. You won't find it in an app or a macro calculator. It's best to listen to your body and pay attention to how it responds to each meal.

When you put together your daily keto plates, look at each ingredient and think of it in terms of what it brings to the team. Does the meal have the right balance of protein, fat, and carbohydrate? Remember, too, that many foods contribute a combination of macronutrients. Avocado has both fat and carbs, for example, so it's best to use only a little. You can't discount the carbs in a food just because it has fat. Combinations of macronutrients can work in your favor, too. A protein that also has fat, like bacon, is a great team member. Lean protein like chicken breast, on the other hand, needs fat added to it to make it a good team player. Get to know your potential team players (foods you like) so that you can put together good teams quickly.

JUST FOR TODAY   I will build a strong team of macronutrients for each of my meals.

Week 1 Review

Welcome to the end of Week 1! You did a great job of learning how to change the way you eat.

Take a look at the Mile Marker Summary that you filled out throughout the week. You might find that you have more energy or less hunger. If you test blood glucose, you might be surprised to find that your numbers are lower. If you're feeling sluggish or having headaches, be sure to add salt to your food, drink broth, and stay hydrated with noncaffeinated beverages. Also take time to record favorite foods, recipes, meals, or strategies that really helped you this week. Make note of what worked well. Likewise, note your struggles or dislikes. What would you avoid in the future? You might also want to jot down any links to websites or useful tips that you discovered. I've included a notes page on my website that you can download and print out for this purpose.

How to Handle a Rough Start

If you weren't 100 percent successful during Week 1, take the time to consider why this first week was difficult for you. For example, if you were hungry, if you weren't prepared with keto foods, or if you struggled with cravings, please use the resources in Part I to troubleshoot. Make sure you have high-fat and low-carb foods that you enjoy. Then begin Week 1 again, better prepared for success. You might also want to think about the reasons why your success is important to you by revisiting the "Know Your Why" section on pages 94 and 95, or to arm yourself with bone broth and adequate sodium to avoid the keto flu. Remember to fight cravings with fat! Read my top ten tips on pages 108 to 110 a second time if you need a refresher on the basics. Keto should be delicious and easy, and your hunger should lessen each day.

Week 2

Welcome to Week 2! Your first week was successful, and you likely are feeling good about having stayed on plan. In my second week, I was fascinated by two things. First, I was never hungry, which was a remarkable feeling. Second, I was eating delicious foods. Unlike other diets that I had followed in the past, the food was enjoyable. Butter on vegetables seemed subversive. No more cardboard low-fat boxed food, and I had more energy than I'd known in quite some time.

During this second week, you might still be struggling to figure out what to eat and how to plan your meals. Although you may spend more time shopping and cooking than you used to, you will find that you eat less food, and you may find yourself eating less frequently. Use Week 2 as a time to explore new ingredients and dishes. One of the primary reasons I was successful in transitioning to a ketogenic lifestyle is that I committed to making at least two new recipes each week. The recipes you try do not have to be elaborate. Instead, focus on recipes that use ingredients you like and are relatively easy to prepare. Becoming familiar with new recipes enables you to replace those old high-carb staples with equally convenient but more delicious and healthy ketogenic meals that you can rely on.

Your primary goal for this week is to develop new habits related to eating—both cooking at home and dining out.

Here are your points of focus for Week 2:

1. Find foods that are easy to prepare and that fit your lifestyle. When planning meals for this week, commit to trying one new recipe, even if it's just a low-carb salad dressing.

2. Continue to explore hunger by paying particular attention to it. Being able to identify and manage true physical hunger will keep you moving forward. A complete discussion of hunger is found on pages 36 to 37.

3. Manage cravings by balancing macronutrients. Fight cravings with more fat, more salt, and good hydration.

4. Learn more about eating keto in restaurants. Using online menus and nutrition information, identify meals that you can eat at local restaurants. See pages 79 to 89 for guidance.

5. Look for less-obvious markers of success. What about this lifestyle is working for you? Refer to your responses on the Week 1 Mile Marker Summary.

The key to success in Week 2 is to focus on food. Continuing to find new low-carb, high-fat options and incorporate them into your meals increases your chances for success. Even when you are eating food that you haven't prepared yourself, you can still enjoy meals that keep you 100 percent on plan as your body adjusts to burning fat instead of glucose for fuel.

Week 2 Checklist

☐ Complete your shopping list and meal prep for Week 2 and decide on your weekly food plan. Review the sample meal plans on pages 60 to 66 for inspiration.

☐ Make or buy bone broth (pages 186 and 187) in case you experience the keto flu.

☐ Identify and commit to making at least one new recipe or meal this week.

☐ Use online menus and nutrition information to identify at least three keto-friendly meals that you can order at local restaurants. Record the name of each restaurant and jot down exactly what you would order. Include any necessary modifications to the menu options. You'll find lots of guidance on making keto-friendly selections at restaurants on pages 79 to 89.

☐ If you're struggling to stay on plan, reread the section "My Top Ten Navigation Tips for Your Ketogenic Journey" on pages 108 to 110.

☐ Take photos, try on clothing, jot down measurements (see pages 98 and 99), and so on and use those mile markers to track your progress.

☐ Throughout the week, use the Week 2 Mile Marker Summary to record your progress.

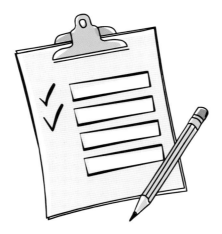

Daily Food Journal

Use a journal like this to record what you ate, what time you ate, how hungry you were when you ate, and how satisfied you felt after eating. Remember to eat only when hungry. For good ketogenic ratios, make sure that each meal has fat grams equal to or higher than protein grams, with carbohydrate grams lower than protein and fat. To print out copies of this chart, go to my website, cookingketowithkristie.com.

First Meal

Time: ....

Hunger level: 1   2   3   4   5   6   7   8   9   10

What I ate: ....

....

Carbs: .... Protein: .... Fat: ....   Satisfaction after meal: 1   2   3   4   5   6   7   8   9   10

Second Meal

Time: ....

Hunger level: 1   2   3   4   5   6   7   8   9   10

What I ate: ....

....

Carbs: .... Protein: .... Fat: ....   Satisfaction after meal: 1   2   3   4   5   6   7   8   9   10

Third Meal

Time: ....

Hunger level: 1   2   3   4   5   6   7   8   9   10

What I ate: ....

....

Carbs: .... Protein: .... Fat: ....   Satisfaction after meal: 1   2   3   4   5   6   7   8   9   10

First Snack

Time: ....

Hunger level: 1   2   3   4   5   6   7   8   9   10

What I ate: ....

....

Carbs: .... Protein: .... Fat: ....   Satisfaction after meal: 1   2   3   4   5   6   7   8   9   10

Second Snack

Time: ....

Hunger level: 1   2   3   4   5   6   7   8   9   10

What I ate: ....

....

Carbs: .... Protein: .... Fat: ....   Satisfaction after meal: 1   2   3   4   5   6   7   8   9   10

Mile Marker Summary, Week 2

Use this summary to record your progress throughout the week. You might also want to record your daily total intake of carbs, protein, and fat so you can begin to understand what works best for you. For a printable version of this worksheet, go to my website, cookingketowithkristie.com.

MONDAY

MACROS FOR ALL MEALS AND SNACKS			MILE MARKERS OF SUCCESS
Daily Total Carbs	Daily Total Protein	Daily Total Fat	

TUESDAY

MACROS FOR ALL MEALS AND SNACKS			MILE MARKERS OF SUCCESS
Daily Total Carbs	Daily Total Protein	Daily Total Fat	

WEDNESDAY

MACROS FOR ALL MEALS AND SNACKS			MILE MARKERS OF SUCCESS
Daily Total Carbs	Daily Total Protein	Daily Total Fat	

THURSDAY

MACROS FOR ALL MEALS AND SNACKS			MILE MARKERS OF SUCCESS
Daily Total Carbs	Daily Total Protein	Daily Total Fat	

FRIDAY

MACROS FOR ALL MEALS AND SNACKS			MILE MARKERS OF SUCCESS
Daily Total Carbs	Daily Total Protein	Daily Total Fat	

SATURDAY

MACROS FOR ALL MEALS AND SNACKS			MILE MARKERS OF SUCCESS
Daily Total Carbs	Daily Total Protein	Daily Total Fat	

SUNDAY

MACROS FOR ALL MEALS AND SNACKS			MILE MARKERS OF SUCCESS
Daily Total Carbs	Daily Total Protein	Daily Total Fat	

Even One Little Hershey's Kiss

The basic science behind a ketogenic diet is that blood glucose remains stable, insulin is lowered, fat can move out of cells, and energy that was previously only stored can be used. The body relies on fat as its primary source of fuel. Fat fuel is called ketones, hence the name *ketogenic diet*.

The process of burning ketones is different from that of burning glucose. While the human body can burn both glucose and ketones for fuel and does make glucose to fuel the brain as needed, it tends to use glucose first because glucose is a quicker source of energy. Just as kerosene thrown on a fire ignites quickly and burns brightly, that fire will die out once the fuel is burned through. Kindling is similar; that's why we use kindling to light larger pieces of wood such as oak that burn more slowly. The heavy oak wood lasts longer in the fire pit than the kindling or kerosene.

Fat is like the oak wood in that it is a more stable and longer-lasting fuel than glucose. In fact, the body has to work somewhat harder to use fat for fuel, so metabolism is higher in a person who is fat-adapted. Fat-adaptation happens over time as the body becomes efficient at using fat as its primary fuel source. When a fat-adapted body is given a surge of glucose, fat burning ceases so that the body can attend to the glucose, which must be used or stored right away. The cascade of hormones necessary to metabolize glucose begins. For a body with metabolic dysfunction, the unhealthy signaling begins anew and disrupts hunger signals along with blood glucose and hormones like ghrelin and leptin.

With the surge of glucose, most people are no longer in ketosis, which means that they are no longer enjoying a state of constant fat-burning, mental clarity, high energy, and controlled hunger. Instead, the metabolic fluctuations can bring cravings back with a vengeance, and you essentially begin again, just as you did when you started a ketogenic diet. This is especially true for people who never reach the point of becoming fat-adapted.

While your body struggles with the surge of glucose, you also struggle with the psychological challenges that come with it. You went off plan. You failed. One more diet and once more you couldn't do it. Failure feels miserable. You're ashamed and angry at yourself, and you fear that nothing will ever work for you. While your body is struggling to regain equilibrium, your mind is weakened. Not only do you lose the mental clarity of ketosis, but now you're defeated, too. Some people become so stressed by it that they binge eat. Some start an unhealthy pattern of restricting food, bingeing, restricting food, and bingeing. Each time they become unhealthier physically and often emotionally as well.

When you go off plan, you regret it because you feel bad physically or you are disappointed in yourself. You're letting yourself be more vulnerable physically and emotionally. In some ways, it's like going shopping for an item you don't really need when you don't have a lot of money. For example, I have a genetic weakness for purses and shoes. I can't help it. When I was younger and living paycheck to paycheck, my fondness for purses was painful at times. I had no credit cards and lived on cash. Once, as I stood in a department store fondling a leather cross-body that I really, really wanted, I had the revelation that if I bought that purse, I would have no money to put in it. Had I bought it, I would have regretted it. I needed my money for other things like paying rent and putting gasoline in my car. Buying the purse would have only made me poorer. Similarly, by eating off plan in a weak moment, we make ourselves weaker. Physically and emotionally we have even less power.

For more than four years, I've watched people try to adapt to a ketogenic lifestyle. Sadly, the people who go off plan within the first month rarely meet their goals. The people who enjoy the most significant progress and post the most extraordinary before-and-after pictures are those who stay on plan for the long haul. They commit, even though they may struggle or may be tempted by high-carb foods. These lucky people fight the carb withdrawals and cravings only once. After they get through those and become fat-adapted, they enjoy all the advantages of ketosis without any of the physical challenges that come with going off plan, and they enjoy psychological success as their confidence increases with pounds shed, inches lost, and health regained.

Those who go off plan constantly struggle. They never feel the benefits of being fat-adapted. They get in the car to begin the journey and then detour, become frustrated, and end up right back where they started. They begin again, hit a small bump in the road, and go back to where they started once more. For many of them, the cravings never stop because they never achieve ketosis. They struggle physically and emotionally because even though they start, they never make much progress. When they see the progress that others are making, they see postcards of where they could be themselves, but they never truly begin the trip.

Imagine this scenario: You leave the house for a trip but forget your wallet, so you go back home to get it. You start out again, but then you can't remember whether you turned off the stove, so you go back to check. At that point, it's late in the day, so you decide to sleep at home and begin again the following day. The next day, you load up the luggage again and hit the road, but two days into the trip, you realize that you left a medication behind. You could call a

pharmacy and see about getting a temporary refill, but you decide to just go home. When you arrive, you decide to do the laundry you have accumulated over those few days. The next day, you put off starting the journey again because you want to visit with friends. You eventually start out again, only to decide that the traffic is too heavy and you should delay the trip yet again.

How many times would you start and stop a journey like that? Most people would eventually give up and just stay home for good. That's what happens with keto sometimes. People see the postcards and get excited about the destination, but they can't stick to the lifestyle changes that help them succeed long term. They start, sputter, stop, start, sputter, stop, and then stop starting. Sadly, some claim, "Keto didn't work for me."

Truthfully, keto does not work if you do not do the work. The most significant work you must do is to choose to stay on plan 100 percent.

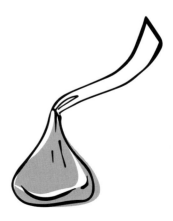

Day 8: Wading into Calmer Waters

Have you ever been to the ocean? If you have, you might have decided to enjoy the water. When you first walk into the water, it is running up to shore and falling in waves over your feet and ankles. As you continue, the water begins to rush up to your knees and thighs. Eventually you reach the area where the waves are breaking. That area can be rough. You might lose your footing. You might get knocked over or pushed back to shore. More than once I've ended up covered in sand after getting stuck in the area where the waves break. It's exhausting to stay in that place where you are both fighting the waves rolling in and standing against the waves pulling you back out. Remaining in that space takes so much energy because you aren't quite safely on shore, but you aren't really out in waters deep enough to swim in.

Once you push beyond the breaking waves, the water is typically calm. If you can get 15 to 20 feet from shore, the waves begin to break behind you. The water is peaceful there, and you can enjoy riding the gentle waves. You can be more relaxed because you don't have to worry about getting knocked down and coming up with a face (or bathing suit) full of sand. In those deeper waters, the ocean gently rocks you—that is, if you can stop worrying about jellyfish and sharks!

If you've been to the ocean, you know that this area where the breaking and receding waves push and pull is to be avoided. Yet many people get "stuck" there. If they aren't strong swimmers or are inexperienced or just short,

like me, they might fear going beyond the breaking waves. Often, they don't really enjoy the ocean because they never make it past the breaking waves.

Too often folks wade into a very-low-carb or ketogenic diet like they wade into the ocean. As they get their feet wet and begin enjoying low-carb foods, they get into the "breaking waves" of cravings or panic over what to eat. Some hurry back to shore, caving to cravings or to social pressure. They give in to high-carb foods at a party or refuse to ditch a high-carb habit. When they try to wade in again, the cravings—those "waves" pushing them off plan—are worse. Some get stuck in that wave-breaking place that is pretty miserable. It's exhausting because they're working to stay upright, but not working to push through. In those moments, they get pushed down and sandy. They never see the progress they want because they're constantly being pushed back to shore. They're tired and often hungry, and many simply give up.

Folks who stay on plan can ride the waves because they take the time to create new habits, embrace new foods, and focus on what they *can* eat. They relax in a state of ketosis that is freeing. It provides a buoyant lack of hunger that enables them to lean in and float! They are further buoyed by better health and weight loss. They swim without exhaustion and without a bathing suit full of sand.

JUST FOR TODAY I will push myself to wade past the cravings and the challenges of eating differently so that I can float and swim in the deeper waters of ketosis. I will learn to swim *with* the tide as I learn to follow a low-carb diet.

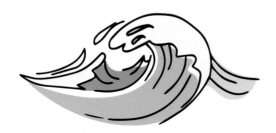

Day 9: No Longer Losing Control

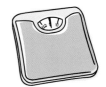

When I opened the freezer, I saw a single low-carb pumpkin spice muffin topped with a sprinkle of cinnamon and brown sugar erythritol. Warmed and smeared with a dollop of mascarpone, those muffins were fantastic, but it wasn't the prospect of eating the leftover muffin that made me smile when I saw it sitting there. I smiled because it was *uneaten*.

That single muffin was one of a dozen that I had baked two weeks earlier. Half of the batch was consumed by others. One muffin left meant that I had eaten five. In fourteen days, I had eaten only five muffins! There was a time when *not one* of those twelve muffins would have been given away. In fact, I likely would have gobbled up nine of them within the first three days, eating them two at a time or between meals or as a bedtime snack. In the past, I made double or triple batches of muffins, cakes, pies, and so on so that I would have "enough." "Enough" meant that I could consume a dozen or more without anyone noticing.

There was a time when I was nearly always hungry. I woke up hungry and had breakfast at around 7 a.m. By 10 a.m. I needed a snack. When noon rolled around, I would eat lunch. Mid-afternoon earned me another snack, and I ate yet another while cooking dinner because I was "starving" by 6 p.m. Feeding time didn't end with dinner, either; I had a bedtime snack, too. The constant feeding was made worse by stress, boredom, joy, disappointment—nearly any emotion was an excuse to eat.

Often, I truly was hungry. My body sent signals telling me to eat. At the time, I did not understand that I was insulin resistant. I had not yet read about the complex interplay of insulin, leptin, ghrelin, or any of the other dozen hormones that regulate hunger, satiety, appetite, mood, and survival. Years of eating the wrong foods for my body had turned those signals into a dysrhythmic Morse Code, pushing my body faster and faster toward foods that would eventually destroy it, not nourish it.

When I consider the "wrong" foods versus the "right" ones, looking back in time gives me the simplest answer. My great-grandparents would have had access to local meats, fish, and vegetables. Their daily lives included working to obtain those real, whole foods. Imagine teleporting those ancestors who lived before the Industrial Revolution into a typical modern-day kitchen. How would we begin to explain Pop-Tarts and Froot Loops and plastic tubs of pasta that are heated in a metal box that dings when dinner is ready? The ways in which we obtain and prepare food have certainly changed, but most importantly, what we call food is vastly different. For most people, food comes from a box or the freezer or a drive-through window; however, real food has real ingredients. Did food even have ingredient lists in 1883? Was there even a place to buy pumpkin spice muffins?

The joy I felt when I spied the single pumpkin spice muffin left in my freezer had nothing to do with warming it, slathering it with butter or mascarpone, and washing it down with fresh French-pressed coffee. That muffin reminded me of the freedom I now have from food. Instead of three meals plus three or four snacks a day, I typically eat two or three meals and no snacks because I am no longer hungry. *No. Longer. Hungry.* By replacing processed and refined foods with real, whole foods, I have helped my body heal, normalized my weight, reduced inflammation, and discovered how true hunger feels. I've broken the ridiculous cycle of diet, binge, hate myself; diet, binge, hate myself; diet binge, hate myself. Eating real food is a solution that works.

JUST FOR TODAY I will choose real, whole foods to nourish my body and enjoy freedom from hunger.

Day 10: Food as Medicine

My husband was sitting on the edge of the bed, letting his back "adjust." He took a deep breath and wondered aloud, "So is this just how aging feels? Will we never again wake without aches and pains?" While I didn't like his conclusion, I couldn't remember days when I awoke and did not feel pain. Heading into our mid-forties, David and I were both obese.

Pain medication had become part of our lifestyle. Before doing yard work, David took naproxen. A trip to the mall for me included ibuprofen both beforehand and afterward to ease the pain associated with so much walking. If I awoke with a twinge in my back, I started the day wondering which medication to take. I was grateful that I could take naproxen, acetaminophen, and ibuprofen at the same time if needed. I kept multiple types of pain medication in my desk drawer at work and never traveled without it. Toothbrush, toothpaste, pain medication—it all went into my toiletry case. David and I had accepted that painful joints, sore muscles, back pain, and low energy were simply to be expected as we aged. In addition to over-the-counter medication, our doctors kept us supplied with prescriptions for muscle relaxers and various narcotics to treat the more severe pain that we experienced a couple of times each year.

I kept my bathroom cabinet stocked with an economy-size bottle of ibuprofen tablets. On some days, I took three pills (or 600 milligrams) every four to six hours. Even at a standard 200-milligram dose, I would use up that entire bottle in less than three months. Buying and taking those pills was routine. My warehouse club shopping list included apples, bananas, bread, cereal, low-fat cheese, and ibuprofen.

Then one day I realized that something had changed. It changed so gradually that I'm not sure when it occurred. When I opened the bathroom cabinet, that economy-size bottle looked huge and sad. It reminded me of the days when I stayed in bed or avoided walking my elementary-aged children into their schools. I checked the expiration date and smiled when it read 2013—the year I discovered keto.

When I began keto, I was laser-focused on the scale and smaller clothes. While I enjoyed significant weight loss, I also discovered better health. Mornings began to greet me without pain. Week over week, I used ibuprofen less and less frequently until it was mostly forgotten. Within four months of changing my diet, I stopped taking all prescription medications.

Now, if I wake up feeling a little sore or if my rings feel tight (which is a sign of inflammation), I no longer lie in bed and wonder which medications to take. I immediately think, "What did I eat yesterday?" Sometimes I can pinpoint that I had too much dairy, peanut butter, or a certain sweetener. Nearly every single time I wake up with what I used to attribute to "feeling my age," I can link the issue to something I ate or something I did, like kayaking, which makes me sore in the most wonderful ways! For a day or two, my arm muscles remind me that I had been paddling along in the cool water while enjoying a warm day.

There are times when I think about my life before and after keto. Not all of the dramatic changes can be captured in a photo. The woman who needed daily pain medications just to shop now takes no medication for pain. In my "before" life, I could not fit into a kayak, nor would I have tried. In my "after" life, I am keenly aware of food and how it affects my health. What I eat is the first thing I consider modifying if I am not feeling well. The idea of good nutrition having the power to heal and strengthen my body is normal to me now. And my new warehouse club shopping list? I buy coffee, butter, full-fat cheese, mushrooms, ribs, beef, and bacon—lots of bacon. What a delicious medicine cabinet!

 JUST FOR TODAY I will focus on how good I feel when I eat low-carb and high-fat, and I will use food to heal my body.

Day 11: Fun without Food

We had been a keto family for nearly two years when we went on a brief weekend vacation. When we stopped to purchase bottled water, I got sidetracked by a display just inside the door—donuts! The children's old favorite beckoned me. My husband and I used to take the kids to the donut shop in their pajamas. Those were such fun times! I started to reach for a box, and then I stopped. We didn't eat donuts anymore.

As I continued toward the bottled water, I saw an enormous display of seasonal flavors of cookies and fillings in various combinations. We could have a taste test! It would be so fun to try the different varieties and pick our favorites. I began to consider which flavors David and each of the children might like, and then I stopped myself again. "We don't eat sugar," I thought. "Why would I even be attracted to that display?" Those cookies would make me sick, and they really weren't good for my family, either.

I finally grabbed a flat of water and headed toward the checkout, but as I rounded the corner, I was greeted by a table holding all the ingredients for s'mores. The chocolate bars, marshmallows, and graham crackers called to me with images of a glowing campfire on the side of the mountain and happy kids gathering sticks to toast marshmallows. Not unlike waking from a dream, I shook my head and headed to the register without the s'mores supplies. What was wrong with me? Three times I had been tempted by sugary foods that my family no longer ate! Three times I had imagined how happy my family would be because of those foods.

While I waited in line, I considered why those high-carb and highly processed foods had caught my attention. I had finally reached the point where I thought of cakes and cookies as poison, yet I was struggling to avoid them because of nostalgia. With each temptation, visions of the children's smiling faces had appeared, but I knew intellectually that we didn't need those sugary foods to have a good time. That's when it hit me: I had to work to find ways to replace food as a way of bonding with my family. It had to be intentional.

I glanced around the checkout aisle. There was gum and candy—no! Then I spied some playing cards. I snatched up two decks just as the clerk was asking, "Will that be all?" I smiled and said, "I'd like these too, please."

When I got to the car, David commented, "That took a while. Is that all you got?" As I loaded the water into the back of the car, I answered, "Well, I also got something fun. I got cards!" Each of the children eagerly took a pack. That evening we laughed together as we played Rummy, War, and Crazy Eights. My son spent much of the weekend teaching himself a card trick and delighted in showing it to his grandfather when we visited him later. We all enjoyed watching as my son went through the "magic" and his grandfather wondered how he did it.

We also started a new tradition with our campfire on that trip. We roasted smoked sausages instead of marshmallows, and they tasted a whole lot better than sugary s'mores! We laughed and told scary stories while we watched the stars emerge and marveled at the still-magical universe. The fun wasn't in the food; it never had been. Vacations are fun because we take the time to go away together. Similarly, a bad movie can't be made better by a tub of popcorn that gives you a tubby tummy, and a football game without beer is still a great way to spend a Sunday afternoon as long as you've got a good team and good friends to help you cheer them on.

JUST FOR TODAY I will look for ways to have fun without food instead of using food to generate happiness for myself and others.

Day 12: Your Problems Are Good Ones

"Your problems are good ones," I said firmly to my son, who was complaining about having to wear hearing aids. "You aren't putting on prosthetic limbs or heading to chemotherapy. You have parents who can afford those hearing aids. You are lucky." He didn't respond or even look at me, but his attitude improved greatly as I drove him to robotics practice.

My son has a genetic hearing loss. While it interferes with his day-to-day life, his hearing aids compensate for much of the loss. His loss is unique in that he hears normally at the top and bottom of the range of sound but does not hear well at 2,000 megahertz, the range at which most conversations take place. Without hearing aids, he often misses bits of conversation, which includes friends talking to him or teachers giving him instruction. In addition to hearing aids, he relies a lot on visual cues and the written word. He struggles in some settings, especially noisy ones, which he tends to avoid.

As a mom, it pains me to see him struggle, but I am grateful for the technology that helps him hear. I am grateful when teachers are understanding and position themselves so that he can read their lips. I am grateful that his loss is not worse and that it has not hindered his speech development. I am grateful that he is still able to work above grade level when many hearing-impaired children fall behind academically. I choose to be grateful.

I could just as easily focus on how hard it is for him. I could ruminate on how hearing loss is an invisible disability that is hard for others to understand. I could lament that the hearing disorder also impacts how his brain processes information and that he needs more time to respond to questions. I could regret that he cannot enjoy parties or large events because the noises and visual stimulation overwhelm him. While knowing those things is helpful as my husband and I assist him in learning to work around his limitations, wallowing in self-pity about what is missing is simply not useful. I choose to be grateful because gratitude helps me focus on what my son *can* do. Grateful people harness the power of what is possible and the power of moving forward.

When people first make the lifestyle changes necessary to begin a ketogenic diet, they sometimes complain about what they can't have: "I miss bread! I miss pasta! I miss pizza!" Instead, try focusing on what you *can* have. You can have bacon! You can have a double bacon cheeseburger with lettuce, tomato, and mayonnaise! You can eat the meat, cheese, and veggies of a Philly cheesesteak! You can have chicken wings! You can have a rib-eye steak! You can have real heavy cream! You can have homemade ranch dressing that tastes so good it will make you cry!

When you focus on what you *can* eat, you approach keto as a diet of opportunity. You can be grateful that high-fat foods taste so good! You can be grateful that you see physical changes and feel healthier! You can be grateful that your lab test results are likely to improve.

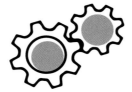

JUST FOR TODAY I will focus on everything that goes right. I will celebrate not feeling hungry, savor the taste of the high-fat foods I've chosen, and be grateful to be working toward better health.

Day 13: The Big Gulp

"You ruined it for me!" The whiny voice on the phone belonged to my husband, who had called me on his way home from work. I wasn't about to apologize until I knew what I'd done, so I asked, a little unsympathetically, "Ruined what?" "My Pepsi," he said. "I waited all week to have one—just one."

Even before going keto, I worried about David's Pepsi habit. To help him limit portions, I started buying it in cans after I saw him guzzle an entire two-liter bottle in one day. I really didn't want our children drinking soft drinks, so after they were born, David often drank Pepsi only at work. We had a small fridge in the garage, and more than once, I'd catch him "cleaning" the garage or working in the yard and sneaking a can or two while the kids weren't looking.

As my husband and I negotiated *his* following a very-low-carb diet, his Pepsi habit was the hardest to break. He willingly gave up bread, but forgoing Pepsi was especially difficult for him. Our compromise was that one day a week, he would treat himself to one can of Pepsi. It wasn't what I preferred, but marriage is based on compromise. And here he was, just a few months into our new diet, declaring that I had ruined Pepsi for him.

"What do you mean?" I asked. He explained, "Well, I'd been thinking about that Pepsi and saving it for when I could savor it. When I went to get it, I was almost skipping down the hall! I took it back to my office, popped the top, took a big swig, and thought, 'Yuck!' Honey, it didn't taste good. It was too sweet! I couldn't even finish it. You ruined it. I'm so mad at you!"

I never apologized. Nope, I gloated. I celebrated! We spent the next few minutes laughing about how wonderful this development was. I remembered seeing a sale on soft drinks that very weekend. I hesitantly asked, "So . . . should I not buy those anymore?" David took a deep breath. "No, don't buy them," he answered. "I don't think I want them anymore." I breathed a huge sigh of relief. This new diet was working,

and my husband had realized it without me badgering him.

I had already stopped drinking diet soft drinks by that point. Water was the only thing that satisfied the thirst that came with my weight loss. I also learned that when I did have an occasional diet drink, I often felt hungrier afterward. Only by eliminating it for several days and then reintroducing it was I able to notice the difference. Less hunger and increased weight loss made it easy to kick the habit. After a long stall, I actually lost more weight by eliminating diet soft drinks.

When people ask me what I drink, I respond, "Water, coffee about once a day, and an occasional glass of wine or low-carb cocktail." (Mojitos, lemon drop martinis, and margaritas are my favorites!) Nearly every time, I hear in return, "I could never give up diet soft drinks!" I smile because I used to say that, too. Then I think about the addiction that David once had and say, "Try cutting down to one serving per day. Have that one serving when you think you 'need' it most. Pay attention to how you feel after you drink it. Are you hungrier later? More agitated? Thirstier? Eventually, you may want to try going three to five days without soft drinks. Then, when you have one, pay close attention to how you feel after drinking it. If you don't notice a difference, then it may not be a problem for you."

More than one person has come back to me to say, "I hated it when you told me that diet soft drinks might be holding me back, but you were right. As soon as I stopped drinking them, the number on the scale went down. Thank you, but I'm still really mad at you for being right!" I just smile.

JUST FOR TODAY I will focus on the foods, drinks, and habits that make me feel better physically and help me feel good about myself.

Day 14: Traveling Differently

"Are you a foodie?" asked the woman sitting next to me. I had woken at 5 a.m. while on vacation to catch a cab at 6 a.m. and stand in line for over an hour and a half at Donut Vault, a specialty bakery in Chicago. I had learned about the shop from a magazine, and I already knew which flavors I wanted to try. David and I ordered two dozen donuts in nearly a dozen gourmet flavors. We sat at a picnic table outside the tiny shop with a bottle of milk and sampled each flavor. With each taste, we compared notes not just with each other, but with the people around us as well. That's when the woman sitting next to me noticed my joy at the conquest and asked, "Are you a foodie?"

I paused. Our entire trip to Chicago had been planned around foods to sample and restaurants to visit. Was I a foodie? One definition of that term is a person who sees food as a hobby instead of eating simply to satisfy hunger. Yep, that sounded about right.

This is what I remember about that trip. Donut Vault is so tiny, only three or four customers can stand inside at a time while the line to order winds around the block. We got there more than an hour before it opened so that we could be among the first in line. We also ate deep-dish pizza at Pizzeria Uno and Giordano's, making sure to arrive early enough to score a table. Another day we took a thirty-minute taxi ride to try a restaurant's signature upside-down pizza in a bowl dish. We had to time that excursion just right to make our flight home. We also discovered one of our favorite restaurants ever—the Purple Pig. It was there that we had pork neck tomato gravy, which later inspired me to make my own low-carb version at home. The Purple Pig was just a few doors down from our hotel, which was important because it meant that I wouldn't have to walk very far. It was July 2012, one year before I began eating low-carb and high-fat. I weighed over 250 pounds. We spent five days scouring the city for foods that I had read about well in advance.

Using magazines and online guides, we had planned the trip around eating. We literally *ate* Chicago!

My family started eating low-carb, high-fat one year later in the summer of 2013, and we travel much differently now. In 2014, we went to Hawaii. We hiked a volcano! We went kayaking in the ocean! We snorkeled, and my husband and daughter went scuba diving! We took a helicopter ride, played in swimming pools, and scouted out the best beaches, where I was not ashamed to wear a bathing suit. We stumbled upon a great seafood restaurant and enjoyed fresh omelets one morning, but the rest of what we ate over those ten days is a blur to me. We did not *eat* Hawaii; we *lived* Hawaii!

Two years later, we traveled to northern California. We hiked Upper Yosemite falls—and I hadn't even eaten! I remember the cheeseburger I devoured afterward, but only because it was so dang expensive. We had a fantastic low-carb meal with friends in San Francisco, and I remember their smiling faces more than the food we ate. We walked Chinatown and tried hot pot there, a fun experience that allowed us to stay on plan. We took a ferry to Angel Island. We visited beaches and rushed to catch sunsets instead of restaurant reservations. In twelve days, we walked everywhere we could, including across the Golden Gate Bridge.

I imagine my next trip to Chicago. While I might enjoy another meal at the Purple Pig, food will not dictate my itinerary. Maybe I will go to the Field Museum or take part in an outdoor yoga class at Millennium Park. I could shop in one of the petite stores on the Magnificent Mile since I no longer have to worry about whether stores carry plus sizes. Whatever I end up doing, I can assure you that I will not wait in line at Donut Vault. I am free!

JUST FOR TODAY I will eat to satisfy hunger, and I will not use food for entertainment or to fight off boredom.

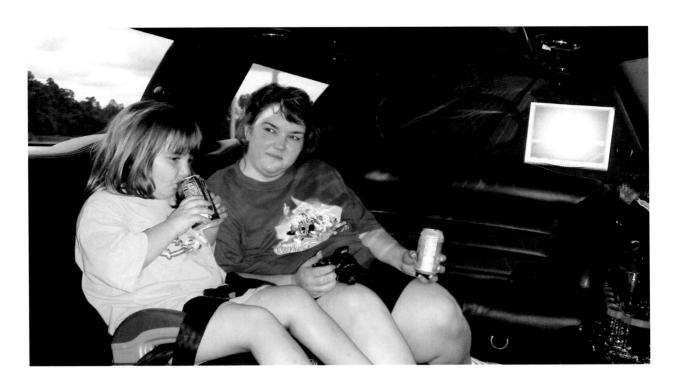

Week 2 Review

Completing Week 2 should leave you feeling accomplished even if you're still learning a lot about the ketogenic lifestyle. Taking what you know and putting it into practice every day is not always easy. It requires you to think and act differently. Fortunately, you are likely to feel increasingly better at this point, and that success make the hard work worth it. High-fat, low-carb eating gets easier at every mile marker. What mile markers did *you* pass this week?

Also take time to record favorite foods, recipes, meals, or strategies that really helped you. Make note of what worked well. Likewise, note your struggles or dislikes. What would you avoid in the future? You might also want to jot down links to websites or useful tips that you discovered. I've included a notes page on my website that you can download and print out for this purpose.

Week 3

You've made it to Week 3. Congratulations! In many ways, the ketogenic way of eating is getting easier for you. You're likely becoming more familiar with the amounts of fat, protein, and carbohydrate in the foods you're eating, and you're probably beginning to pass a few mile markers of progress that make it all seem worthwhile. Your clothes may be looser, and you may notice that your hunger has diminished. You might even be well on your way to reducing or eliminating your use of some medications.

Use the successes of the past two weeks to help you navigate Week 3. You are still creating new habits, and that takes focus. Real-life challenges can be disruptive, but the work you did before you started—learning about macronutrients, planning meals, and looking at ways to modify your pre-keto foods—will help you. When you feel tired or the route gets rough, take a look back at your "Know Your Why!" worksheet (see pages 94 and 95). Remember why you started this journey. This path isn't one you chose only to lose weight; it is about wanting to be healthier, too. You're still learning how to read the road signs, so be patient with yourself. Don't forget that the scenic overlooks are there for a reason. In a few more weeks, everything that seems like hard work now will seem easier and more natural, but only if you stick with it.

Remember that following a ketogenic path is not a journey you ever complete, only a journey that you start. You begin each day with the decision to stay on plan. Your primary goal for this week is to keep moving forward, even if the journey that was once new and exciting is becoming tedious. Even if you're feeling a bit homesick for familiar foods and the easy comfort of old habits, remember why you started and *keep going*.

Here are your points of focus for Week 3:

1. Keep developing new shopping and cooking habits. Every time you try a new recipe, you are expanding your options. Each time you meal plan, you are building in success for yourself.

2. Eat when you are hungry and avoid eating when prompted by triggers, such as eating to the clock or because others around you are eating. Eliminate snacking out of habit.

3. Develop strategies for coping with eating differently when dining with others.

4. Work to expand your options for dining out.

5. Celebrate mile markers of progress. Look for the rewards associated with staying on plan. In addition, think about what you *enjoy* about eating low-carb and high-fat.

The key to success in Week 3 is to create new habits. You want to expand your food options for when life gets busy and you're tempted to resort to old ways of cooking and eating. You also want to develop new methods for coping with challenges such as stress eating and dining with others who do not eat low-carb.

Week 3 Checklist

☐ Reread your "Know Your Why!" worksheet. Remind yourself why you started this journey.

☐ If you're struggling to stay on plan, reread the section "My Top Ten Navigation Tips for Your Ketogenic Journey" on pages 108 to 110.

☐ Review the food lists on pages 43 to 47. Which foods do you enjoy? Which of those foods have high fat and moderate protein? Which vegetables are the lowest in carbs? Be sure to pay attention to portion sizes and carb counts.

☐ Complete your shopping list and meal prep for Week 3 and decide on your weekly food plan. Review the sample meal plans on pages 60 to 66 for inspiration.

☐ Use online menus and nutrition information to identify at least two additional keto-friendly meals that you can order at local restaurants. Record the name of each restaurant and jot down exactly what you would order. Include any necessary modifications to the menu options. You'll find lots of guidance on making keto-friendly selections at restaurants on pages 79 to 89.

☐ Review your Mile Marker Summaries for Weeks 1 and 2. Consider what good things might be in store for Week 3.

☐ Take photos, try on clothing, jot down measurements (see pages 98 and 99), and so on and use those mile markers to track your progress.

☐ Throughout the week, use the Week 3 Mile Marker Summary to record your progress.

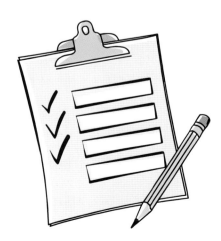

Daily Food Journal

Use a journal like this to record what you ate, what time you ate, how hungry you were when you ate, and how satisfied you felt after eating. Remember to eat only when hungry. For good ketogenic ratios, make sure that each meal has fat grams equal to or higher than protein grams, with carbohydrate grams lower than protein and fat. To print out copies of this chart, go to my website, cookingketowithkristie.com.

First Meal

Time: ....   Hunger level: 1   2   3   4   5   6   7   8   9   10

What I ate: ....

....

Carbs: .... Protein: .... Fat: ....   Satisfaction after meal: 1   2   3   4   5   6   7   8   9   10

Second Meal

Time: ....   Hunger level: 1   2   3   4   5   6   7   8   9   10

What I ate: ....

....

Carbs: .... Protein: .... Fat: ....   Satisfaction after meal: 1   2   3   4   5   6   7   8   9   10

Third Meal

Time: ....   Hunger level: 1   2   3   4   5   6   7   8   9   10

What I ate: ....

....

Carbs: .... Protein: .... Fat: ....   Satisfaction after meal: 1   2   3   4   5   6   7   8   9   10

First Snack

Time: ....   Hunger level: 1   2   3   4   5   6   7   8   9   10

What I ate: ....

....

Carbs: .... Protein: .... Fat: ....   Satisfaction after meal: 1   2   3   4   5   6   7   8   9   10

Second Snack

Time: ....   Hunger level: 1   2   3   4   5   6   7   8   9   10

What I ate: ....

....

Carbs: .... Protein: .... Fat: ....   Satisfaction after meal: 1   2   3   4   5   6   7   8   9   10

Mile Marker Summary, Week 3

Use this summary to record your progress throughout the week. You might also want to record your daily total intake of carbs, protein, and fat so you can begin to understand what works best for you. For a printable version of this worksheet, go to my website, cookingketowithkristie.com.

MONDAY

MACROS FOR ALL MEALS AND SNACKS			MILE MARKERS OF SUCCESS
Daily Total Carbs	Daily Total Protein	Daily Total Fat	

TUESDAY

MACROS FOR ALL MEALS AND SNACKS			MILE MARKERS OF SUCCESS
Daily Total Carbs	Daily Total Protein	Daily Total Fat	

WEDNESDAY

MACROS FOR ALL MEALS AND SNACKS			MILE MARKERS OF SUCCESS
Daily Total Carbs	Daily Total Protein	Daily Total Fat	

THURSDAY

MACROS FOR ALL MEALS AND SNACKS			MILE MARKERS OF SUCCESS
Daily Total Carbs	Daily Total Protein	Daily Total Fat	

FRIDAY

MACROS FOR ALL MEALS AND SNACKS			MILE MARKERS OF SUCCESS
Daily Total Carbs	Daily Total Protein	Daily Total Fat	

SATURDAY

MACROS FOR ALL MEALS AND SNACKS			MILE MARKERS OF SUCCESS
Daily Total Carbs	Daily Total Protein	Daily Total Fat	

SUNDAY

MACROS FOR ALL MEALS AND SNACKS			MILE MARKERS OF SUCCESS
Daily Total Carbs	Daily Total Protein	Daily Total Fat	

Day 15: No Yielding

Each day is guided by the things you will do, the things you will not do, and the things you hope to accomplish. Here's a typical day for me:

Today I will: brush my teeth, get dressed, attend two morning meetings, finish a report, run errands at lunch, meet with a colleague to troubleshoot a project, make dinner, help the kids with homework, and text my mom.

Today I will not: rob a bank, lick a sidewalk, plant flowers, go dress shopping, check the post office box, or bury money in the backyard.

Today I hope that: my family stays safe, I can devise good solutions at work, my kids don't have a lot of homework (and I can help them with it), my family likes the dinner I prepare, and it doesn't storm.

Consider these three categories:

1. **What I will do** includes those tasks that I have chosen to prioritize.

2. **What I will not do** is a list of personal boundaries or decisions that I control.

3. **What I hope happens** contains some wishes or prayers that I can't control directly.

Each of us has similar categories. What we *can* control falls under Category 1 or 2. For example, I can change my mind and decide to lick a sidewalk, but I'm in control of that decision. I can cancel a work meeting, but I decide whether to do so.

There's no need to hope, wish, pray, or ask friends and family for luck in regard to those things we can control (except for those times when I pray I will get it all done!). What if I said, "Wish me luck that I can put my clothes on so I don't leave the house naked!" Barring the existence of any medical conditions, sheer will helps a person accomplish this sort of task. Yet people who are beginning a ketogenic diet frequently say, "Wish me luck!" or "I hope I can do this!"

You do not need hopes and wishes to stay on plan. Staying on plan has to be non-negotiable. Eating keto is something that you *will* do today, tomorrow, the next day, and the day after that. If you're only wishing and hoping that you can do it, then you need to stop right there. Eating keto has to be in Category 1. It has to be something you *will* do. Wishing will not make it happen.

Going off plan goes in Category 2. It is not something you will do, even in an emergency. Yes, I've been called to the hospital for a loved one at 3 a.m. Yes, I've been in meetings or at social gatherings where there was no keto-friendly food. In those situations, I simply didn't eat; I chose to wait until I had better food options. The longer you stay on plan, the easier it becomes to navigate challenging circumstances. The keys to success are a little creative problem solving and a lot of determination. (See pages 76 to 78 for tips for staying on plan in challenging situations.)

In spite of my list, my days do not always go as planned. There are times when I've missed a meal, but because of keto, I just powered through and burned the fat from my butt (at least I hope it came from there!).

Look at your categories. What *will* you do? What will you *not* do? Take wishing and hoping off the table.

 JUST FOR TODAY I will stay on plan. Eating off plan is not an option.

Day 16: Intersections

Recently, I was thinking about a time when my husband came home from a work trip. Although he hadn't been away long, he brought me a bouquet of flowers and greeted me with a big wrap-your-arms-around-me-tight kind of hug. As my head rested on his chest, I realized that his arms were truly wrapped around me. We were facing each other, and his left arm went around my right side, across my back, and rested on my left side, with his fingers pointing toward him! His right arm wrapped around me in the opposite direction—all the way around! Both of his arms were wrapped completely around me. My arms were on his shoulders and my hands were around his neck. I felt completely wrapped up in his embrace.

I took a breath and realized that before I had lost 120 pounds, he could not have held me like that. When I was obese, his hands would have rested on my sides and not wrapped around my back at all. In fact, his hands would have rested just above my waist on that area where back fat hangs, because that's what he would have been able to reach.

I remember cringing every time he touched me there. He felt me cringe, but I don't know that he knew I was cringing because of *me*. Was I repulsive to him? I worried about that when other people hugged me, too. When someone touched my arm, did it feel jiggly? More than once after being hugged, I would reach to touch the same part of me that the other person had touched—back, arm, waist—and wonder what he or she had felt. Was it as bad as I feared?

Quantum physics insists that we can never really touch anyone else, nor they us; it has to do with the structures of atoms, electrons, neutrons, and electromagnetic fields. Regardless of what those physicists say, we *perceive* touch. A hug or touch is one of the few ways in which we can connect with others emotionally and show that we care for them. A hug should convey warmth and support. Hugs are meant to reassure others and to share joy, not to bring our self-worth into question.

For all those years, I was cringing and worrying about whether others were disgusted by touching me. I could not enjoy their embraces because I found myself unembraceable. I did not want to be touched and rejected. I was so focused on what they felt of me that I could not accept the warmth and love that they wanted to convey. I was untouchable in ways that had nothing to do with the laws of physics.

After losing so much weight, I no longer cringe when my husband—or anyone else—hugs me. I don't stop to worry whether the hugger is put off by my fat rolls. While I'm not buff or muscular, and I have more body fat than I'd like, I can touch and be touched. In fact, I can be *embraced,* and it feels amazing!

 JUST FOR TODAY I will choose foods that make me feel better about who I am so that I can feel better about connecting with others.

Day 17: Using Your Gauges

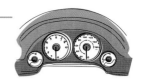

As I drove into my neighborhood, I took my foot off the gas pedal and coasted down the gentle slope. If I coasted just 1,000 feet, I could turn right onto my street without ever hitting the gas. If I was lucky, no one else would be coming, and with a little careful steering, I could continue to coast onto our driveway and into the garage. As I navigated, I watched the display that reports how many miles per gallon the car is getting. When you coast, you aren't using any gas, and the gauge reports that you are getting 50-plus MPG. Accelerate and your performance drops to less than 12 MPG! Watching that gauge has become like a game to me. I've learned to coast on hills to increase my average MPG. Over time, I've learned that many variables impact fuel economy. For example, it is generally better on longer trips at steady speeds than on short jaunts around town or while idling in traffic. Acceleration, deceleration, and the amount of weight in the car all impact fuel economy, too.

The way my car uses gas is similar to the way my body uses fuel. On some days I use more calories and on other days I use fewer. Age, gender, hormones, stress, activity level, and other factors can impact our metabolic rate, which is, in essence, our fuel economy. Moreover, as we now know from research, not all calories are created equal. The body treats a calorie of fat and a calorie of carbohydrate differently. Carbs are burned more quickly than fat or protein, and a different balance of hormones is required to process (metabolize) them. It's the process and the hormones your body uses to metabolize food that matter most. Some of us have dysregulated or dysfunctional responses to carbohydrate. In some ways, carbohydrate is like a food allergy for me; my body simply cannot process it efficiently.

So, if you want to lose weight, how do you account for those variables? Unlike a car, your body doesn't have a fancy-pants gauge to calculate your metabolism, or CPM (calories per minute). Or does it? Maybe you've always had a gauge, and over time the "noise" from metabolic dysregulation, insulin resistance, and obesity built up and kept you from reading it properly. That gauge is hunger. Before keto, my body was so challenged that I couldn't rely on my hunger gauge. It was always stuck on empty, even though my tank (fat cells) was full. Eating keto enables me to trust my hunger gauge, even though it took me years to learn to trust it. At first, my horrible eating habits, including eating from boredom, stress eating, and eating by the clock, kept me from identifying true hunger. In many ways, food was one of my few pleasures.

While I used food as a psychological crutch, there was also a physiological basis for my hunger. Keto experts Gary Taubes, Peter Attia, Stephen Phinney, and Jeff Volek all describe obesity as a condition in which the body can't access stored fat for fuel, so hunger is ever-present. When we eat keto consistently, blood sugar levels should remain stable, and insulin levels are likely to normalize over time. Then our bodies can access that stored fuel, and the hunger gauge becomes more reliable. When I was new to keto, I remember the incredible feeling of being not hungry. For the first time in my life, I forgot to eat! I was being fed from stored fuel—my body's fat reserves. I wondered, "Is this how 'normal' people feel?"

Certain foods and ingredients can make that hunger gauge less effective. Carbohydrates distort my gauge; diet soft drinks interfere with my CPM; and coffee (which I adore) impacts my calibration. Stress affects my gauge, too. An important part of this journey is being able to read your gauge, which begins with giving your body the best fuel you can. It also means avoiding foods and ingredients that interfere with your gauge, even when you crave them.

JUST FOR TODAY I will concentrate on my hunger gauge and choose the foods that help my gauge function best.

Day 18: Mama Said Start Counting

Yep, Mama said there'd be days like this. She didn't say there would be *weeks* like this, but she did say there would be days! There are times when we feel as if we can't get anything right. The kids don't like the meal we cooked, or we forgot to make or cancel an appointment. We hurry and scurry, but we always seem to be late. We get tired even when eating keto because we are human. When we think, "I can't," some of us think first of comfort food—salty, sweet, crunchy, soft, gooey. When the stress piles on, it often brings up old coping mechanisms, which can include unhealthy habits like eating too much, eating the wrong types of foods, or both.

Even during times of high stress, we have choices. One option is to dive headfirst into a high-carb food. Afterward, you feel sick, heavy, and tired. Your body literally feels bad because you've raised your blood glucose and triggered a cascade of hormones related to metabolic dysfunction. When there is sugar in your fuel tank, your body simply cannot run as efficiently. Eating high-carb slows you down. Moreover, the cravings come back, often stronger than ever, at a time when you are especially vulnerable.

High-carb foods weaken us physically and emotionally. We feel even more defeated because we have failed yet again. There is no true comfort in many of the foods that we call comfort foods. After an indulgence, not only will the stressors you're trying to avoid still be there, but you will suffer even more emotional stress from letting yourself down, along with physical stress caused by high-carb foods. True comfort comes from *avoiding* high-carb foods.

Your second option is to stay on plan. Even when stress has you by the throat—when you don't know how you will get it all done, your feelings have been hurt significantly, you don't know where the money will come from, or you've received crushing news—even then you can choose to give your body low-carb foods. When you choose the bacon over the cookie, the stressor remains, but the food choice is far healthier. The result is pride in your decision to do what is best in the long term and not choose what you think you want in the moment. Your confidence is renewed because you didn't fail this time, even in the face of considerable pressure. Your body gets what it needs, and you enjoy continued health that leaves you better equipped to handle whatever stressors come your way.

How do you consistently make the best choice? It's easy to say that you won't binge-eat or go off plan on a calm day without temptations, but making the right decision in the heat of the moment can be harder. The solution is to decide *in advance* how you will cope. For me, the best relief for stress is a brief walk. Taking a walk always calms me down. I often start at a rapid pace, as if I am walking quickly away from my worries. As I walk, the obligations hanging from my arms, wrapped over my shoulders, and attached to my legs feel like leaden weights. I imagine those worries falling away, and I leave them by the side of the path. Many of those worries fall away because they really weren't that important. By the time I finish my walk, I'm left carrying only what really matters, and the load is far lighter. I can then face whatever has to be done, and I feel empowered because my head is clear, my blood glucose is stable, and I am in control. While I cannot control much of the craziness around me, I *can* control what I eat, which impacts my health. In times of stress, I need to control my food choices the most so that I can face those challenges at my very best.

Another strategy for coping with stress is to reach out to a friend who will just let you rant. A physical release of energy from punching a pillow or screaming into the air might help, too. A long, hot bath or shower helps me escape stress because it's one of the few times I can be alone without anyone talking, texting, or emailing. It gives me time to gather my thoughts and renew my resolve.

Lastly, a strategy that never fails me is to count my blessings. Never in my life, not even in the darkest moments, did I not have at least one blessing to count. I have healthy children, a warm bed, a husband who leaves toothpaste drops on the mirror over the sink, and a job that pays my bills. Once you start counting, the blessings start tumbling out, just waiting to be counted. So many blessings that we tuck away and forget about line up and remind us how fortunate we really are. Counting my blessings is one of my favorite ways to de-stress these days. So far I'm up to 1,896,432,783, and I'm just getting started.

 JUST FOR TODAY I will count my blessings and remember that of all my choices, the best choice is to stay on plan, even in times of stress.

Day 19: Say Cheese!

David and I were excited to take family photos. Our daughter was three and a half, and our son was just six months old. He had been a very sick premature infant, and we were still celebrating that he had survived a serious illness. We coordinated our clothing and went to our photo session with our favorite photographer. But when we reviewed the photos, we were mortified. The photographer had captured us exactly as we were. David and I were both obese. We were ashamed, shocked, embarrassed, and disappointed in how we looked. We were so unhappy with ourselves that we purchased only photos of the children, and not a single picture of all four of us together.

As a mom, I second-guessed our decision not to purchase family poses, but I could not even look at those photos. I wondered aloud to David, "Do you think we might ever look back on the current photos of us and think, 'Man, we were younger and thinner then'?" We both chuckled, but the underlying truth was grim. As unhappy as we were with our current weights, what if this wasn't the worst of it? What if we grew older and wider? The thought was so troubling that I remember exactly where I was when I posed this question. I thought about how I often looked back at photos from college and marveled at how young I was and, though I was already overweight, how much thinner I was then.

We spent the next several years hiding from the camera. I declared myself the official family photographer. In that capacity, I could stand on the sidelines and out of focus. During that time, we had one family photo taken for our church directory. The children were three and six at the time. We all dressed in black. Black is slimming, right? Our faces were full and round. We are smiling, but I dreaded that day. We did not have another professional photo taken until 2015, when the kids were twelve and nine years old.

In 2015, however, things were very different. Not only did we spend three hours having our photos taken on a farm that is very special to our family, but we purchased nearly all of the poses the photographer took! We loved them—all of them! David and I posed and smiled and even laughed during the session, and we continued smiling and giggling as we approved the proofs. What a difference keto makes. Between the two of us, we had lost nearly 175 pounds.

The photo session was a gift I had requested from my husband. I recognized those lost years for which there will be no family portrait for our wall. There is no record of me as a younger mother with toddlers. In the few candid photos we do have, I am hiding behind something or someone and cringing at having my picture taken. No longer. I'm still the mom with the camera, but I'm not shy about asking others to take photos with me in them. One day my children will sort through my things, including the family photos. I wonder what they will think of the pictures they find. I wonder whether they will judge their obese mom. I wonder if they will be ashamed of her, and I wonder if they will care as much as I did about how obese I was. I suspect that they will love Obese Mom just as much as they love Healthy Mom. My children have never expressed embarrassment over my weight. That privilege was always left to me.

If I could get back the past fourteen years, I would take more photos this time around. I would look at myself as an obese mom of young children, and I would thank my younger self. Instead of cringing and being embarrassed, I would recognize her bravery. It was she, that obese woman in so much pain, who made the difficult decision to try once more to lose weight. It was she who did the work to learn about the ketogenic diet. It was she who cooked the meals and made the right choices. Every. Single. Day. She is my hero, and I wish I had her portrait, with her young family, to hang on my wall.

JUST FOR TODAY I will be my own hero by doing the work necessary to give my future self the chance to be proud of me.

Day 20: Right Turns

After struggling so much to walk from a parking lot into a store that I had considered asking my doctor for a handicapped parking sticker, I now enjoy a walk through my neighborhood every chance I get. Except for Wednesdays. I don't like to walk on Wednesdays. Wednesday is trash day. It isn't the sight or smell of the garbage that I find particularly offensive; it's the recycling bins. Those bins are filled with pizza boxes, ice cream cartons, and low-fat cereal boxes. My neighbors are mostly kind and wonderful people, but they are carbivores.

Before you accuse me of being judgmental, let me describe my own recycling bin before I began keto. Empty soft drink bottles, whole-grain cereal boxes, low-fat cracker boxes, granola bar boxes, and frozen waffle cartons. Those last four were the "healthy," low-fat foods that I fed my growing children. Our pediatricians had instructed us to give our toddlers whole-grain Cheerios because those little O's helped them develop their fine motor skills. By the time our daughter was three, though, her doctors were berating us because her weight was increasing exponentially. She had gone from a preemie whose weight didn't register on the growth chart to an obese toddler whose weight was off the growth chart, and it was my fault. The pediatricians told us, "No juice!" She didn't drink juice, only water. "Switch to skim milk!" We did. "Give her only low-fat foods!" Each morning I toasted a frozen waffle, smeared it with low-fat peanut butter (with its added high-fructose corn syrup) and high-sugar grape jam, and topped it with a second toasted waffle. She ate that waffle sandwich in the car on the way to daycare. I dutifully filled her sippy cup with skim milk to go with it.

My young daughter was always hungry, and I figured she had the same horrible metabolism that I had. We moms make a lot of mistakes even when we are trying really hard. From the time she was four years old, I packed her lunches: low-fat cheese and lean deli meat on low-fat bread, with fruit. She dipped her broccoli in bottled low-fat ranch dressing. A preschool teacher once criticized her lunch and told her that she should not be eating high-fat cheese. It was the only time I ever requested a meeting with the school headmaster. I began to dread taking her for well visits because the doctors always worried about her weight. They told us, "Put her in sports!" We did. We tried soccer and swimming and even a fitness class for kids. She continued to gain weight more rapidly than her peers. She enjoyed swimming, but we found that she was ravenous afterward. I fed her fruit. "No soft drinks!" said the pediatrician. She was the *only* child at the end-of-year kindergarten party who willingly chose water instead of a soft drink from the beverage cooler. She was also the only child who was overweight.

As I planned meals for my family, I worked to provide "five a day" fruits and veggies, often relying on canned fruits because of our busy schedule. When I could, I went to the farmers' market and bought watermelon and cantaloupe. We nearly always had apples, bananas, and grapes on hand. At the time, I had no idea that the fructose and sugary canned fruits were only perpetuating the problem. When I consider the foods I used to buy, I cringe. Frozen chicken tenders and lean frozen meals were staples. I fed my kids frozen fries and hot dogs with buns and ketchup—lots of ketchup. They ate not-so-happy meals as we scurried about. Pizza, frozen or delivery, was not an uncommon choice.

I added fruit and some raw broccoli or carrot sticks with ranch dressing to get in those "healthy" five-a-day options. I didn't know any better.

After David and I started following a very-low-carb diet, our hunger was tamed, and the weight seemed to melt away effortlessly. I wondered if keto might help our daughter as well. She was nine when I started keto and ten when I began to consider it for her. I remembered all the "diets" and food restrictions that I'd tolerated as a child and struggled with how to help her. I decided that she needed to know what I knew. She needed to be empowered to make her own choices. She was entering a time in which body image becomes important, and she had already endured fat shaming. I could only help her by supporting her. She needed to know that I was on her side.

I decided to help my daughter in three ways. First, I would help her learn what I had learned. Second, I would provide delicious foods so that she never felt deprived. Third, I would give her the grace and latitude to choose for herself. Yet my "mama's heart" worried.

Even though she was a pretty precocious ten-year-old, I knew she needed concrete examples that were easy to understand. Going keto had to be her idea. I had just finished reading Dr. William Davis' book *Wheat Belly*. I showed her my copy and suggested that she might want to read through it. If nothing else, I told her, it includes some interesting recipes. She could pick out something she liked. I left the book in her room and never mentioned it again. Within a week, she told me that she had read it. She also said that she wanted to test her blood glucose. I showed her how. We were both surprised by the high number. Knowing that

her grandmother is diabetic provided her with extra motivation, and she said, "Mom, I want to try this." Sure thing, baby girl, sure thing.

She joined us on our ketogenic journey and was amazed at how much better her hunger was managed. I bought her a meter so that she could continue to monitor her blood glucose. I never asked her to weigh herself. She did so from time to time, but I respected her privacy and never monitored her weight. Navigating food wasn't always easy for her. There were times when I made "suggestions" and times when I said nothing. My job was to come up with recipes that kept her from feeling deprived and to provide good options for when she was with her friends—all of whom seemed to gorge on packaged foods and still wore the smallest clothing sizes available. At her last well visit, her pediatrician said to me, "I'm happy with her weight! She's not built to be a skinny Minnie, but she's in a good range." To my daughter, she said, "You're healthy and you're smart and you're awesome in every way!" Finally, her doctor got the diagnosis right!

As I walk by those recycling bins on Wednesdays, the low-fat cereal boxes haunt me a little. Along with the pizza boxes, they remind me of all the meals I got wrong. The ice cream cartons take me back to the milkshakes I used to make on Fridays to "celebrate" the weekend. I shake my head at that as I circle through the neighborhood and back to my own recycling bin and look at what's in there now: an empty coconut oil bottle kept company by an empty carton of heavy cream. Sometimes I wonder what those carbivore neighbors think of us!

JUST FOR TODAY   I will be an example to those around me who may be helped by following a ketogenic diet.

Day 21: Well Fed

It was a subtle disruption—a slight gnawing in the pit of my belly that disturbed my concentration. I was sitting at my desk at work and checking off the three items I really needed to complete when hunger came knocking. I smiled as I looked at the clock. It was nearly 2:30 p.m. I'd eaten breakfast seven hours earlier, and these were the first twinges of hunger I felt. Instead of feeling weak or fighting mad with hunger, I had just a pleasant little knock on the walls of my stomach, followed by a polite "We could use a little food in here."

In the past, my desk drawers and credenza were always stocked with low-fat snacks. In my high-carb heyday, I had more packages of crackers, granola bars, and other snacks than any respectable convenience store. In addition, I kept hard candy on hand in case I had a bout of hypoglycemia. My daily routine was to eat breakfast before leaving home at 7:30 a.m. and then have a snack between 9 and 10 a.m. Although I tried to avoid eating again before lunch at noon, I often did. By 2 p.m., I was having a second snack, and often I grabbed one more before leaving the office at 5 p.m. so that I wouldn't be ravenous before dinner with my family at 6 p.m. The entire time I was cooking dinner, I was also eating. By the time we had finished dinner and the kitchen had been cleaned, I was thinking about a bedtime snack, which I ate dutifully by 10 p.m. On a typical day, I ate at least six or seven times.

Not only did I eat frequently, but I was eating sizable portions. After all, there were two Pop-Tarts to a package despite the nutrition label telling me that just one pastry was a serving. Eating two granola bars for a snack was not atypical for me. I bought four boxes at a time. Regardless of serving size, I didn't know that those packaged, processed, high-carb, and low-fat foods were not really feeding me. If anything, they were making me hungrier because they kept my blood sugar in a constant state of extreme highs followed by extreme lows. They fed my insulin resistance and metabolic disorder. They fed the inflammation that limited my mobility and put me on pain medications. I was hungry, obese, and sick, and I was constantly eating.

Now, four years later, my desk drawers are stocked with coconut oil, coffee, canned salmon, pork rinds, and coconut vinegar and avocado oil to make a fatty salad dressing. On that day when hunger disrupted my work at 2:30 p.m., I had a decision to make: stop and eat or push through the rest of my checklist before I had to leave the office early to pick up my children at 3:30. In another couple of hours I could eat a real, full meal at home with my family. My blood glucose was stable because I have been eating high-fat and low-carb for so long that I am truly fat-adapted. With no worries about hypoglycemia, I grabbed a bottle of water and pushed through.

I am grateful that I am no longer desperately hungry nearly every hour of the day. When life is more hectic than usual or plans get disrupted, my focus is not on food. When you are fat-adapted, you have easy access to stored energy. The fat on my thighs can feed me well for quite some time! I finally know how true hunger feels, and I am not tethered to food or to eating by the clock.

I had mostly finished my checklist by the time I walked to my car in the parking lot that day. The sun felt warm on my face. My tummy had stopped grumbling as I considered making dinner for my family, and I looked forward to hearing about their day as we ate a meal together.

JUST FOR TODAY I will avoid snacking and will wait for real hunger cues before enjoying healthy keto meals.

Week 3 Review

By the end of Week 3, you may be passing mile markers of progress so frequently that you may no longer notice them. This way of eating is becoming a little more automatic. As you review your Mile Marker Summary for this week, think back to the days when you felt less hungry and the days when staying on plan was easier for you. What did those days have in common? Look for patterns in the macronutrient ratios of your meals, the times and places you ate, and the people with whom you ate.

Also take time to record favorite foods, recipes, meals, or strategies that really helped you. Make note of what worked well. Likewise, note your struggles or dislikes. What would you avoid in the future? You might also want to jot down links to websites or useful tips that you discovered. I've included a notes page on my website that you can download and print out for this purpose.

Week 4

Welcome to the final week of your guided journey! Your hard work over the first three weeks will make this week easier. You likely are no longer fighting cravings, your energy level has likely increased, and your clothes are probably looser. You are passing mile markers of progress at high rates of speed, and the view is looking pretty good.

Throughout Week 4, you might feel as if you're alternating between sailing along on cruise control and slowing down for intermittent speed bumps. Some days will be easier than others; selecting meal options has become more automatic, yet you may still find that you need to double-check carb counts, portion sizes, or ingredient lists sometimes. Remember that each day completed and each challenge met will erode future speed bumps.

Your primary goal for this week is to enjoy the keto lifestyle as your new normal so that every decision about what and when to eat becomes truly automatic.

Here are your points of focus for Week 4:

1. Work toward sustaining this lifestyle for the rest of your life by making sure that you have the tools and resources you need to continue the journey with confidence.

2. Establish boundaries for yourself that help you stay on plan every day.

3. Consider which ketogenic foods and meals work best for your body, your lifestyle, and your preferences.

4. Reflect on the challenges you have faced while following this plan and focus on finding solutions that will help you stay on plan for the long term.

The key to success in Week 4 is to make keto mundane. Eating this way must become automatic, like brushing your teeth—something you simply do without fail. Following the plan becomes an extension of who you are such that you will not compromise, even if others do not understand or support your way of eating.

Week 4 Checklist

☐ Record your favorite keto meals (see pages 51 to 53). Be sure to include meals that keep you feeling full for longer periods and meals that are easy for you to prepare. Note whether your family or other dining companions also enjoy those foods. If you monitor your blood glucose, be sure to check whether it remains stable after you eat those foods.

☐ Make a list of what you enjoy about following a ketogenic lifestyle, and then create a second list of what makes this lifestyle difficult for you. For each struggle, brainstorm potential solutions.

☐ Review the strategies on pages 76 to 78 for staying on plan when others are not supportive of your choices.

☐ Complete the shopping list and meal prep for Week 4 and decide on your weekly food plan. Review the sample meal plans on pages 60 to 66 for inspiration.

☐ Use online menus and nutrition information to identify at least two additional keto-friendly meals that you can order at local restaurants. Record the name of each restaurant and jot down exactly what you would order. Include any necessary modifications to the menu options.

☐ Review your Mile Marker Summaries for Weeks 1, 2, and 3. What differences do you notice between Week 1 and Week 3?

☐ Take photos, try on clothing, jot down measurements (see pages 98 and 99), and so on and use those mile markers to track your progress.

☐ Throughout the week, use the Week 4 Mile Marker Summary to record your progress.

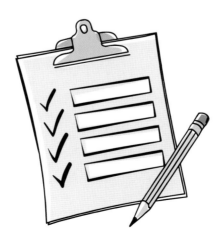

Daily Food Journal

Use a journal like this to record what you ate, what time you ate, how hungry you were when you ate, and how satisfied you felt after eating. Remember to eat only when hungry. For good ketogenic ratios, make sure that each meal has fat grams equal to or higher than protein grams, with carbohydrate grams lower than protein and fat. To print out copies of this chart, go to my website, cookingketowithkristie.com.

First Meal

Time: ....

What I ate: ....

....

Carbs: .... Protein: .... Fat: ....

Hunger level: 1   2   3   4   5   6   7   8   9   10

Satisfaction after meal: 1   2   3   4   5   6   7   8   9   10

Second Meal

Time: ....

What I ate: ....

....

Carbs: .... Protein: .... Fat: ....

Hunger level: 1   2   3   4   5   6   7   8   9   10

Satisfaction after meal: 1   2   3   4   5   6   7   8   9   10

Third Meal

Time: ....

What I ate: ....

....

Carbs: .... Protein: .... Fat: ....

Hunger level: 1   2   3   4   5   6   7   8   9   10

Satisfaction after meal: 1   2   3   4   5   6   7   8   9   10

First Snack

Time: ....

What I ate: ....

....

Carbs: .... Protein: .... Fat: ....

Hunger level: 1   2   3   4   5   6   7   8   9   10

Satisfaction after meal: 1   2   3   4   5   6   7   8   9   10

Second Snack

Time: ....

What I ate: ....

....

Carbs: .... Protein: .... Fat: ....

Hunger level: 1   2   3   4   5   6   7   8   9   10

Satisfaction after meal: 1   2   3   4   5   6   7   8   9   10

Mile Marker Summary, Week 4

Use this summary to record your progress throughout the week. You might also want to record your daily total intake of carbs, protein, and fat so you can begin to understand what works best for you. For a printable version of this worksheet, go to my website, cookingketowithkristie.com.

MONDAY

MACROS FOR ALL MEALS AND SNACKS			MILE MARKERS OF SUCCESS
Daily Total Carbs	Daily Total Protein	Daily Total Fat	

TUESDAY

MACROS FOR ALL MEALS AND SNACKS			MILE MARKERS OF SUCCESS
Daily Total Carbs	Daily Total Protein	Daily Total Fat	

WEDNESDAY

MACROS FOR ALL MEALS AND SNACKS			MILE MARKERS OF SUCCESS
Daily Total Carbs	Daily Total Protein	Daily Total Fat	

THURSDAY

MACROS FOR ALL MEALS AND SNACKS			MILE MARKERS OF SUCCESS
Daily Total Carbs	Daily Total Protein	Daily Total Fat	

FRIDAY

MACROS FOR ALL MEALS AND SNACKS			MILE MARKERS OF SUCCESS
Daily Total Carbs	Daily Total Protein	Daily Total Fat	

SATURDAY

MACROS FOR ALL MEALS AND SNACKS			MILE MARKERS OF SUCCESS
Daily Total Carbs	Daily Total Protein	Daily Total Fat	

SUNDAY

MACROS FOR ALL MEALS AND SNACKS			MILE MARKERS OF SUCCESS
Daily Total Carbs	Daily Total Protein	Daily Total Fat	

Day 22: Objects in Mirror Are Closer Than They Appear

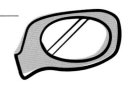

"Oh gosh! I see carbs!" The filter between my brain and my mouth temporarily malfunctioned. I didn't realize it until I noticed that three people had turned to look at me. We were gathered at a mutual friend's house, preparing foods for the buffet table. The menu was supposed to be low-carb, yet here I was staring at loads of vegetables. My reaction required an explanation.

With a nervous giggle, I said, "I'm sorry. After so many years of keto, I no longer see foods; I see macronutrients. I automatically start calculating the nutrient content of the dish. Foods are made up of fat, protein, or carbs and often some of each. When I see a salad with lettuce and lots of veggies, a warning light goes off in my brain. That dish," I pointed, "would be low-carb, but it wouldn't give me the essential nutrients of fat and protein." I giggled again, "My brain looks for fat first!" Instead of defusing the awkwardness, I had drawn the attention of six others. "Wait, you see a salad and think that's bad?" one guest asked. "Not exactly," I tried to explain. "The vegetables aren't bad, but I need some fat and protein to eat with them. Meat, eggs, cheese, and a wonderfully fatty dressing would make the salad a better low-carb option."

"What about this dish? What do you see?" asked a second guest, pointing to a serving bowl that contained a lot of vegetables and a little lean chicken. While they looked at me like a diviner who can see into the beyond, I carefully explained that I saw a dish with more protein than fat and a too-high ratio of carbs to fat. Just guesstimating, I'd say that a serving of the dish had an equal number of grams of protein and carbohydrate and less fat than protein or carbs. To be ketogenic, fat grams should be equal to or higher than protein grams, and carbohydrates should be very low.

"Would you not eat that?" chimed in a third guest. The awkwardness intensified. They had designated me the expert on all things ketogenic based on my personal success and longevity on the plan. I was uncomfortable because I wouldn't dare proclaim a food "bad," but it was not a dish that I would have chosen as a low-carb option. My dilemma was worsened by the fact that the guest who had prepared the dish was waiting with bated breath for my answer. I replied as diplomatically as possible, "If I was eating that, I would look for ways to add more fat. Perhaps some butter or sour cream, or maybe bacon. It would work well with a fatty meat." Everyone relaxed a little.

"How do you balance a meal? What do you look for?" quizzed the first guest. Before I could answer, another person asked, "How do you learn to see carbs?" I smiled. In a way, it seemed as if they were asking a magician to reveal the secrets behind a sleight-of-hand illusion.

"It's a curse." I smiled. "It's rooted in fear. I'm terrified of going back to that place of hunger, sickness, pain, and obesity. When I see carbs, I see all those things. I remember my back hurting, the plus-sized clothes, and all the things I couldn't do. Someone else looks at a piece of cake or a croissant and thinks it looks good; I feel repulsed. High-carb food represents everything I don't want to be anymore. It means poor health and loneliness and limitations." Their expressions were difficult to read, but I'm pretty sure I saw a mix of surprise, confusion, and sympathy. "So, a big slice of chocolate cake doesn't look good to you?" someone asked.

"Not at all! How can being sick and feeling bad taste good? I can't have that cake without the high blood glucose and inflammation that come with it. Poor health is baked right in! Instead, I can have a juicy hamburger on leaf lettuce with cheese, bacon, mayonnaise, and mushrooms sautéed in butter and enjoy better health.

"In short, carbs generally bring all the negative things that I want to avoid. Fat and protein make my body healthier and stronger. I've spent the last several years learning roughly how many carbs are in every food, and I've built a visual hierarchy in my brain. Leafy vegetables, other than kale, are low in carbs. When I see those on a plate, they look good. Tomatoes, onions, and peppers are higher in carbs. I always limit those, especially if they are together in a dish. Broccoli and asparagus are good options, and mushrooms are very low in carbs as well. There's no magic to it; you just repeatedly look up the carb counts from a reliable source. Over time, you learn."

"So, basically, you do the work?" asked a lady standing nearby. "Yes!" I replied. "I didn't know any of this a few years ago. All I had was determination and the USDA database to look up macronutrients. I made a lot of mistakes, which is exactly how most of us learn anything." "So there really is no magic?" she asked. "Oh yes, there is magic! Have you ever tasted a juicy hamburger on leaf lettuce with cheese, bacon, mayonnaise, and mushrooms sautéed in butter? There's your magic! And don't forget that the bunless burger is served with a side of smaller skinny jeans."

JUST FOR TODAY   I will look at foods as fat, protein, and carbs so that I can make good choices.

Day 23: Traveling Companions

"Are you going to eat the cookie?" I overheard the lady sitting across from me ask her coworker. The other woman nodded as she took a drink of her diet soft drink. We were attending a professional conference and had been served the typical boxed lunch: sandwich, pasta salad, pickle, and cookie. Having been low-carb for about six weeks, I chose to eat the meat, cheese, and lettuce from the sandwich with the pickle and a packet of mayonnaise and discarded the bread and pasta salad. I did not eat (or even want) the cookie, but I was fascinated by the exchange between the two women sitting near me. While I did not know them, they obviously knew each other.

From the context of the conversation, I guessed that one or both of the women was "dieting." They spent time comparing notes on what they were eating. The woman who asked, "Are you going to eat the cookie?" seemed hesitant and maybe a little embarrassed, but she asked nonetheless. When her colleague responded yes, the first woman appeared to be given permission somehow. She relaxed and then proceeded to eat her cookie, too.

Imagine if the second woman had said that she was *not* going to eat the cookie. Would the first lady have eaten her own dessert? I'd bet you a pound of bacon that she wouldn't have. Whether it was permission or approval or comradery, the first lady needed someone else to tell her that it was okay to eat the cookie. She had to know that eating the cookie was not a good option for her, or she wouldn't have asked. She had to have felt torn about whether to eat it. Clearly, it mattered to her whether she was alone in eating that cookie. She didn't want to be different.

There I sat, eating the innards of my sandwich and throwing away the high-carb components. Even if anyone had noticed, and some of the people around me may have, do you think they cared? Probably not. And even if they did, I would not have cared that they cared, not even a little. What if it had been one of my coworkers asking me, "Are you going to eat the cookie?" My response likely would have been, "No. Do you want it?" I choose my food based on my convictions. What anyone else eats is irrelevant to me.

You need permission about what to eat from only one person—yourself! It doesn't matter what anyone around you chooses to eat. Unless someone else is force-feeding you, you are solely responsible for your own food choices. The choices in front of you may not always be optimal, but make the best of them.

Now that I am fat-adapted, I skip boxed lunches entirely and either eat ahead of time, eat later, or bring my own food for lunch. Most frequently I drink water, enjoy talking with others, and look forward to a high-fat meal later in the day. If someone asks why I'm not eating, I say that I am not hungry or have food sensitivities or that I'm looking forward to a big meal later. I often avoid saying that I eat low-carb, and I *never* say that I'm trying to lose weight. (See pages 76 to 78 for more tips on eating with others.)

If you know that eating keto is best for your body, then use the courage of that conviction. You don't need permission from anyone else.

JUST FOR TODAY I will take responsibility for my food choices without looking for permission from others.

Day 24: Automatic Transmissions

"How long have you had that shirt?" I tried to ask casually, but David saw right through me. "I don't know, but it's still in good shape. Good enough to wear," he responded. My husband's shirt had to have been circa 1990. He'd bought it before we met, of that much I was certain.

As I considered various strategies to get him to change clothes, our daughter walked in. "Um, Dad, what are you wearing?" she asked. "This nice shirt. I'm wearing *this* nice shirt." He folded his arms. I knew that tone. I worried that he might have to be buried in *that* shirt because there was no getting him to change out of it now.

"Mom, are you going to let him wear that?" she asked. My children obviously overestimate me if they think I *let* their father wear any particular piece of clothing. Trying to be diplomatic, I replied, "Well, I was just wondering myself whether that shirt was a good choice for him." He was not having my feigned diplomacy. "This is a *great* choice, and I'm wearing *this* shirt, and you two can just get over it."

David is one of those people who believes that clothing lasts as long as it comfortably fits. His criteria for discarding clothes are vague. If a garment is threadbare or has holes, then he saves it for yard work. If it has paint on it, then he saves it for the next painting project. Grease stains? It will do for puttering around the house. If he has one pair of pants for each day of the week, then he has plenty of pants. He is a creature of habit.

Many of us are creatures of habit, and those habits serve us well when we need to do things quickly and efficiently. When parts of life become automatic, we can focus on other tasks that require our attention, like a project at work or a leaking toilet. Many of us have developed food habits over the years. We eat at certain times of the day, or we eat certain foods with certain people or certain foods on certain occasions. Certainly, not all of those habits are good ones.

When we switch to a low-carb lifestyle, many of those habits are challenged. Because high-fat foods are satiating, we find ourselves not hungry, but faced with the custom of eating breakfast before work or school or eating dinner with others in the evening. We might eat lunch at midday because that is simply what we have always done, but should we eat just because of the clock? Nearly every physician who advocates for low-carb eating seems to agree that we should eat to hunger. Eating to the clock is a habit that still catches me at times, though, especially because I look forward to sitting down to dinner with my family.

Another habit that folks who are new to low-carb often struggle with is associating high-carb foods with certain meals. For example, a standard American breakfast is a bagel, a muffin, cereal, or toast. None of those options is low-carb, but all of them are quick. Often folks tell me that they don't have time to fix breakfast, so they reach for a low-carb protein bar or a smoothie or some other fast fix that isn't ideal in terms of ingredients or macros. When my family began eating a ketogenic diet, I started spending Sunday evenings making frittatas and cooking bacon for the week. The key to not falling into "easy" and "quick" high-carb eating habits is replacing those high-carb foods with easy and quick keto-friendly foods.

A third habit to kick relates to socializing. I used to have a favorite shopping buddy who always wanted to share a cinnamon roll at the mall food court. Those rolls were the size of dinner plates! The first time we went shopping together after I started eating low-carb, I worried about hurting her feelings when I chose not to eat the cinnamon roll. Things got awkward when she wanted one and really wanted me to have one, too. Somehow my not eating that roll became her guilt. Moreover, it became me rejecting her. That shared cinnamon roll somehow bonded us. I didn't want to reject her, but I knew that I couldn't enjoy the cinnamon roll. Unfortunately, she could not enjoy one without me. We decided that coffee was a better option and then got distracted by a shoe sale. Shoe shopping is a much better way to bond!

I had to think about who my "eating friends" were, and I had to be intentional about suggesting things we could do together that did not involve high-carb foods. It took time, but in most cases we were able to change our routines while maintaining our friendships.

Like comfortable old clothing, we tend to hold on to habits, especially when we are stressed or we don't know what else to do. When there's nothing else in the closet, we wear the old shirt that fell out of fashion a decade ago. To successfully exchange those habits that didn't serve us well for new habits that do, we must be intentional about it. We must clean out the closet and the dresser drawers and then replace those outdated items with new pieces that match our new lifestyle. We need comfortable clothing that slips on easily, like a well-prepped meal that keeps us out of the fast-food drive-through. We need satisfying meals that keep us from diving face-first into sugary treats.

I've heard it said that most people can build a wardrobe around a few essential pieces. Similarly, most people can build a ketogenic lifestyle around a few "essential" meals. Start by identifying five of your favorite keto meals. Next week, add one or two more favorites. Keep adding to your list week after week, and a month later you will have a dozen or more new meals to keep you on plan and feeling great. Before long, you won't even have to think about what to eat because your new routines will have become old habits. The good news is that unlike my husband's wardrobe, delicious low-carb meals never go out of style!

 JUST FOR TODAY   I will intentionally form new habits to help me create a new, healthier lifestyle.

Day 25: Blocking Out Road Noise

"OMG! This task has me so stressed out that I want to eat potato chips!" I was laughing, and I was talking more to myself than to my colleague, but I was acknowledging the stress of piecing together one coherent document edited separately by five other administrators. Potato chips? I don't even like potato chips, but that's what I said.

I wondered why I had even thought of potato chips. After committing to a very-low-carb lifestyle, I hadn't eaten a chip in more than four years. I wasn't overly fond of them before going low-carb, to be honest. The fatty ranch dressing that I liked to dip them in was sublime, though; that was the best part of eating chips. I could have ranch dressing and stay low-carb, so why did I holler to my coworker that I wanted potato chips?

As I took a minute to breathe, I started to negotiate with myself as a child negotiates with a parent. "If I don't have chips, can I have a Diet Coke?" I reasoned. Then I sat there wondering why I would want a diet soft drink, knowing that those artificial sweeteners only make my cravings worse. Since I'd stopped drinking them some time ago, their taste was no longer appealing to me. What did I *really* want? What did the chips or the soft drink represent?

The word *escape* bounced around in my brain. I wanted to escape the task. I wanted the cessation of pain. Walking out of my office to grab a snack or a soft drink would get me away from my desk. Even a temporary reprieve is a reprieve. There was nothing I really wanted in chips or a soft drink. In fact, even if I had buried my face in a bag of salty avoidance, the difficult project would still be waiting for me. Not only would I continue the hair-pulling process of wrangling different thoughts and writing styles into one professional and polished piece, but I would have lost time to work on it while I was chasing down chips. Perhaps more importantly, I would have then sat at my desk with an empty bag of chips, grease-stained fingers, a document that still needed a great deal of work, and a guilty conscience, along with the heavy, lethargic feeling that comes from too many carbs and a stomach that feels like it's filled with lead.

The act of indulging in those chips would have left a lingering taste of regret and failure that no diet soft drink could wash away. Beyond that, my blood glucose would have soared and, with my history of hypoglycemia, potentially crashed until I was tired and sleepy and even less capable of crafting the document that required my full attention. It would have pushed me further from my professional goal of completing the task as well as further from my personal goal of staying healthy.

I took a deep breath and decided to escape by completing another item on my to-do list—contacting another colleague to arrange a meeting. As I looked up her extension, I thought, "I've never regretted something that I didn't eat." I chuckled. That thought has rescued me more than once, always helping me choose to walk away from some high-carb temptation. I hear that statement in my grandmother's voice. Maybe it's because she, too, struggled with obesity, and because she knew my struggle all too well. She desperately wanted me to lose weight. She wanted to see me happy.

My grandmother passed away in 2003, shortly after Grace was born, but she has stayed with me. In many ways, she is my good conscience and my sense of determination. It was she who taught me, "If wishes were horses, beggars would ride," and the similar phrase, "Wishing don't make it so." In other words, if you want to make something happen, you have to act on it. Doing something—controlling the action—is more valuable than sitting back and wishing.

I could munch through that bag of chips and wish that the document were completed or sat on someone else's desk, but the job had been given to me by folks who deemed me competent to do it. Many times I wished my struggle with obesity belonged to someone else, too, but this burden also was given to me, and I knew that if I was going to meet the challenge, wishing wouldn't make it so. Each day, I have to do the best I can for my body. I must choose foods that leave me with no regrets, empower my body with better health, and embrace the confidence that I can accomplish the task at hand, even if that task is as simple as refusing a bag of chips.

JUST FOR TODAY I will *be* different because I *am* different. I no longer wish for success; I *choose* success.

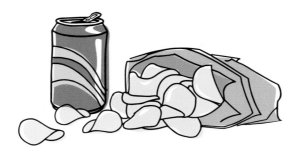

Day 26: Installing a GPS

"I'm sorry, honey, I can't today." It nearly broke my heart to say it, but my daughter had called me from school three times that week because she had forgotten something. Each time she called, I had left work or made myself late as I stopped to retrieve what she needed from home, run it to her at school, and then return to work. In previous weeks, she had forgotten at least one thing per week, which was frustrating to us both and embarrassing to her. While I could have taken the forgotten item to her once more, I knew that she had to take responsibility. Mom could not keep rescuing her. Her dad and I agreed that making her deal with the repercussions was an important lesson, but we also worked with her to build in additional support.

After school that day, she and I sat down and talked about the consequences of her forgetfulness. We took the time to discuss *why* she had forgotten some of the items I had recently taken to her. Much of her struggle was related to disorganization. She forgot the binder because she'd left it on her desk instead of packing it in her backpack. She forgot her lunch because she was looking for the shoes she had left outside. She didn't remember to turn in a permission form because she had put it in her backpack instead of in her folder for homeroom.

As we talked about why she had forgotten various items, two things became clear. One, she had a lot to remember! Two, mornings were harder when she didn't follow a routine. Once we knew *why*, we set about changing *how*. I showed her how I use checklists to help me remember things. She liked the idea and decided to make two checklists, one for the morning and one for the evening. We went to the computer and typed up her evening list: pack backpack with homework (binders) and notes to turn in, charge laptop, pick out clothes, find shoes, put lunch box on kitchen counter. Then she created a morning list: brush teeth, apply deodorant, pack laptop, pack lunch box. She (and we) began using these lists, and the panicked phone calls stopped. We both were very pleased!

She relied on the lists for the first few weeks, but eventually she no longer had to stop and mentally check off each item. She was creating good habits. Those visual reminders became routine tasks. She was still using the checklists, but she had internalized them. Her brain had needed to create and remember a routine to make her successful. What took a little extra time in the beginning—making the lists and checking them twice—actually saved her time and saved all of us some stress over things she really needed being forgotten.

Even more important, my sweet G felt accomplished. I overheard her one day talking to a friend who was visiting. Her checklists were pinned to the wall just outside her room so that she could review them before heading downstairs, and she explained, "Yeah, I used to need those because I was forgetting stuff. Now I don't forget those things, but I like to leave the lists there anyway because they remind me of how much better I am at remembering." Her pride was apparent. She had taken what was embarrassing for her and frustrating for us both and turned it into an achievement. With only a little extra effort, she set herself up for success.

If you're struggling to stay on plan or to figure out the carb counts in foods or to create balanced keto plates, consider these two things: one, you have a lot to learn and remember; and two, new habits are hard to create if you don't work to make them routine. Figure out why you struggle and then consider changing how you approach it. Once you take the time to do that, you'll experience the pride of accomplishment rather than struggle with embarrassment and failure. You'll find a lot of information in Part I to guide you.

 JUST FOR TODAY I'll consider why I struggle, and then I will focus on how I can make things easier for myself.

Day 27: Adjusting the Driver's Seat

We all get them—those reminders of the past that propel us back in time and remind us of who we used to be. I got one recently in the form of a reminder text from my neurologist's office. I was instantly catapulted back to 2012. We had moved into our new house that January. Because of my back, we had built the house to be handicapped accessible, with a raised dishwasher. During the build, we discussed whether to purchase disability insurance for me.

While I'd had multiple surgeries for scoliosis in 1994, the fusion had been successful; I had been pretty healthy and active afterward. When I began having ongoing pain in 2012, my physician referred me to a neurologist. The neurologist reviewed my most recent imaging results with surprise and called to colleagues to "look at this!" One of them said to me, "Did you know that you have a second curve above the spinal fusion? Not only is the spine curving, but it's twisting. We need to look at your lung function." The diagnosis codes on my chart looked like advanced math taught in Latin, with accompanying medical terminology that described issues from the bottom of my spine to the top.

Shortly after that, at the pain management clinic, an anesthesiologist used a fluoroscope to administer my first epidural steroid injection. A fluoroscope is like a real-time X-ray and provides a visual guide so that the needle can inject the pain medication in just the right spot. The doctor left me under the fluoroscope, backside up and barely draped, to wait for two different colleagues to come and view the hardware, curvature, stenosis, and so on. "You don't see that every day!" he exclaimed. One asked, "Is this patient mobile?" Yes, and the patient was lying right there under the fluoroscope, praying for someone to adjust the draping over her hind end and to find an intervention to manage her pain.

The pain was incessant. Each morning I took three different medications for pain. My company had purchased a desk that I could raise and lower so that I could stand as needed during the workday. By the time I arrived home after work, pain was shooting down my left leg and across my lower back. Cooking dinner was often difficult, but I nearly always had dinner on the table by the time my husband got home at 6 p.m. Most nights I tried to sit at the table with my family, but the pain was often so severe that I only wanted to lie down. On the worst nights, I didn't even try to cook. Instead, David brought me dinner in bed. With few exceptions, by 7 p.m., I had taken more pain medication and was in bed. My children were nine and six years old at the time, and their bedrooms were upstairs. David had to help me walk from the kitchen to our bedroom on the main floor. Climbing the stairs to tuck my children into bed was not possible. My littles would climb into my bed with me for snuggles and reading and help with homework. Then they kissed me goodnight and went upstairs and waited for Daddy to tuck them in.

Even our weekends were framed by Mom's bad back. I couldn't get on the trampoline, but I could sit and watch everyone else jump. I waited in the car while David took them for a hike to see a waterfall. Hearing them describe their hike with such joy was as painful as being left behind, but I never told them that. Instead, I asked questions and encouraged them to draw pictures for me. When they had their first snow skiing lessons, I was safely inside where no one had to worry about me falling and hurting my back further. No water slides with Mom. No roller coasters, either. The children knew I had to be let out at the door of the shopping center because walking too much would hurt my back. Some days it seemed that the list of what Mom couldn't do was longer than the list of what she *could* do. I was the mom who couldn't.

Until I began losing weight, that is. Almost one year after that first steroid injection, I discovered the ketogenic diet. Let's be honest: at that point, I only wanted to wear smaller clothes and not be obese. After losing the first 30 pounds, though, I realized that my back pain was decreasing. The mega bottle of ibuprofen (see "Day 10: Food as Medicine") was the first to go. Instead of taking ibuprofen several times daily, I took it only after exertion. Gradually, my definition of exertion changed. A few hours of shopping no longer qualified as exertion. Walking to the end of the cul-de-sac and vacuuming the great room had previously required pain meds, but no more. Slowly I stopped taking pain meds even while becoming more active. By June 2014, on a family trip to Hawaii, this mom was hiking up a volcano and kayaking in the ocean—med free and pain free! I was not the mom I used to be.

In 2015, I decided to follow up with the neurologist, wondering if more recent imaging might be warranted. We never had tested my lung function, and I wasn't getting any younger. At that appointment, the neurologist looked at my chart, and then he looked at me. "You're not taking any meds or getting steroid injections anymore?" he asked. I confirmed that I wasn't. "You've lost a lot of weight since you were here last, over 100 pounds. Tell me what you're doing." He needed to understand why the old chart didn't match the patient sitting in front of him. He needed to know who this new woman was.

I explained my very-low-carb diet. He became animated, telling me that a ketogenic diet was a wonderful way to eat. He said that he wished all his patients would eat that way because it is anti-inflammatory. Encouraged, I eagerly asked, "Do you follow a ketogenic diet?" He shook his head and said, "No, it's too damn hard. I like beer and potatoes too much!" He encouraged me to stay the course, but he didn't see a need for imaging unless I was still having pain. He said that we could do the lung function testing if I wanted to since it couldn't hurt to have a baseline. He wished me well and told me how proud he was of my progress. I left and haven't followed up with him since.

Two years later, the text from his office that disrupted my day was a simple one. "Kristie, you may be overdue for an appointment. Please call to set up an appointment if needed." No, thank you. I'm not that woman anymore.

JUST FOR TODAY I will remember how my life is different when I eat keto: I feel better.

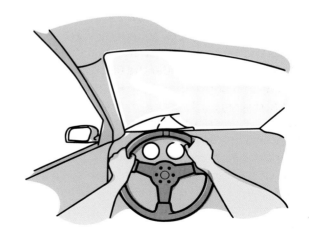

Day 28: It's the Journey, Not the Destination

"I don't know if we're gonna make it on time!" My stress level was rising by the second. My son and I both had appointments in a larger city. Depending on the time of day and a half dozen other variables, it generally took an hour and a half to two hours to drive there from our house. Since the first appointment was at 9 a.m., I decided we should leave by 7:15 because of the morning traffic. We didn't leave the house until 7:22.

Just thirty minutes into our trip, traffic was much worse than I anticipated. About halfway into the journey, I started to panic that we were going to be late. Looking at the road signs, I started trying to predict how late we might be. Five minutes? Ten minutes? Twenty? As the anxiety began to build, I reached for my phone to turn on Google Maps so that I would know our *exact* anticipated arrival time. Reason found me at the last minute, and a quiet, calmer voice inside my head said, "Stop! What will you do if the GPS predicts you will be five minutes late?"

My thought was, "Well, I'll keep heading to the appointment and watch for crazy drivers and stay in the 'best' lanes and avoid accidents and go as fast as I can."

The voice of reason wondered, "What will you do if the GPS predicts you will be ten minutes late?"

I gave myself the same answer: "Well, I'll keep heading to the appointment and watch for crazy drivers and stay in the 'best' lanes and avoid accidents and go as fast as I can."

"And if you're twenty minutes late? You're not gonna turn around and head home, are you?" The voice of reason was starting to make sense.

"No. I could call the doctor's office and let them know, but they don't open until 9 a.m., so I'll still keep heading to the appointment and watching for crazy drivers and staying in the 'best' lanes and avoiding accidents and going as fast as I can."

Realizing that my anxiety was not going to help me arrive any earlier, I took a deep breath and decided to focus on driving safely, looking for funny vanity plates, wondering at the strange clouds, and talking with my son. My destination would be there regardless, and I would arrive as long as I kept moving forward and didn't stop to look for pork rinds at every exit, as I've been known to do.

Our low-carb journey is very similar. We become anxious about the weight loss that we monitor on the scale or the inches that we feel we aren't losing quickly enough. We fixate on the goal because we want to arrive at our destination as soon as possible, but it is the drive, the journey, that matters most. The destination will always be there. Some folks may arrive fifteen minutes earlier than they expected, and others might arrive thirty minutes later than they wanted to. The most significant thing to remember is that if you stop driving, you will *never* arrive. You can obsess over weighing and measuring, but most folks make progress simply by controlling their carbohydrate intake and eating real, whole foods that they enjoy.

After all the worry about being late, we arrived at the doctor's office at 8:59 a.m. What a waste of adrenaline! At 9:25, I was still waiting to see the doctor and laughing with my son as we waited together. It's the journey, right?

 JUST FOR TODAY I will concentrate on enjoying my new lifestyle and better health without worrying about arriving at my destination at a particular time. I will remember that keto is a journey that we begin but never complete.

Week 4 Review

The conclusion of Week 4 brings us to the end of our twenty-eight-day journey together, and it is an excellent time to reflect on the entire four-week period. After completing the Mile Marker Summary for this week, I challenge you to look back to your Mile Marker Summary for Week 1 to see how far you have come. You may want to go through this day-by-day guide again, treating Week 1 as Week 5, Week 2 as Week 6, and so on.

As in previous weeks, take time to record favorite foods, recipes, meals, or strategies that really helped you. Make note of what worked well. Likewise, note your struggles or dislikes. What would you avoid in the future? You might also want to jot down links to websites or useful tips that you discovered. I've included a notes page on my website that you can download and print out for this purpose.

Please continue to use the tools in this book to help you along your journey. Remember that keto is a journey you start, but never finish. It is a lifelong commitment to better health.

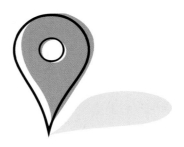

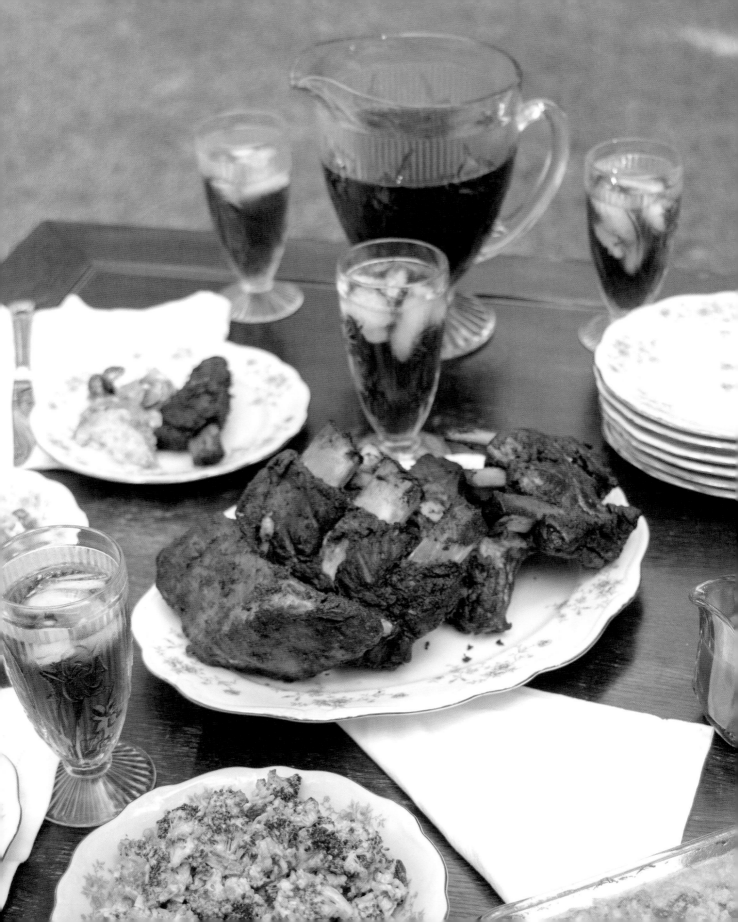

PART III:

The Recipes

Guide to Using the Recipes

I've chosen the recipes in this book specifically for those of you who really do not enjoy cooking but do enjoy eating! If you're unsure about cooking most of your own meals, do not fear; you will find these recipes easy to follow and quick to prepare. I use straightforward cooking techniques to create dishes that are tasty yet completely keto. By the end of twenty-eight days, you will be completely at ease in the kitchen.

Key Recipe Components

To make the recipes easier to use and provide you with all the information you need to follow a keto lifestyle, I've included nutritional information as well as icons and tips.

Yield

Many of my recipes are designed to feed a family of four and, ideally, to leave you with leftovers for later meals or the freezer. Others are designed for entertaining, so the yield is larger. Most of these recipes intended to feed a crowd can be easily halved if you need a smaller yield. A few recipes, such as certain breakfasts and beverages, make just one serving. These recipes are quick to prepare and work well when family members are eating on different schedules or have varying food preferences.

Icons

Icons are provided at the top of each recipe to give you at-a-glance guidance for recipes that avoid allergens or that provide guidance to how quickly a recipe can be made. Look for the following icons to help guide your meal plans:

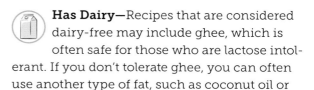 **Has Dairy**—Recipes that are considered dairy-free may include ghee, which is often safe for those who are lactose intolerant. If you don't tolerate ghee, you can often use another type of fat, such as coconut oil or bacon fat.

Has Eggs—If you are sensitive to eggs or have an allergy, please look for this icon to avoid recipes that include eggs.

Has Nuts—Only two recipes in this book use nuts. These recipes are flagged as having nuts so that if you have a nut allergy, you can easily avoid them. For the purpose of this icon, I do not consider coconut to be a nut because most people with nut allergies can tolerate coconut.

Slow Cooker—When possible, I've included options for using a slow cooker, which makes prepping dinner far easier. I especially enjoy walking into the house after a long day to a warm dinner that typically requires no more than my reaching for plates and utensils.

 30 Minutes or Less—Recipes marked with this icon can be made from start to finish in 30 minutes or less. This includes prep and cook time.

One-Pot Wonder—Not only are these recipes usually quick to make, but all of them are complete meals and nearly all are made in one pot, skillet, or dish, making cleanup a breeze.

Useful tips and suggestions

In addition to the icons, where appropriate, I've included notes following the recipes to provide strategies for making the recipes faster, offer appropriate substitutions, or warn you about ingredients that may add carbs when used in larger amounts.

- **Time-Saver Tips**—Look for these tips for making recipes more quickly to save your time for what matters most.

- **Substitution Suggestions**—Whether it's a product that can be difficult to find or an ingredient that many people avoid, such as dairy or pork, where practical, I've tried to provide substitutions to make your life easier.

- **Carb Check**—Carb creep, those pesky carbs that sneak up on us, can be a real problem for some people. One way to avoid carb creep is to shop smart. Some products or brands can be carby land mines; I provide guidance on label reading and offer other pointers. Some ingredients, such as tomatoes and onions, naturally have a surprisingly high number of carbs and can cause carb creep if eaten in too great quantities; in the Keto Carb Checks, I point out these potential pitfalls.

Nutritional information

While I have provided nutritional information for each recipe, please understand that this information is based on the nutritional information for the particular ingredients that I use. The macronutrients in ingredients can vary widely. For example, cream cheese varies from 1 gram of total carb per serving to 2 grams of carbs per one 1-ounce serving. Because I use only the brands of cream cheese that have 1 gram of total carb per ounce, when a recipe calls for 8 ounces of cream cheese, I count that as 8 grams of total carbs. Keep in mind that you should count it as 16 grams of total carbs if you are using a higher-carb brand of cream cheese. In addition, different brands of chorizo, sausage, tomato sauce, dairy products, and coconut-based products are likely to have widely varying nutritional information. Please use the information that I have provided as a guide; however, it is not intended to be a substitute for calculating your own nutritional information based on the ingredients you use and the portions you eat.

I do not count sugar alcohols for erythritol because it does not raise blood glucose for most people; however, if you are diabetic or have other health concerns, please test your blood glucose to determine whether it affects you. Finally, there are several good online recipe calculators that allow you to select the brands and nutritional information for the products you use. I would encourage you to use those if you have any questions about the nutritional content of these recipes.

Making Substitutions

Where possible, I have provided suggested substitutions, particularly for dairy or pork. I often suggest using ghee instead of butter since many people who cannot tolerate dairy can enjoy ghee. You can use other fats if ghee is problematic for you. If you find that you need to make substitutions, consider whether you are varying the carb, fat, or protein content. In addition to thinking about macros, consider whether you have affected the moisture, texture, or yield of the finished product. For example, turkey bacon will add less fat to a dish than pork bacon, and the dish might be drier as a result.

Ingredient Guide

Because I wrote this book for people who are just starting out on keto, I worked hard to ensure that nearly all of the ingredients used in the recipes are easy to find. With very few exceptions, a major retailer or grocery store chain should have everything you need. As you stock your keto kitchen, here are a few things to note about some of the key ingredients used in this book.

Fats and Oils

Bacon fat—A personal favorite, bacon fat works well for frying, baking, and roasting because it holds up to high heat. Unfortunately, rendered bacon fat is not available commercially. To get bacon fat, you will have to cook bacon and render the fat yourself. It's a win-win, actually, because you're left with bacon to eat! You'll find my method of baking bacon and rendering the fat on page 188.

Butter—Butter definitely makes life better. I use it for low-carb baking and to season foods. I don't often use it for frying, however, because butter burns at high temperatures. In these recipes, please use unsalted butter unless a recipe specifically calls for salted butter. Using unsalted allows you to adjust salt to taste.

Ghee—With the casein, or milk solids, removed, ghee is a good option for most people who avoid dairy. Ghee doesn't burn like butter, so it can be an excellent choice for frying or roasting.

Avocado oil—A mild-tasting oil, avocado oil can be used for both hot and cold applications. I keep some on hand to use on salads and to make mayonnaise. Because of its mild flavor, it works well in a variety of dishes.

Coconut oil—Refined coconut oil is another good option for cooking at high heat. I use it for baking, roasting, and frying. The two basic types are refined and unrefined. Although some people swear by the health benefits of unrefined coconut oil, I tend to use refined because it has little to no coconut flavor, and that's what my family prefers. Coconut oil is often a good option for those who avoid dairy.

Olive oil—While there are many types of olive oil, I tend to use a light-tasting olive oil for most applications. If you like a heartier, more robust olive oil flavor, you can use extra-virgin olive oil.

Sesame oil, toasted—Most sesame oil is intended as a finishing oil and not meant for cooking. Just a tablespoon adds great flavor to Asian-inspired dishes.

Dairy

Heavy cream—My fridge usually houses at least a pint or two of heavy cream. We use it in coffee as well as in many different dishes. An excellent source of fat, heavy cream also gives foods a fantastic creamy texture. I prefer to use heavy cream rather than heavy whipping cream because it has a higher fat content, but heavy cream can be more difficult to find. (See page 45 for a discussion of the different types of cream.) You can always ask your favorite store to stock it.

Another tip related to heavy cream has to do with its carb count. Despite nutrition labels saying that cream has 0 carbs, it actually has 0.6 gram of carbs per tablespoon, meaning that ¼ cup has 2.4 grams of carbs, which can quickly put you over your carb limit. Just be sure to count all of the carbs!

Sour cream—Sour cream is a great thickener and makes a wonderful base for dips, sauces, and casseroles. Be sure to buy the full-fat type and to check the ingredients. Some brands have added food starches; therefore, they also have a higher carb count.

Crème fraîche—While pricey, crème fraîche is worth every penny. Similar to sour cream in texture, crème fraîche has a much higher fat content, is lower in carbs, and has moderate protein. You can use it like sour cream or to make a healthy full-fat alternative to yogurt (see page 236).

Cream cheese—Another staple in my house. I use cream cheese with deli meat and pickles or olives for quick lunches and add it to dishes to create a creamy gravy. Just be sure to read labels and select a brand that has 1 gram of carbs per serving; avoid those brands with 2 grams per serving.

Mascarpone—Mascarpone is similar to a soft cream cheese but has a higher fat content and less protein than cream cheese. It can be used in sweet or savory dishes and pairs well with crème fraîche to make a high-fat, low-carb faux yogurt (page 236).

Ricotta—Here, too, nutritional values vary greatly among brands. When buying ricotta, search for full-fat versions and check the ingredients for food starches. Always compare labels to find the brands with the lowest carbs and highest fats. Interestingly, store brands are often the best option because they have the fewest additives.

Other cheeses—After decades of searching for low-fat cheeses, keto lets me enjoy the fattiest kinds! Double cream Brie, Gouda, Gruyère, and fresh goat cheese are just a few of my favorites. Be aware that you generally want to avoid processed cheese, such as American cheese or anything labeled "cheese product." There are just a few brands of American cheese that do not include vegetable oils in their lists of ingredients. Avoid anything that contains food starches or added oils; be sure to check the labels.

General Pantry Items

Almond milk—A popular dairy-free option. Be sure to purchase unsweetened almond milk and be vigilant about finding brands without added ingredients.

Coconut milk—If you avoid dairy, coconut milk is an excellent option, but you must read labels. Too often sugar and thickeners are added to coconut milk.

Coconut cream—Like coconut milk, coconut cream is often adulterated with sugar and thickeners. In particular, you want to avoid the coconut creams used to make cocktails and other beverages, as they almost always have added sugars. If you can't find coconut cream, you can place a large can of full-fat coconut milk upside down in the refrigerator overnight. When you remove it from the refrigerator, turn the can right side up, use a can opener to remove the top, pour off the coconut water, and use the fatty cream that remains.

Ketchup—As someone who doesn't care for ketchup, I never dreamed I would make my own. Who does that? After reading the carb counts and seeing the ingredients in commercial ketchup, I hope you do, too! Homemade ketchup (page 190) is super quick to make and actually tastes better than the high-carb commercial options. Be careful about using "sugar-free" brands, as many have undesirable sweeteners and are higher in carbs than homemade.

Mayonnaise—My favorite condiment by far; however, commercial brands can be problematic because they are often made with canola oil or vegetable oils that are known to be inflammatory and suspected of contributing to cardiovascular disease. In addition, many brands have added sugars. With the exception of Primal Kitchen's mayo, which I'll purchase when pressed for time, I prefer to make my own mayonnaise with avocado oil. The recipe is on page 192. Don't be intimidated to try it. Making mayonnaise is very quick and truly tastes good.

Mustard—Low in carbs, mustard is a good keto condiment. I keep prepared yellow mustard on hand for burgers and deli meats and Dijon and spicy mustard for salad dressings and other sauces and condiments. Just read labels to avoid added sugar.

Pickles—As they contain no sugar, pickles are a great low-carb staple. The salt often helps with the keto flu, and some people swear that pickles are perfect for combating cravings.

Pork rinds—Don't underestimate the humble, inexpensive pork rind. I've used pork rinds to make everything from nachos (page 260) to pancakes to casseroles (pages 357 and 368). Ground pork rinds make a great substitute for breadcrumbs and can even be used as a "breading" for meats (as in my Pickle-Brined Chicken Tenders recipe on page 318). When one of my recipes calls for "pork rind dust," you can make your own by pulverizing whole pork rinds into a fine powder in a blender. Furthermore, you can use ground pork rinds as a low-carb, high-fat flour substitute. My husband refuses to eat them straight out of the bag, but he has never refused them in a cooked dish. Don't be afraid to try them in different ways. Also, pork rinds vary by type. There are fluffy, crispy versions and smaller, harder, crunchier types. I tend to use the fluffy versions for cooking. These are also the ones that I pulverize to make pork dust to use as breadcrumbs or as a baking flour.

Balsamic vinegar—Just a splash provides a lot of flavor. Like other pantry staples, the carb counts in balsamic vinegar vary greatly by brand because of the sugar content. Buy with caution and use sparingly.

Rice wine vinegar, unseasoned—Some brands are sweetened, so use caution when buying rice wine vinegar. There are a few brands that are very low in carbs.

Salt—I use basic table salt in the recipes throughout this book; however, you may choose to use a form of sea salt if you prefer.

Seasoning salt (Jane's Krazy Mixed-Up Salt)—Many brands of seasoning salt have added sugars or starches. This is one brand that does not, so that is why I refer to it by name. You may use your preferred seasoning salt, but be aware of variations in ingredients and carb counts.

Coconut aminos—An excellent alternative to soy sauce. My favorite brand is Coconut Secret, which has a lower carb count than others. Coconut aminos are slightly sweet and not as salty as soy sauce or tamari (a wheat-free kind of soy sauce). Adjust salt in dishes that use coconut aminos if you use soy sauce instead.

Fish sauce—Provides an excellent flavor in Asian dishes, but some commercial brands have added sugars. Red Boat is one brand that does not, so I prefer it.

Tomato products—Not all tomato products are created equal. Many have added sugars or sweeteners. The best advice I can offer is to read every label and to compare nutritional values among brands. I tend to use diced tomatoes or tomato sauce, as these forms are less concentrated and provide flavor without adding too many carbs.

Whey protein isolate—Of all the ingredients you will use to make the recipes in this book, whey protein isolate is probably the most important to buy with caution. Whey protein isolate is different from whey protein; the isolate has lactose and casein removed. Look for a brand that has 0 carbs and no added sweeteners. There are only two brands that I recommend: Isopure Zero Carb

Whey Protein Isolate (Unflavored) and Jay Robb. These brands are more expensive than the whey protein powders you might find in many stores; however, those are full of really bad ingredients. Please use good judgment when purchasing whey protein isolate.

Meats and Eggs

Bone broth or bouillon—Homemade broth is super easy to make (see pages 186 and 187) and easy to keep stocked in the freezer. If you have difficulty sourcing bones or chicken feet to make your own broth, use caution when buying it. Look for brands that have no added sugars or corn syrup solids. Not only do manufacturers tend to add these, but they also remove the fat, so store-bought versions are lower in fat than homemade broth, making it less keto-friendly. If you buy broth that is low in fat, you can add some butter or your favorite fat.

Chorizo, Mexican-style fresh (raw)—Mexican chorizo is high in fat and high in flavor! I love it in anything with a Southwestern flavor. Supremo brand is easy to find and does not have added sugar and fillers, which you must be careful to check for when sourcing chorizo.

Deli meat—Often deli meat has added fillers and sugars. Check the ingredients and purchase brands without either or with less than 2 percent dextrose.

Ground beef—Not only is ground beef relatively inexpensive, but it's easy to cook quickly, making it a staple in my kitchen. I've indicated the percent lean that I used in each recipe. Often, I use 93 percent lean in dishes that would shrink in size too much if a fattier ground beef was used, such as meatloaf or meatballs. (Burgers are an exception to that rule; I want my burgers as fatty as possible!) I also use 93 percent lean ground beef in recipes that have other sources of fat, such as heavy cream or cheese or, to avoid wasting fat, in recipes that involve draining off the excess fat after cooking the meat.

Sausage—For some reason, manufacturers like to add fillers and sweeteners, particularly corn syrup, to sausage. You can easily make your own breakfast sausage with ground pork (see my recipe on page 224) or look for brands that do not have added ingredients. Jimmy Dean Naturals is a relatively clean brand that I favor.

Eggs—A standard large egg is what I use throughout this book. I prefer pastured eggs, but if I can't find those, then I buy whatever is on sale.

Sweeteners

There are many options for ketogenic sweeteners and many opinions about which ones are best. As a general rule, I prefer the natural sweeteners erythritol, monkfruit, and stevia. I also like xylitol. Artificial sweeteners such as aspartame, phenylalanine, and acesulfame potassium (Ace K) often raise blood glucose and cause cravings, so I avoid them. In addition, some sugar alcohols that are ubiquitous in sugar-free products, including maltitol, sorbitol, and mannitol, not only raise blood glucose but also cause intestinal distress. Sucralose is an artificial sweetener that I use from time to time; however, pure sucralose, which is 600 times sweeter than sugar, is not the same as Splenda. Splenda uses maltodextrin to give bulk to sucralose and make it easier to use Splenda in recipes; with the addition of maltodextrin, it measures cup for cup like sugar. The problem is that maltodextrin is a food starch and has a higher glycemic index than pure sugar! I do not recommend Splenda for that reason.

For the purpose of helping you determine which (if any) sweetener to use, I'll describe their use by texture, form (liquid, powder, or granulated), and intensity. Regardless of which sweetener you choose, be mindful that sweeteners affect each of us differently. Especially if you have diabetes, please use your meter to monitor your blood glucose to see whether a sweetener affects you adversely.

Liquid sweeteners—Most liquid sweeteners are very intense, with just a few drops providing the equivalent of ¼ to ½ cup of sugar. The liquid sweeteners with which I am most familiar are liquid sucralose and liquid stevia. The intensity of liquid stevia seems greater than that of liquid sucralose, but it varies widely by brand. Start with just a drop or two and add a drop at a time until the taste is sweet enough.

Granulated sweeteners—Granulated sweeteners can add bulk as well as sweetness. Bulk can be important in baked goods. Granulated erythritol and xylitol are examples of bulk sweeteners. Pure sucralose and powdered stevia are other non-liquid options, but they do not provide the bulk that the other types add. When I need to bulk up a recipe, I often use erythritol or xylitol, and then add powdered pure sucralose or stevia to achieve the desired sweetness. If you're using stevia, look for brands with 90 percent or higher steviosides to avoid the bitter aftertaste that can be common in stevia products.

Powdered sweeteners—Sometimes recipes call for powdered sweeteners. This can be important when you need a smooth texture, as in a ganache, "buttercream" frosting, chilled creamy dessert, or sauce. If a recipe calls for powdered sweetener, simply run your preferred granulated sweetener through a blender or coffee grinder until it is powdery.

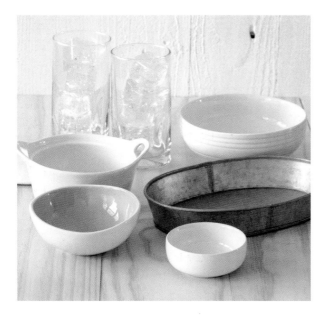

Baking for Success

My grandmother's handwritten recipes are among my most treasured possessions. She jotted them down on scraps of paper, listing each ingredient and then providing written directions for preparing them. Nearly all of her recipe instructions end with "Bake until done." That's it. No baking times or guidelines such as "Bake until the center is set." Due to variations in ingredients, oven temperatures, pan sizes, altitude, and so on, baking times may vary from my house to yours. For this reason, in many cases I offer a range of baking times as well as guidelines for how the finished product should look or feel. I hope you find this guidance helpful so that over time you can learn how to intuitively "bake until done."

Cooking Tools and Equipment

The tools and equipment used in most of the recipes in this book are very basic and, in most cases, inexpensive. I've included a short list of basic tools or equipment needed to make the recipes in this book.

Pots and pans—A basic set of pots and pans is essential. I prefer stainless steel because it holds up well over time. The essential pieces include a 2-quart saucepan with a lid, a 9-inch sauté pan, a 10-inch skillet, and a 5-quart casserole (aka soup pot). While I use a variety of skillets, I am partial to cast iron and enameled cast iron, both of which easily transition from cooktop to oven. Oven-safe skillets offer flexibility and allow for a dish to be finished in the oven without dirtying an extra pot.

Bakeware—In addition to oven-safe skillets, a couple of baking sheets (aka cookie sheets) and rimmed baking sheets (aka sheet pans) are essential. The baking sheets I use are 18 by 13 inches and 13 by 9½ inches. Also useful is a set of glass baking dishes, ramekins, and ceramic baking dishes that can be used in the oven or microwave to serve multiple functions.

Slow cooker—I confess to owning two! Slow cookers typically have a low and high setting and often have a timer function. They come in handy for cooking meals without supervision as well as for keeping foods warm. A 6-quart slow cooker will be large enough to make all of the slow cooker recipes in this book.

Food processor—This appliance is really useful for shredding large quantities of cheese or slicing lots of vegetables quickly.

Hand mixer—Very inexpensive and useful for mixing a variety of dips, sauces, or desserts. Essential for whipping cream.

Ice cream maker—Prices vary. Newer models often have bowls that must be frozen 12 to 24 hours before use but require no ice or rock salt. More expensive models often include a compressor freezer that does not require advance refrigeration and can make ice cream in about 45 minutes from start to finish.

Immersion blender—I use this tool to make mayonnaise (page 192) quickly and with minimal effort. You can also use an immersion (or stick) blender to froth coffee drinks.

Rubber spatulas—I have at least three sizes, and I use them to blend ingredients quickly and to scrape the sides of bowls to get all the goodness out.

Silicone baking mat—Use a silicone mat to line a baking sheet to help foods brown evenly and to make cleanup easy. Parchment paper is a good substitute.

Spiral slicer—There are many different spiral slicers to make vegetable noodles, and they come at a wide range of prices. Because I don't make vegetable noodles frequently, I use a small handheld tool that costs less than $10.

Whisk—A whisk is handy for beating eggs and for blending dry ingredients.

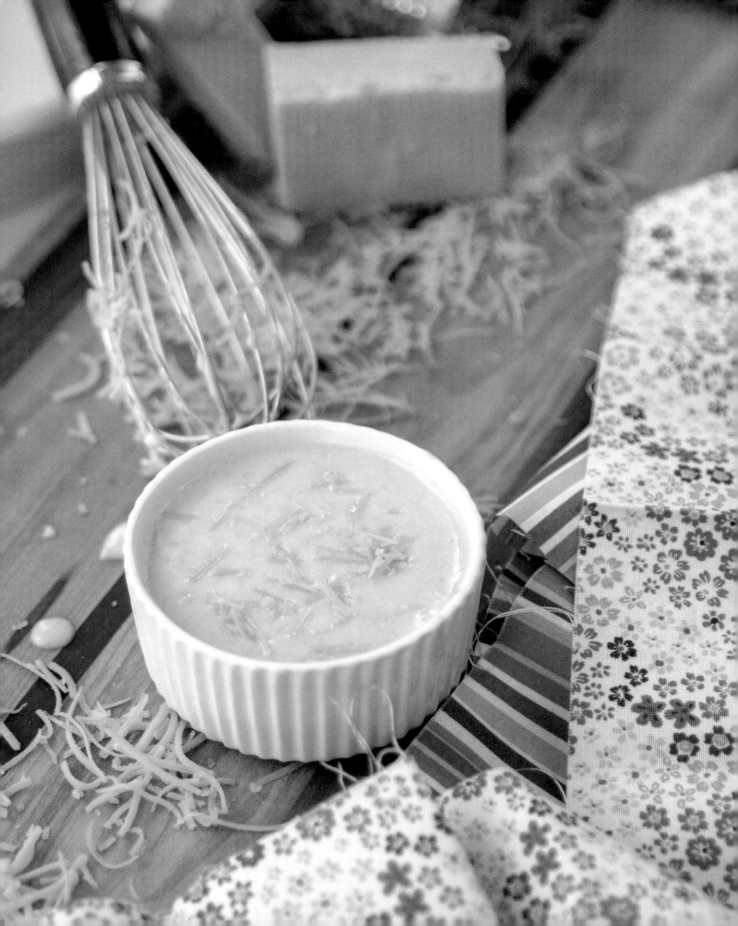

Chapter 6

The Basics

This chapter includes simple but flavorful recipes that you can use to create hundreds of meals. These sauces, condiments, and other basic recipes provide some of the most flavorful parts of any good keto meal.

Beef or Chicken Bone Broth

Bone broth can be your best friend when you first start a ketogenic diet. While there are a lot of store-bought options, including bouillon cubes and powders, nearly all of them have added sugar and/or food starches. While I've used them in a pinch, I try to make my own broth instead. Once you understand how simple it is and how amazing the flavor can be, you won't mind dem bones! Broth is believed to be healing to the gut and is certainly something you want to keep on hand to fight the keto flu, which is common in the first few weeks of a ketogenic diet. Bone broth also makes some of the best soups and stews.

Some folks believe that you should use only bones from grass-fed cattle or pastured chickens. While the way the animals were raised may be important, the evidence is anecdotal at best. If you can find and afford bones from grass-fed cattle or pastured chickens, then feel free to use them. If you only have access to bones from conventionally raised cattle or chickens, those will work, too.

There is also some debate over whether it is important to roast the bones first and whether apple cider vinegar should be added. If there is some meat or fat on the bones you're using, you may want to roast them first. In my experience, though, roasting the bones really isn't necessary and does not result in a richer broth. With regard to adding vinegar, some people believe that it helps leach the minerals from the bones. I don't know for certain whether it does, but it can't hurt. I pour just a tablespoon over the bones before adding water. That small amount does not impact the flavor of the broth but should be enough to help break down the bones.

Bone broth can be made in several ways. Some people use a pressure cooker so that the broth cooks quickly. Others simmer it on the stovetop, and still others prefer to use a slow cooker for even slower cooking. I have made bone broth using all three methods. The slow cooker method is the easiest and results in the heartiest broth. With a slow cooker, you don't have to monitor a pot on the stove, and the broth seems richer after it simmers slowly over time. I tend to start my bone broth on Friday evening and let it cook until Sunday evening when I have time to use some in a fresh batch of soup. I put the rest in containers and freeze it.

Beef bone broth is excellent for making hearty soups and stews. I use it as a base for chili and for most tomato-based soups and stews. For the best beef broth, use a variety of bones. When possible, include marrow and knuckle bones and joints for collagen. Neck bones and even hooves are excellent, too, if you can find them.

Chicken bone broth is a versatile base for chicken soups or meat and veggie stir-fries. It is excellent to sip when you're feeling under the weather. You can also use it for egg drop soup, which is perfect for fighting a cold or a queasy stomach. Like beef broth, good chicken broth requires a variety of bones—necks, backs, wings, and feet. The carcass of a roasted chicken (see page 316) is great, but you also want to add neck bones and some chicken feet if you can find them. Using feet may seem off-putting, but they add the wonderful healing collagen that makes chicken broth so healthy. If your broth doesn't jell when it cools, try adding chicken feet to your next batch.

CHICKEN BONE BROTH

NUTRITION FACTS (PER SERVING):	Calories: 40	Fat: 6g	Protein: 3.6g	Carbs: 0.5g	Fiber: 0g

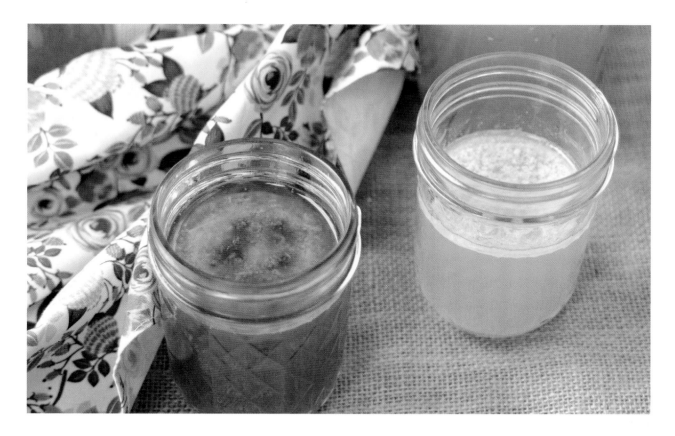

MAKES: about 2½ quarts (1 cup per serving)

3 to 4 pounds beef or chicken bones

1 tablespoon apple cider vinegar

1 tablespoon salt

3 quarts water, or more as needed

1. Place the bones in a 6-quart or larger slow cooker. Pour the vinegar over the bones, then sprinkle in the salt. Add enough water to cover the bones. Place the lid on the slow cooker and simmer on low for a minimum of 24 hours or up to 48 hours.

2. When the broth is done, remove and discard the bones. Use a fine-mesh sieve or coffee filter to strain the broth into jars. When the broth is cool, a layer of fat should form on the top. You can remove the fat or stir it into the broth when you use it. Store the jars of broth in the refrigerator for up to 1 week or in the freezer for up to 6 months.

Time-Saver Tip:

Whenever you have beef or chicken bones left over after cooking a meal, toss them into a gallon-sized freezer bag. Keep the bag in the freezer, and when the bag is full, use the bones to make broth.

BEEF BONE BROTH

NUTRITION FACTS (PER SERVING):   Calories: 55 | Fat: 8g | Protein: 4g | Carbs: 0.5g | Fiber: 0g

Baked Bacon and Rendered Bacon Fat

Bacon is one of the most delicious foods you can enjoy on a ketogenic diet. It has nearly perfect macros, with equal amounts of protein and fat and just a trace of carbohydrate. If you have ever spent hours standing over the stove frying bacon, however, it may not seem like such a perfect food. Frying bacon can be a chore. The grease splatters all over the cooktop and sometimes on your clothes or skin. Frying enough bacon for several days can take quite a while, and the pan needs to be watched closely. That's why I rarely fry bacon. The nirvana of cooking bacon is to bake it! Baking results not only in better bacon but also in far easier cleanup, while giving you the perfect way to collect bacon fat for other uses.

There are at least two schools of thought on baking bacon. The first, my way, is to bake it low and slow. I set the oven to around 300°F and bake the bacon in a single layer until it is well browned. The texture is somewhat softer and chewier than fried bacon, yet well done. It can become crispy, but it still has a softness that I really enjoy. A second popular method is to bake it quickly at higher heat. Oven temperatures of 375°F to 400°F result in crispy bacon that cooks much faster. Either way works well—it's still delicious bacon, after all! The cooking time will vary according to your preference, so if you haven't baked bacon before, you will want to monitor it closely to figure out how long it takes your bacon to reach nirvana.

Baking bacon is also a simple way to render the fat, which is like a perfect little gift left behind after the bacon is devoured. Bacon fat adds wonderful flavor to dressings and sauces and is great for frying and roasting. I could not cook keto without it.

MAKES: **about 18 slices of bacon and 2 ounces of rendered fat**

---

1 pound sliced bacon

1. Preheat the oven to 300°F. Line a 13 by 9-inch baking dish with parchment paper or aluminum foil.

2. Lay the bacon in a single layer in the lined baking dish. The slices can be touching but should not overlap. Bake for 45 to 50 minutes, until the bacon is cooked to your liking.

3. Remove the dish from the oven and use kitchen tongs to move the cooked bacon to a serving plate or tray. Let the fat cool in the baking dish for at least 10 minutes.

4. When you are ready to bottle the fat, hold one corner of the baking dish over a wide-mouth jar and pour the fat into the jar. (Recycled pickle jars and mason jars work well.) While I don't think it's necessary, you may want to cover the top of the jar with a coffee filter to catch any remaining bits of meat. If you do, use a rubber band to hold the filter in place. Create enough slack in the filter so that the bacon fat can seep through without spilling over the rim of the jar. Store the rendered fat on the countertop or in the refrigerator. I keep my jar of bacon fat right by the stove so that it is always handy.

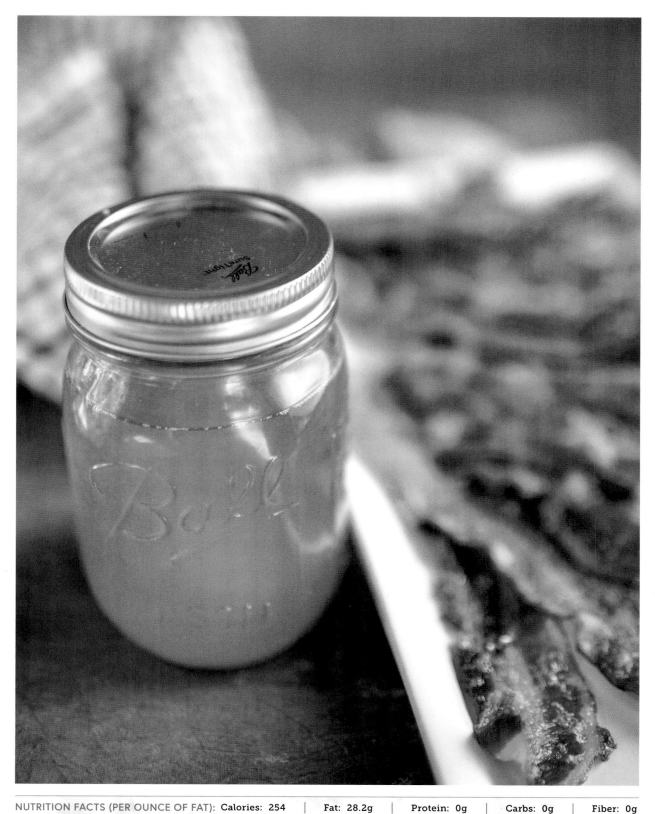

NUTRITION FACTS (PER OUNCE OF FAT): **Calories: 254** | **Fat: 28.2g** | **Protein: 0g** | **Carbs: 0g** | **Fiber: 0g**

NUTRITION FACTS (PER SLICE OF BACON): **Calories: 44** | **Fat: 3.5g** | **Protein: 4g** | **Carbs: 0.1g** | **Fiber: 0g**

Kristie's Ketchup

Yes, there are "low-carb" commercial ketchups. I used to use them, but when I started paying attention to the quality of ingredients, I decided to make my own instead. Not only is making ketchup far less expensive than buying it, but the homemade version truly tastes better!

1 (8-ounce) can tomato sauce

2 tablespoons apple cider vinegar

$\frac{1}{3}$ cup brown sugar alternative or your preferred granulated sweetener

1 teaspoon garlic powder

1 teaspoon onion powder

$\frac{1}{8}$ teaspoon ground cinnamon

$\frac{1}{8}$ teaspoon ground cloves

$\frac{1}{8}$ teaspoon salt

Mix all the ingredients together in a small saucepan. Simmer over low heat for 10 to 15 minutes, until thickened. Store in the refrigerator for up to 2 weeks.

Carb Check:

Be sure to check the ingredient list and nutrition label on the tomato sauce you buy. The carb count varies considerably from brand to brand. *Tip:* The store brand often has the fewest added ingredients and the lowest carbs.

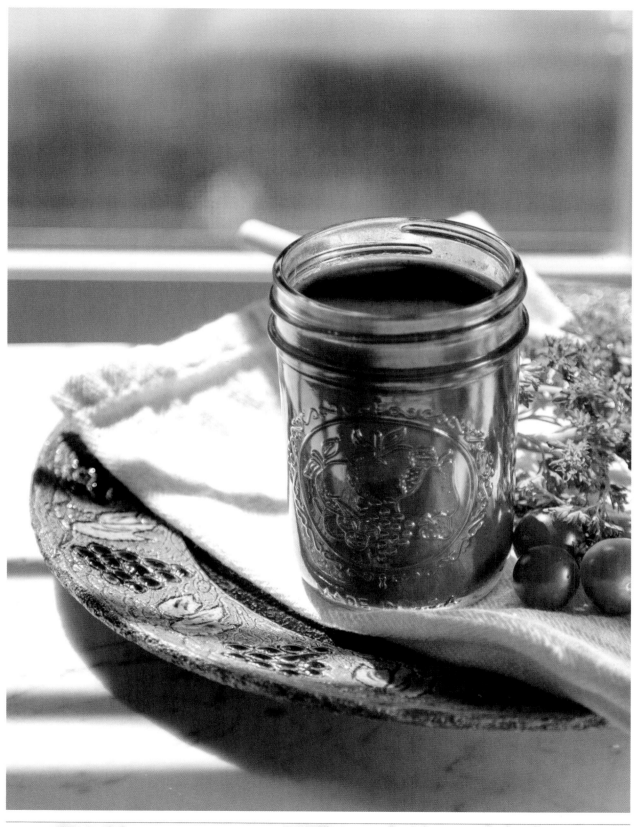

NUTRITION FACTS (PER SERVING):   Calories: 12 | Fat: 0g | Protein: 0.6g | Carbs: 2.2g | Fiber: 0.6g | Erythritol: 2g

Mayonnaise

I confess: I tried several different mayonnaise recipes over the course of three years until I finally found one that I actually liked. Until then, I paid close to $10 per jar for the kind made with avocado oil! (Please don't tell my husband.) I knew that most store-bought mayonnaise includes added sugar, and even the brands that don't are made with inflammatory soybean oil or canola oil, but when I tried making my own mayo, it was bitter or not as thick as I wanted. Eventually I found that the secret is to use avocado oil or a combination of avocado oil and bacon fat and to make it in a wide-mouthed mason jar with an immersion blender. You want to use a jar that's just wide enough to insert the blender; if you use a wider container, like a bowl, the ingredients will spread out and you won't be able to blend them fully. Once you try making your own mayo, you will discover that it is just as tasty as the high-quality store-bought options, and far less expensive.

MAKES: about 1 cup (2 tablespoons per serving)

1 large egg

1 large egg yolk

2 teaspoons lemon juice

1 teaspoon apple cider vinegar or white wine vinegar

1 teaspoon prepared yellow mustard

½ teaspoon salt

¼ cup bacon fat, melted but not hot

¾ cup avocado oil

1. Place the whole egg and egg yolk in a wide-mouthed mason jar. Add the lemon juice, vinegar, mustard, and salt, then add the bacon fat and avocado oil.

2. Push the immersion blender to the bottom of the jar and hold it steady. Begin blending. You will see the mixture begin to emulsify and start to turn white at the bottom. You may need to move the blender up and down to emulsify the entire contents of the jar evenly. Keep blending until the mayonnaise is thick and creamy and all the oil is incorporated. It will thicken as you continue to blend.

3. Store in the refrigerator for up to 10 days.

Note:

I like this mayonnaise best when it's made with a combination of avocado oil and bacon fat, but you can omit the bacon fat and use 1 cup of avocado oil if you prefer.

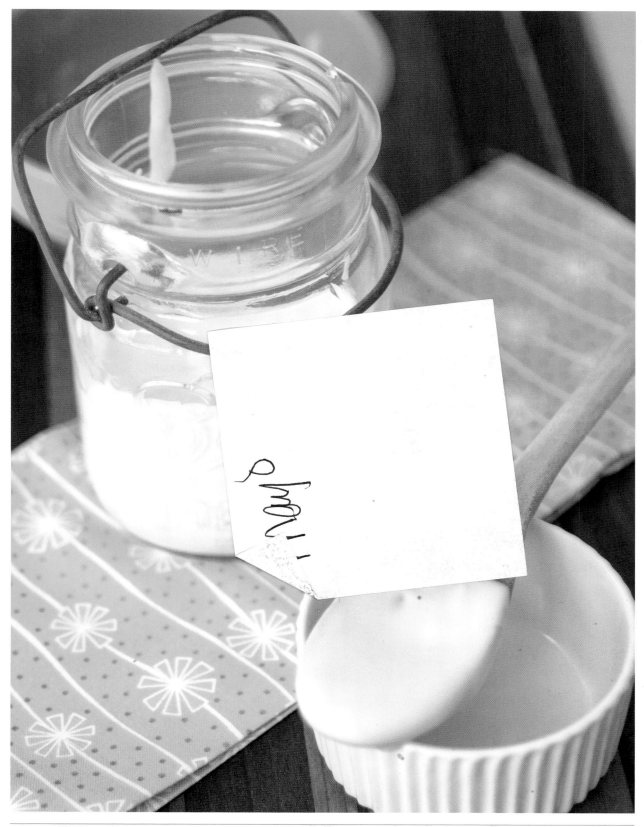

NUTRITION FACTS (PER SERVING):   Calories: 252 | Fat: 28.1g | Protein: 0.4g | Carbs: 0.3g | Fiber: 0g

Eastern NC BBQ Sauce

I often tell people that David and I have a mixed marriage. While he grew up in eastern North Carolina, I grew up in western North Carolina, where BBQ slaw is supposed to be red, like a classic tomato-based BBQ sauce. He grew up in a land where BBQ slaw is white and vinegar-based. Somehow we make it work! That's because we often compromise and have a little bit of everything on the table. I used to buy his favorite bottled vinegar-based barbecue sauce, but those eastern North Carolina folks are prone to slipping a little sugar into the bottle. We've found that this homemade sauce is equally tasty with no sugar added, but you can add sweetener if you like.

This vinegar-based sauce is lower in carbs than a traditional tomato-based sauce but packs a lot of great flavor. It should be made at least 12 hours in advance to allow the spices to flavor the vinegar.

MAKES: about 1 cup (2 tablespoons per serving)

1 cup white vinegar

1 teaspoon hot sauce

1 tablespoon salt

1 teaspoon ground black pepper

1 teaspoon red pepper flakes

1 teaspoon smoked paprika

2 teaspoons granulated sweetener, or 2 drops liquid sweetener (optional)

Mix all the ingredients in a jar or bottle with a tight-fitting lid. Store in the refrigerator for up to 3 weeks. Shake well before using.

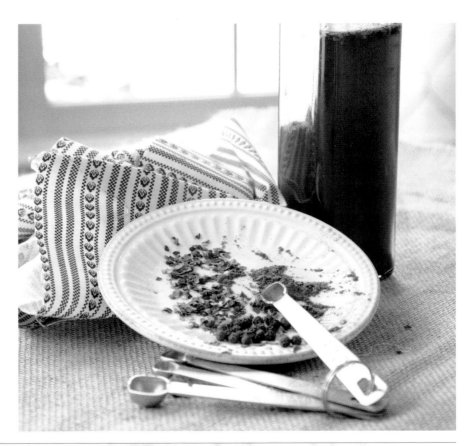

NUTRITION FACTS (PER SERVING): | Calories: 0 | Fat: 0g | Protein: 0g | Carbs: 0g | Fiber: 0g | Erythritol: 0g

Classic BBQ Sauce

If you're looking for a simple and versatile BBQ sauce to enjoy with barbecued or grilled meats, this is it! I use it on pulled pork, ribs, and wings. This classic tomato-based sauce is what I grew up eating in western North Carolina; but it's no longer just a regional style—it's the default BBQ sauce for most Americans. The addition of cinnamon and cloves is what really makes this sauce special. Maple extract and liquid smoke also kick this recipe up a notch or two. Be sure to make plenty to use as a dipping sauce at the table. Our non-low-carb family members and friends always ask for the recipe, and that's high praise!

MAKES: **about 1¼ cups (2 tablespoons per serving)**

1 tablespoon bacon fat

1 (8-ounce) can tomato sauce (no sugar added)

2 tablespoons apple cider vinegar

1 tablespoon prepared yellow mustard

1 tablespoon Worcestershire sauce

½ teaspoon maple extract

¼ teaspoon liquid smoke (optional)

1 teaspoon garlic powder

1 teaspoon onion powder

½ teaspoon mustard powder

½ teaspoon salt

¼ teaspoon cayenne pepper (optional)

⅛ teaspoon ground cinnamon

⅛ teaspoon ground cloves

Sweetener, to taste

1. Melt the bacon fat in a small saucepan. Add the tomato sauce, vinegar, mustard, and Worcestershire sauce and bring to a low simmer. Simmer for 4 to 5 minutes.

2. Add the remaining ingredients and continue to simmer over low heat for 10 to 15 more minutes to allow the sauce to thicken. It keeps well in the refrigerator for at least 2 weeks.

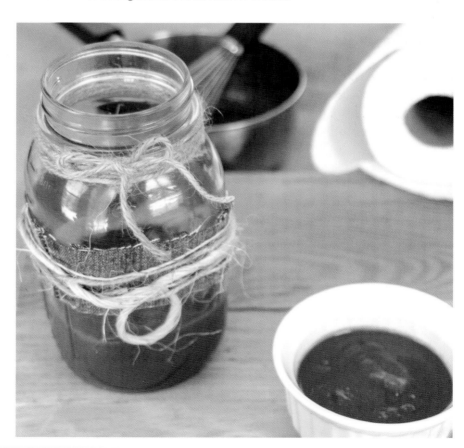

NUTRITION FACTS (PER SERVING):	Calories: 14	Fat: 0.8g	Protein: 0.3g	Carbs: 1.2g	Fiber: 0.3g

White BBQ Sauce

White BBQ sauce, which also goes by the name "Bama sauce," was created in northern Alabama to accompany barbecued chicken. It is popular in only a few Southern states, and that's really a shame. Based on mayonnaise instead of tomatoes or vinegar, white BBQ sauce is a perfect keto accompaniment because it is naturally higher in fat and lower in carbs than tomato-based sauces and higher in fat than vinegar-based sauces. I'm partial to using it on grilled chicken, but it's tasty on beef and pork as well. It is also excellent on raw or roasted vegetables.

MAKES: about 2 cups (2 tablespoons per serving)

1½ cups mayonnaise, homemade (page 192) or store-bought

¼ cup plus 1 tablespoon white wine vinegar

2 teaspoons spicy mustard

2 teaspoons prepared horseradish

1 clove garlic, minced

1 teaspoon ground black pepper

1 teaspoon granulated sweetener, or 1 drop liquid sweetener

1 teaspoon salt

Use a whisk to mix all the ingredients together until smooth. Store in a jar or container in the refrigerator for up to 2 weeks.

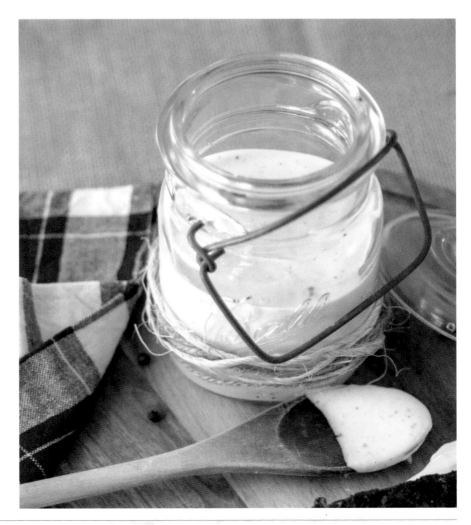

NUTRITION FACTS (PER SERVING): | Calories: 115g | Fat: 13.6g | Protein: 0.1g | Carbs: 0.4g | Fiber: 0g

Tartar Sauce

When I was younger, I loved tartar sauce. I remember being told to limit how much I used because it is high in fat and being encouraged to use lower-in-fat cocktail sauce instead. I always hated that tangy red sauce! Even before I had the words, my body knew that fat was what it craved.

Tartar sauce is simple to make. The mayonnaise base adds excellent fats, but the key is to avoid seed and vegetable oils. In general, I avoid mayonnaise made with canola oil or soybean oil because those oils are thought to contribute to inflammation. While it's often healthiest to make your own mayonnaise, there are a few good brands made with avocado oil. Whichever mayonnaise you choose, tartar sauce is a tasty way to add delicious fats to seafood dishes.

MAKES: about 1 cup (2 tablespoons per serving)

½ cup mayonnaise, homemade (page 192) or store-bought

⅓ cup chopped dill pickles

½ teaspoon lemon juice

¼ teaspoon onion powder

⅛ teaspoon salt

⅛ teaspoon ground black pepper

In a small bowl, mix all the ingredients until thoroughly combined. Chill for 30 to 60 minutes before serving. Store in the refrigerator for up to 5 days.

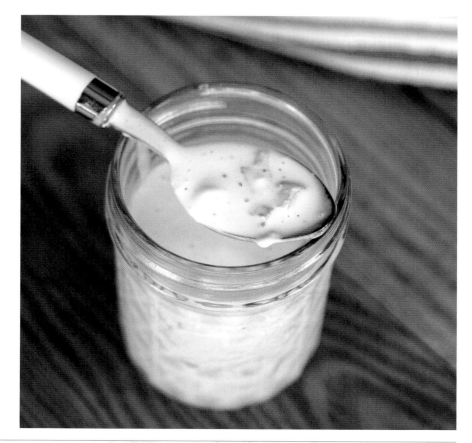

NUTRITION FACTS (PER SERVING): Calories: 66 | Fat: 7g | Protein: 0.2g | Carbs: 0.6g | Fiber: 0g

Cocktail Sauce

Even though it isn't my favorite sauce, some people enjoy this mildly spicy red sauce, which adds a nice kick to the milder flavor of shrimp. While you can use a sugar-free brand of ketchup, I strongly encourage you to make your own for this recipe. Not only is homemade ketchup lower in carbs than store-bought ketchup, but it is also less expensive and much tastier to boot.

MAKES: about ⅔ cup (2 tablespoons per serving)

½ cup ketchup, preferably homemade (page 190)

2 tablespoons prepared horseradish

1 tablespoon lemon juice

1½ teaspoons Worcestershire sauce

Dash of hot sauce (optional)

Mix all the ingredients in a small bowl. Refrigerate for at least 30 minutes before serving. The sauce will keep in the refrigerator for at least 1 week.

Carb Check:

Be sure to read labels when purchasing Worcestershire sauce. Buy the brand with the least carbs. Another word of caution is to look for horseradish that does not contain added sugar or high-fructose corn syrup.

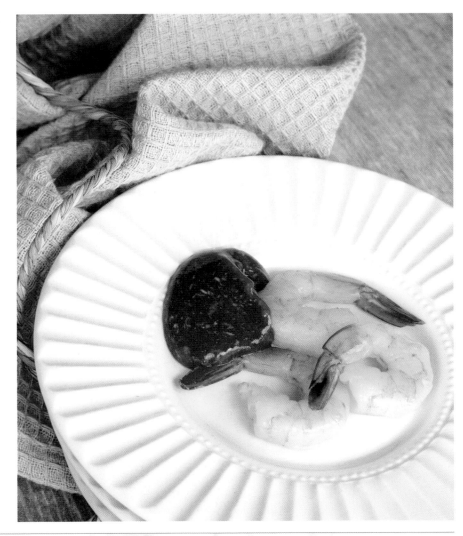

NUTRITION FACTS (PER SERVING): | Calories: 14 | Fat: 0g | Protein: 0.4g | Carbs: 2.8g | Fiber: 0.4g

Simple
Cheese Sauce

Cheese sauce is a quick and tasty way to add fat and protein to your plate. My family is particularly fond of pouring it over steamed or roasted cauliflower or broccoli, although I'm pretty sure that any vegetable would benefit from a healthy smothering of cheese sauce. The secret to a delicious and silky-smooth sauce is to use a cheese you love and whisk it in after removing the pan from the heat. If the cheese gets too hot, the proteins in it will become stringy.

MAKES: about 2 cups (¼ cup per serving)

½ cup (1 stick) salted butter

½ cup heavy cream

Pinch of cayenne pepper (optional)

Pinch of garlic powder (optional)

5 ounces cheddar cheese or other semi-firm cheese, shredded (about 1¼ cups)

Salt and pepper

1. Bring the butter and cream to a simmer in a heavy saucepan over medium-low heat. Simmer for 2 to 3 minutes, whisking constantly. Add the cayenne pepper and garlic powder, if using, and remove the pan from the heat.

2. Whisk in the cheese and continue whisking until the cheese is melted and the sauce is creamy. Season to taste with salt and pepper. The sauce will thicken as it cools.

3. Store leftover sauce in the refrigerator for up to 4 days. Reheat on the stovetop. Add a little heavy cream or bone broth to thin it, if desired.

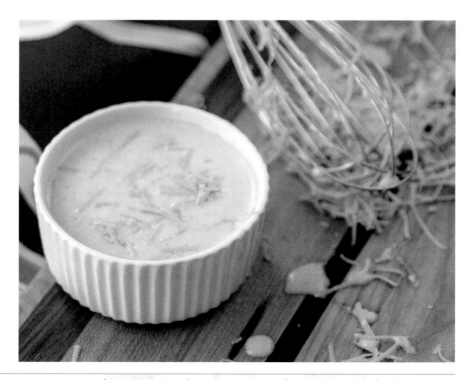

NUTRITION FACTS (PER SERVING): | Calories: 199 | Fat: 19.4g | Protein: 4.4g | Carbs: 0.8g | Fiber: 0g

Chile con Queso
(Mexican Cheese Dip with Chilies)

Don't tell my kids, but I always enjoy a little of this dip before I call them to the kitchen! Both of them really enjoy queso. They spoon it over Mexican dishes, dip pork rinds in it, or eat it straight from a spoon! The hardest part of this recipe is finding a good-quality white American cheese; see the Carb Check below for details. When made with a good white American cheese, you will want to pour this queso over everything! It really is that good!

MAKES: about 2 cups (¼ cup per serving)

3 tablespoons unsalted butter

1½ cups heavy cream

1 pound good-quality white American cheese, diced

1 (4-ounce) can green chilies

¼ teaspoon chili powder

¼ teaspoon ground cumin

¼ teaspoon garlic powder

¼ teaspoon onion powder

⅛ teaspoon salt

1. Melt the butter in a heavy saucepan over low heat. Stir in the cream. Add the cheese in small pieces and whisk until the cheese is melted. Add the remaining ingredients and whisk until smooth and creamy. Serve warm.

2. Refrigerate leftovers for up to 4 days. Reheat in a saucepan over low heat. Add a little bone broth or heavy cream to thin it, if desired.

Carb Check:

I hesitated to share this recipe because many white American cheeses contain food starches and/or inflammatory oils. Be sure to use a brand that has less than 1 gram of carbohydrate per serving, with ingredients that include only milk or cream—no food starches, canola oil, or soybean oil. Although it is pricey, Boar's Head is one of the cleanest brands I have found.

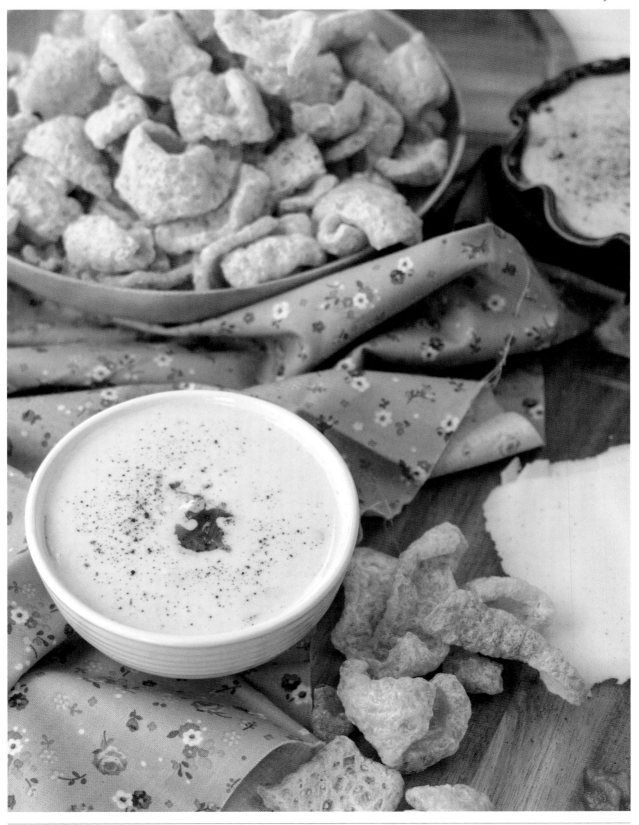

NUTRITION FACTS (PER SERVING): Calories: 227 | Fat: 21.4g | Protein: 7.7g | Carbs: 1.2g | Fiber: 0g

Lemon-Herb
Compound Butter

Compound butter can be made in hundreds of flavor combinations. Because I use it to add fat and flavor to a variety of cooked vegetables and meats, especially leaner cuts of chicken, beef, and pork, I keep my version fairly basic. You can use fresh or dried herbs, although fresh herbs generally provide more flavor. If you grow them yourself, making compound butter is an excellent way to preserve them. On the other hand, dried herbs are often easier to find and work almost as well. My recipe uses fresh herbs. If you use dried herbs instead, reduce the amounts by half. The olive oil is included to make the butter easier to spread. You can omit it if you prefer.

MAKES: about 1 cup (1 tablespoon per serving)

1 cup (2 sticks) unsalted butter, softened

1 tablespoon chopped fresh oregano

1 tablespoon chopped fresh parsley

1 tablespoon chopped fresh thyme

1½ teaspoons finely chopped fresh rosemary

1 teaspoon salt

½ teaspoon ground black pepper (optional)

1 teaspoon lemon juice

2 teaspoons olive oil (optional)

1. Use a fork to combine the softened butter, herbs, and seasonings. When well blended, add the lemon juice and olive oil, if using. Stir to combine.

2. Place the butter mixture on a sheet of parchment paper and roll into a log. Wrap tightly and refrigerate until firm, then slice crosswise into rounds to serve.

3. Store tightly wrapped in the refrigerator for up to 1 week. You can also freeze the compound butter and slice as needed. It will keep in the freezer for up to 1 month.

Time-Saver Tip:

If you're using fresh leafy herbs, kitchen shears are a great tool for snipping them finely and quickly.

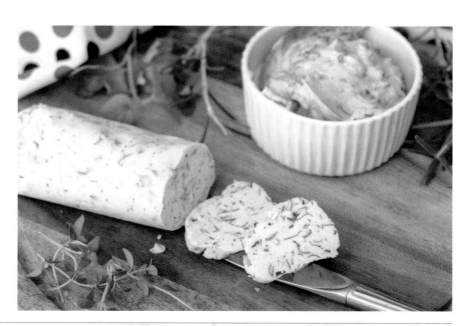

NUTRITION FACTS (PER SERVING): Calories: 102 | Fat: 12g | Protein: 0.2g | Carbs: 0.2g | Fiber: 0.1g

Marinara Sauce

Marinara is a basic Italian sauce that can be used as a base for pizza sauce or as a dipping sauce. It is made mostly of tomatoes and without meat, so it can be high in carbs. Adding olive oil helps increase the fat content, but you will want to use this sauce sparingly to minimize your carbohydrate intake.

MAKES: 2 cups (⅓ cup per serving)

2 (8-ounce) cans tomato sauce

¼ cup olive oil

1 tablespoon Italian seasoning

2 teaspoons garlic powder

1 teaspoon onion powder

½ teaspoon salt

In a heavy saucepan, warm the tomato sauce. Add the remaining ingredients and simmer for 10 minutes, stirring occasionally. Serve warm. Store leftovers in the refrigerator for up to 5 days.

Carb Check:

Be sure to check tomato sauce labels for added sugars. Carb counts vary widely by brand, so shop carefully for the brand with the lowest carb count per serving. Also, spices add carbs, so be sure to account for those if you use more seasonings than called for.

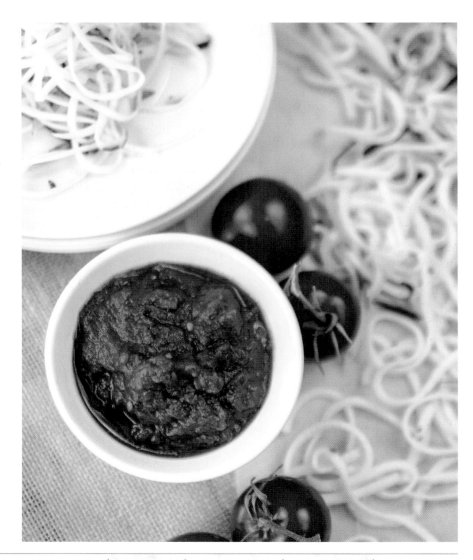

NUTRITION FACTS (PER SERVING):   Calories: 104 | Fat: 9.3g | Protein: 1.2g | Carbs: 5.4g | Fiber: 1.4g

Creamy Alfredo Sauce

As classic as a string of pearls, this versatile Alfredo sauce goes with everything! There is no vegetable or meat that would not taste better with a little of this rich, fatty sauce drizzled over it. Kick it up with a pinch of cayenne pepper or upscale it even more by adding crispy bacon pieces. You might want to make a double batch to have on hand for adding fat to lean proteins like chicken breast or pork tenderloin. Grab a whisk and learn to make this easy staple without flour!

MAKES: 1½ cups (¼ cup per serving)

½ cup (1 stick) salted butter

2 ounces cream cheese (¼ cup)

¾ cup heavy cream

1 teaspoon minced garlic

Dash of ground nutmeg (optional)

Freshly cracked black pepper

5 ounces Parmesan cheese, grated (about 1½ cups)

1. In a heavy saucepan over low heat, whisk to combine the butter and cream cheese as they melt. Add the cream and continue whisking over low heat until smooth and creamy.

2. Add the garlic, nutmeg (if using), pepper, and Parmesan cheese. Continue whisking until the sauce is creamy and well blended, keeping the heat low so that the sauce doesn't break or separate.

3. Refrigerate leftover sauce for up to 4 days. Reheat in a saucepan over low heat, stirring constantly. Add a little heavy cream or bone broth to thin it, if needed.

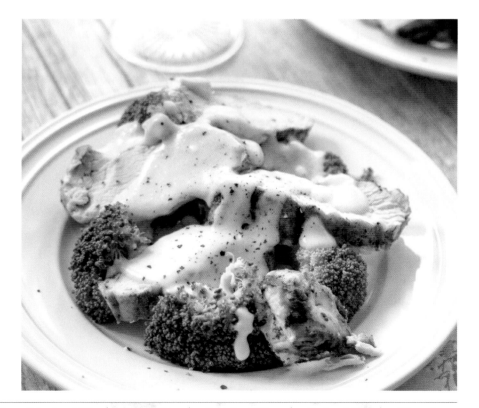

NUTRITION FACTS (PER SERVING):   Calories: 387 | Fat: 36.3g | Protein: 10.7g | Carbs: 1.2g | Fiber: 0g

Guacamole

The lime juice in this guacamole gives the avocado a bright hit of flavor. My family likes a creamier guacamole, but if you prefer a chunkier style, then cut the avocado into pieces and stir it after all the other ingredients have been blended. Though it's not traditional, I add sour cream to up the fat content and for the extra creamy and luxurious texture it provides. Because we adore cilantro, we typically set some aside to use for garnish.

OPTION

1 large Hass avocado, cut in half and pitted

1½ tablespoons lime juice

1 tablespoon sour cream

¼ cup chopped fresh cilantro

2 tablespoons finely chopped red onions

2 tablespoons seeded and finely chopped jalapeño peppers

¼ teaspoon salt

⅛ teaspoon ground black pepper

Substitution Suggestion:

To make this guacamole dairy-free, omit the sour cream.

MAKES: about 1 cup (¼ cup per serving)

Scoop the avocado flesh into a small bowl. Add the lime juice and sour cream and mix with a fork until smooth. Add the remaining ingredients and stir until thoroughly mixed. Serve immediately. Refrigerate leftovers for up to 3 days.

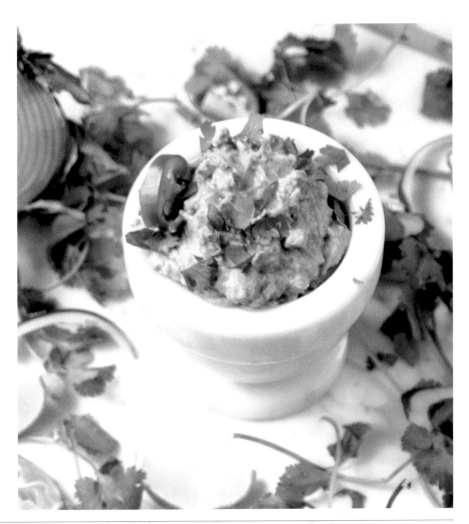

NUTRITION FACTS (PER SERVING): | Calories: **51** | Fat: **4.3g** | Protein: **0.7g** | Carbs: **3.7g** | Fiber: **2g**

Simple
Salsa Fresca

Not quite salsa and not quite pico de gallo, salsa fresca is a delicious combination of fresh flavors that complements any Southwestern dish. Using cucumbers keeps the carb count lower than using all tomatoes. The cucumber lends a refreshing crunch and absorbs the flavors of the spices. Altogether, it's a unique blend that's fun to share or keep all to yourself.

MAKES: about 1½ cups (¼ cup per serving)

¾ cup peeled and diced cucumbers

¾ cup seeded and diced tomatoes

¼ cup fresh cilantro leaves, chopped

2 tablespoons diced green bell peppers

1 jalapeño pepper, seeded and finely chopped

1 tablespoon finely chopped onions

1 tablespoon minced garlic

2 tablespoons red wine vinegar

1 tablespoon lime juice

1 teaspoon ground cumin

Dash of salt

Dash of ground black pepper

Mix all the ingredients in a glass bowl and refrigerate for 20 to 30 minutes before serving. Store in the refrigerator for up to 3 days.

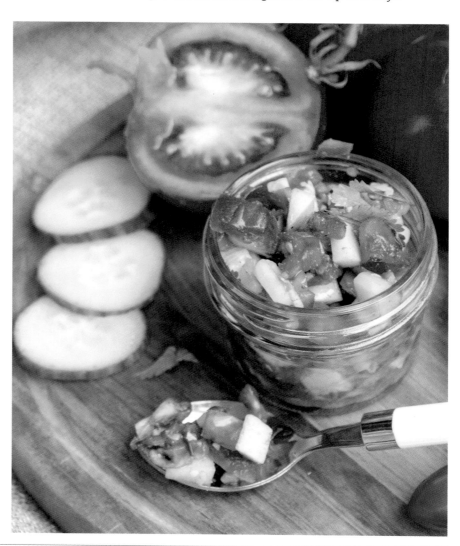

Carb Check:

Peeling the cucumber reduces the amount of carbohydrates in this salsa.

NUTRITION FACTS (PER SERVING):   Calories: 15 | Fat: 0.1g | Protein: 0.7g | Carbs: 3.4g | Fiber: 0.9g

Taco Seasoning

Yes, I know that premade taco seasoning exists. Did you know that most brands are full of food starches and sugars? Since my body has never met a carb it liked, I do everything I can to avoid them! Spices naturally contain some carbohydrates, so I like to make my own seasoning mixes to minimize carbs and maximize flavor.

MAKES: ⅓ cup

2 tablespoons chili powder

1 tablespoon ground cumin

1 tablespoon paprika

1 teaspoon garlic powder

1 teaspoon onion powder

1 teaspoon dried oregano leaves

½ teaspoon salt

Mix all the ingredients well and store in an airtight container in the pantry, away from direct sunlight, for up to 6 weeks.

Time-Saver Tip:

This recipe makes just over 5 tablespoons of seasoning. I typically use 2 tablespoons per pound of ground beef. Because my family really enjoys taco flavor, I tend to double this recipe so that I have some on hand whenever I need it.

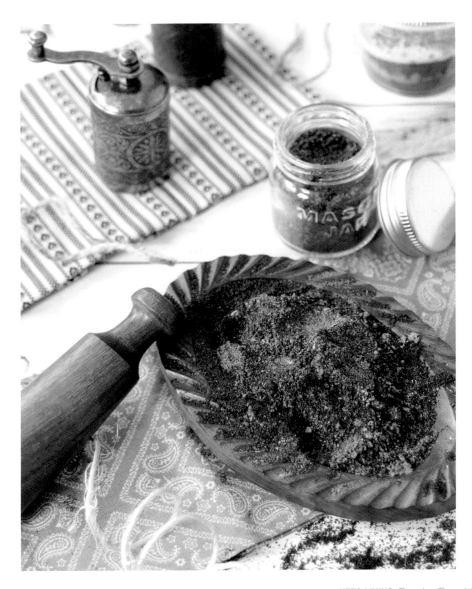

Parmesan Peppercorn Dressing

This fatty dressing works well with Roasted Chicken Wings (page 259) or any grilled meat. It is also delicious on salads; its peppery flavor makes it especially good with tomatoes and cucumbers. The Parmesan cheese gives the dressing a hint of Italian flavor, but it isn't really an Italian dressing. Grating the Parmesan into different sizes gives it a nice texture if you want to use it as a dipping sauce. I love to serve it this way with a tray of raw vegetables.

MAKES: about 1½ cups (¼ cup per serving)

¾ cup mayonnaise, homemade (page 192) or store-bought

½ cup sour cream

⅓ cup heavy cream

1 teaspoon white wine vinegar

1 teaspoon Worcestershire sauce

½ teaspoon salt

1 tablespoon coarsely ground black pepper

½ teaspoon garlic powder

½ teaspoon onion powder

½ teaspoon dried parsley

1 ounce Parmesan cheese, grated (about ⅓ cup)

1. In a bowl, stir together the mayonnaise, sour cream, and heavy cream until smooth and creamy. Add the vinegar, Worcestershire sauce, salt, and spices and mix well. Stir in the Parmesan cheese.

2. Place in the refrigerator to chill for 20 to 30 minutes before serving. Store in the fridge for up to 1 week.

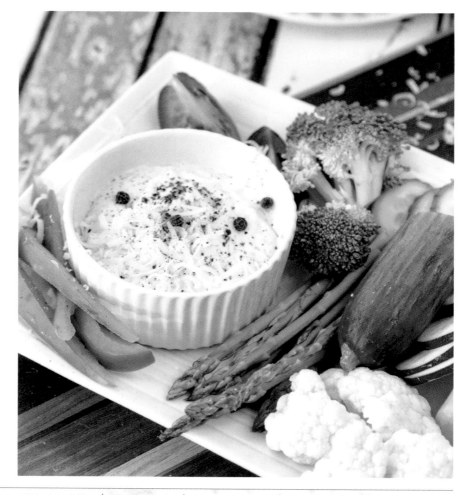

Carb Check:

Be sure to use a block of Parmesan that you grate yourself or use a pregrated Parmesan from the refrigerated cheese section of the grocery store. Shelf-stable canned Parmesan frequently contains fillers and does not have the flavor or low-carb value of real Parmesan cheese.

NUTRITION FACTS (PER SERVING):   Calories: 310 | Fat: 32.6g | Protein: 2.7g | Carbs: 2.8g | Fiber: 0.3g

Thousand Island Dressing

Thousand Island is a classic sweet dressing that many people love, and it can be part of a low-carb lifestyle. This dressing is fantastic over salad or as a dip for crudités, but I use it primarily for the Big Mac Salad on page 283. It's the "special sauce" that reminds you there is no deprivation in a ketogenic lifestyle.

MAKES: about ¾ cup (¼ cup per serving)

½ cup mayonnaise, homemade (page 192) or store-bought

2 tablespoons ketchup, homemade (page 190) or store-bought

2 tablespoons sugar-free dill pickle relish

2 teaspoons dried minced onions, or ½ teaspoon onion powder

2 teaspoons white vinegar

¼ teaspoon garlic powder

¼ teaspoon salt

8 drops liquid sweetener, or to taste

Mix all the ingredients together in a small bowl. Place in the refrigerator to chill for 20 to 30 minutes before serving. Store in the fridge for up to 1 week.

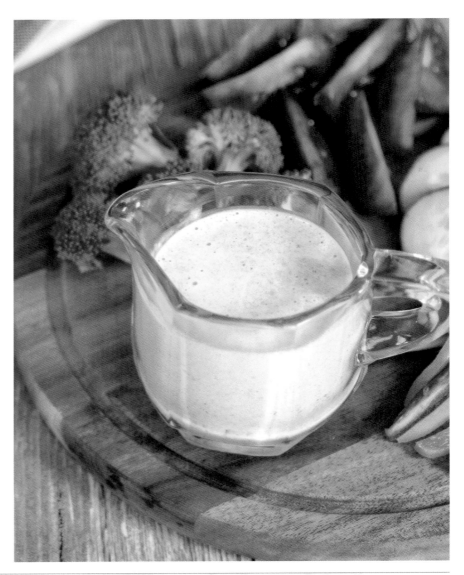

Carb Check:

Be sure to look for a relish that has no added sugar or high-fructose corn syrup.

NUTRITION FACTS (6 SERVINGS): | Calories: 216 | Fat: 25.6g | Protein: 0g | Carbs: 1g | Fiber: 0g

Hot Bacon Fat Dressing

My maternal grandmother always had bacon fat by the stove—at least until she listened to her doctor and went low-fat. Before that, back in the good ol' days, she would heat up a couple spoonfuls of bacon fat, toss in some vinegar and seasonings, and pour it warm over salad greens. It was so good that we licked the plate clean even though she pretended to fuss about it! I serve this dressing over spinach salad with boiled eggs and bacon (see page 353) for a meal with nearly perfect ketogenic macros. Quite frankly, Hot Bacon Fat Dressing is the only civilized way to dress a spinach salad.

MAKES: about ¾ cup (2 tablespoons per serving)

½ cup bacon fat

¼ cup apple cider vinegar

1 tablespoon Dijon mustard

Dash of salt

Dash of ground black pepper

6 drops liquid sweetener

Heat the bacon fat in a small saucepan, then whisk in the remaining ingredients. Serve warm and mix again just before pouring. Store in the refrigerator for up to 10 days. Reheat on the stovetop or in the microwave.

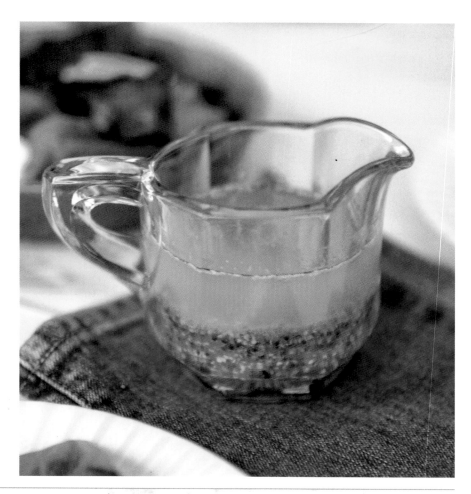

NUTRITION FACTS (PER SERVING):   Calories: 152 | Fat: 16g | Protein: 0g | Carbs: 0g | Fiber: 0g

Blue Cheese Dressing

You might wonder why anyone would take the time to make something that can easily be bought from a store. Trust me when I say that after the first bite of this dressing, you will know exactly why! Some things simply cannot be bottled, and a good blue cheese dressing is one of them. Serve this dressing over salad or with Roasted Chicken Wings (page 259) or crunchy pork rinds, but don't blame me if you find yourself licking it off your fingers!

MAKES: about 1 cup (¼ cup per serving)

⅓ cup mayonnaise, homemade (page 192) or store-bought

¼ cup heavy cream

¼ cup sour cream

3 teaspoons lemon juice, or 2 teaspoons white vinegar

¼ teaspoon garlic powder

¼ teaspoon salt

4 ounces blue cheese, crumbled (about 1 cup)

In a small bowl, whisk together the mayonnaise, heavy cream, sour cream, lemon juice, garlic powder, and salt until well blended. Add the blue cheese crumbles and stir well to combine. Place in the refrigerator to chill for about 45 minutes before serving. Store in the fridge for up to 1 week.

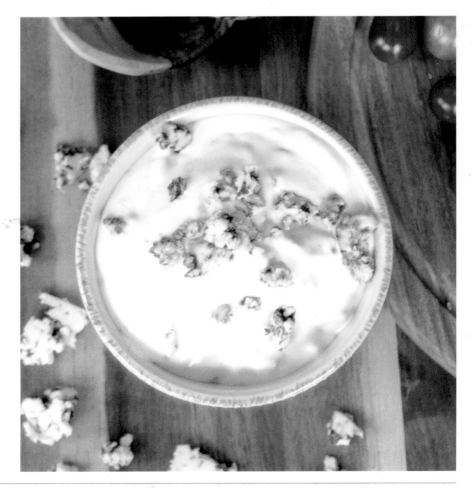

NUTRITION FACTS (6 SERVINGS): | Calories: 169 | Fat: 15.7g | Protein: 4.3g | Carbs: 0.8g | Fiber: 0g

Basic Vinaigrette

This simple vinaigrette is so easy to make that I keep the ingredients in my office at work so I can make up a small batch whenever I need it. When stored separately, the ingredients are shelf stable. I use this vinaigrette when I want a dressing with a neutral flavor so that the salad ingredients can shine through. It is especially good over salads that include fresh tomatoes.

MAKES: about ⅔ cup (2 tablespoons per serving)

⅓ cup olive oil or avocado oil

¼ cup white wine vinegar or apple cider vinegar

¼ teaspoon dried minced garlic (see Note)

½ teaspoon Italian seasoning

¼ teaspoon salt

Put all the ingredients in a jar with a lid. Secure the lid and shake the jar vigorously. Pour the vinaigrette over your favorite salad. Store in the refrigerator for up to 2 weeks. Shake before using.

VARIATION: Creamy Vinaigrette

To make a creamy vinaigrette, add 2 tablespoons homemade (page 192) or store-bought mayonnaise or sour cream to the jar with the rest of the ingredients before shaking.

Note:

I use shelf-stable dried minced garlic for this dressing so I can keep the ingredients on hand and ready to mix together at a moment's notice. If you prefer, you can replace it with ½ teaspoon minced fresh garlic.

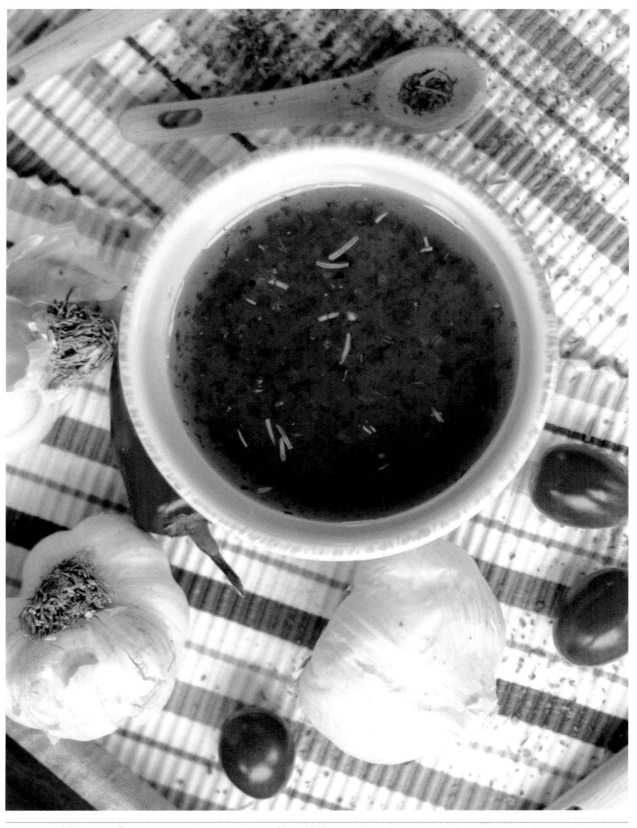

NUTRITION FACTS (PER SERVING):   Calories: 107 | Fat: 12.5g | Protein: 0g | Carbs: 0.2g | Fiber: 0g

The Sullivans'
KeDough Pizza Crust

A handheld keto pizza crust is a rarity. This crisp crust is perfect for holding in your hands—no fork or plate required. We love it enough to put the family name on it! Not only is it just like "real" pizza crust, but it can also be used to make a Breakfast Pizza (page 238). I've even been known to bake this versatile dough in a donut pan to make low-carb bagels! It requires no melting of cheese in advance. You can mix the batter with a spatula and smooth it out with a wooden spoon without getting your hands dirty. My favorite low-carb toppings include pepperoni, sausage, bacon, bell peppers, onions, black olives, and shredded mozzarella. For the sauce, you can use the homemade marinara on page 203 or make an amazing white pizza using the Creamy Alfredo Sauce on page 204. If you don't have time to make your own sauce, canned tomato sauce or softened cream cheese will work just fine.

MAKES: one 13 by 9-inch rectangular crust, one 9-inch round crust, or four 5-inch round crusts (4 servings)

½ cup unflavored whey protein isolate

½ teaspoon baking powder

½ teaspoon granulated garlic

½ teaspoon Italian seasoning

½ teaspoon salt

5 ounces mozzarella cheese, shredded (about 1¼ cups)

1 ounce Parmesan cheese, grated (about ⅓ cup)

2 ounces cream cheese (¼ cup), softened

¼ cup olive oil

1 large egg

1. Preheat the oven to 375°F. Line a pizza stone or baking sheet with parchment paper.

2. Put all the ingredients in a large mixing bowl and, using a rubber spatula, mix until combined. The mixture will be more like a thick batter than a workable dough.

3. Place the dough on the lined stone or baking sheet and use a wooden spoon or spatula to smooth it into a 13 by 9-inch rectangle or a 9-inch circle. Alternatively, you can divide the dough into fourths and create four 5-inch round crusts.

4. Par-bake the crust(s) for 9 to 12 minutes, until golden brown, then remove from the oven.

5. To make a pizza, top the par-baked crust(s) with your favorite sauce and toppings, or freeze the crust(s) for later use. Return the topped crust(s) to the oven to bake until the toppings are browned and the cheese is melted, 6 to 8 minutes.

Time-Saver Tip:

The par-baked crust freezes well and can be pulled from the freezer, piled with toppings while still frozen, and baked until hot for a quick meal.

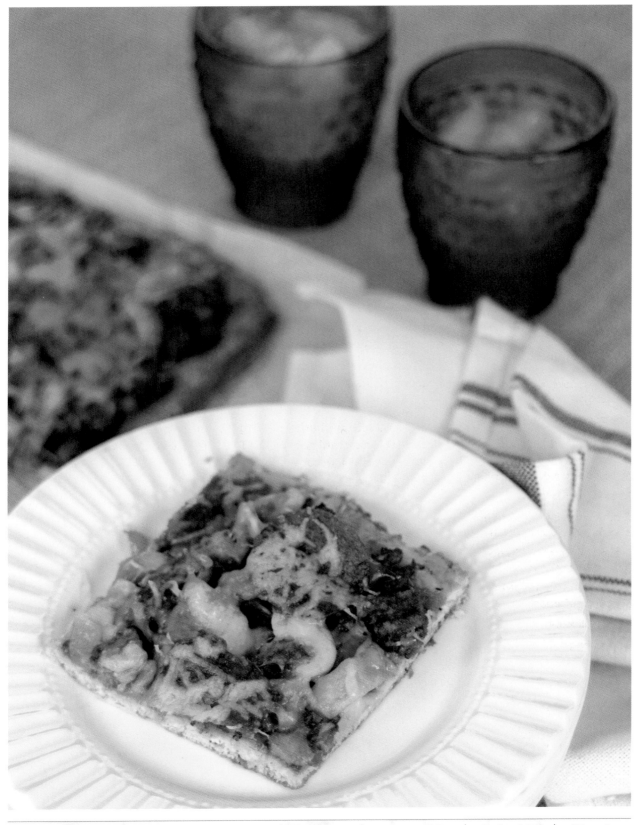

NUTRITION FACTS (PER SERVING):   **Calories:** 414 | **Fat:** 48.7g | **Protein:** 22.5g | **Carbs:** 1.5g | **Fiber:** 0g

Unsweetened Iced Tea

Iced tea is known as the table wine of the South. I suspect that its ubiquitous nature might be linked to the prevalence of obesity and diabetes across the land I love, since it is traditionally served as a highly concentrated sweet elixir. Fortunately, iced tea is not off the table on a ketogenic diet. When made properly, unsweetened iced tea is smooth and refreshing and not at all bitter. The emphasis here is on making it properly. If you can boil water, you can make a superior iced tea. Just promise me that you will never, ever boil the tea bags. That tragedy results in a bitter, undrinkable brew. Another tip is to use a glass pitcher. Plastic is said to make iced tea bitter, and it truly does taste smoother in a glass or ceramic pitcher.

You may choose to sweeten your iced tea with a keto-friendly sweetener; however, after a few weeks of following a ketogenic diet, you may find that you prefer it unsweetened.

MAKES: 1 gallon (8 ounces per serving)

4 cups water

6 tea bags

1. Place the water in a saucepan and bring to a rolling boil. Remove from the heat and wait a full minute, then add the tea bags. Place the lid on the pan and set aside to steep for 1 to 2 hours. I wait at least 2 hours.

2. After the tea has steeped, remove the tea bags and pour the tea into a gallon-sized pitcher. The concentrated tea will not fill the pitcher, so add cold water until the pitcher is full. Refrigerate for at least an hour before serving over plenty of ice. Best used within 6 days.

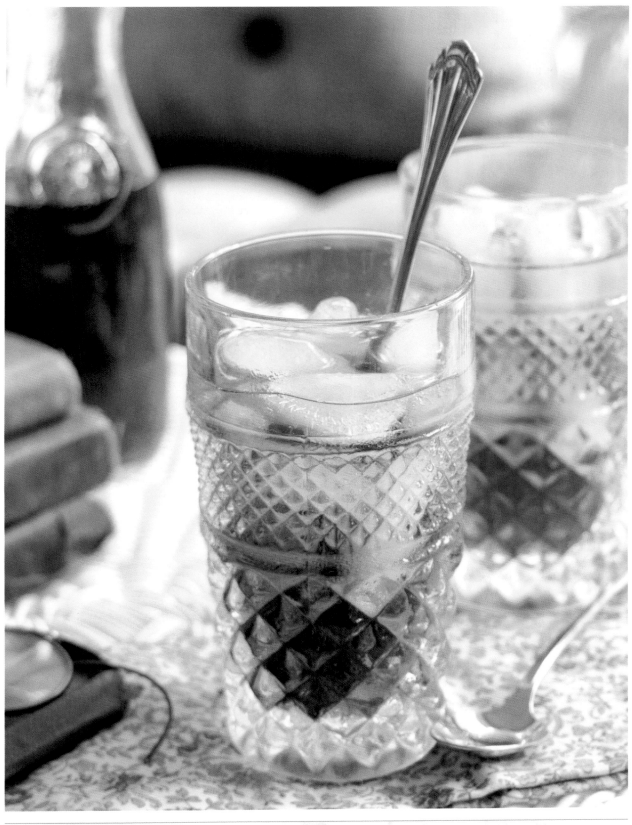

NUTRITION FACTS (PER SERVING):   Calories: 0 | Fat: 0g | Protein: 0g | Carbs: 0g | Fiber: 0g

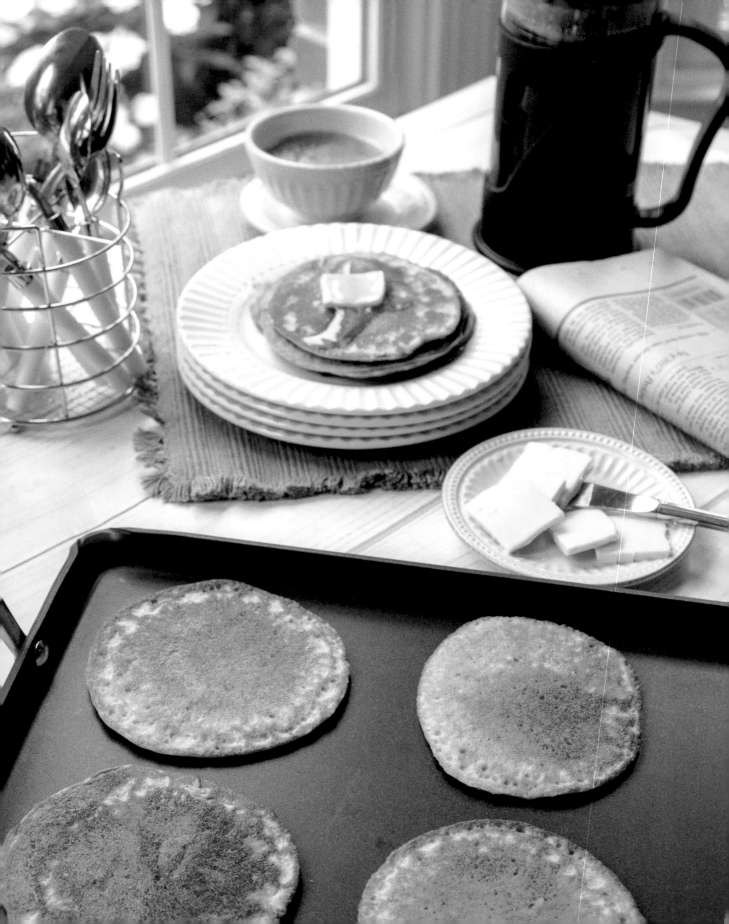

Chapter 7
Breakfast

For most of us, breakfast, especially on week-days, must be fast and easy or made ahead of time. Truthfully, my family is more likely to eat leftover dinner for breakfast than they are to eat a traditional egg-based dish, because none of us really loves eggs. For that reason, the egg recipes in this chapter are designed for people who are not big fans of eggs or who might become easily bored by them. I feature some nontraditional combinations along with some dishes highlighting other flavors that mask the egg taste.

While this chapter does include some sweet options, I encourage you to make your first thirty days on keto sweetener-free. Still, if you find yourself flipping for pancakes, I have given you a suitable low-carb recipe.

Minute Mug Omelet

Many folks complain that they don't have time to cook breakfast, and the thought of washing dishes while getting everyone out the door is enough to keep the skillet tucked away. Because mornings tend to be hectic, many of us become accustomed to grabbing a high-carb option and eating on the run. This Minute Mug Omelet is a super low-carb alternative. First, it's fast because it uses ingredients you already have on hand that don't have to be cooked. If you choose the right ingredients, it has nearly perfect macros! Second, it requires minimal cleanup. You mix, cook, and eat from one mug. Third, if you have a house full of people with varying food preferences, then everyone can choose ingredients according to their tastes.

OPTION

MAKES: 1 serving

1 large egg

⅓ cup meat(s) of choice

¼ cup veggie(s) of choice

2 tablespoons cheese(s) of choice

Fresh or dried herb(s) or other seasoning(s) of choice

Pinch of salt

Crack the egg into a 10-ounce microwave-safe mug and use a fork to beat the egg until frothy. Add the meat(s), veggie(s), cheese(s), and seasoning(s) of your choice, along with the salt, and stir to combine. (See my suggested additions below.) Microwave for 1 minute, or until the egg is set. Let sit for 1 minute before serving.

Substitution Suggestion:

To make this omelet dairy-free, omit the cheese.

Carb Check:

If you add veggies to your omelet, be sure to balance the carbohydrates with fat and protein. Meats typically provide mostly protein and fat, while cheese provides fat and some protein. Vegetables add carbs almost exclusively.

Meats	Veggies	Cheeses
Bacon, cooked and crumbled	Bell pepper, diced	Cream cheese, softened
Ham, diced	Broccoli florets, steamed and chopped	Cheddar cheese, shredded
Pepperoni, chopped	Mushrooms, sliced	Goat cheese
Breakfast Sausage (page 224), cooked and chopped	Spinach, chopped	Smoked Gouda, shredded

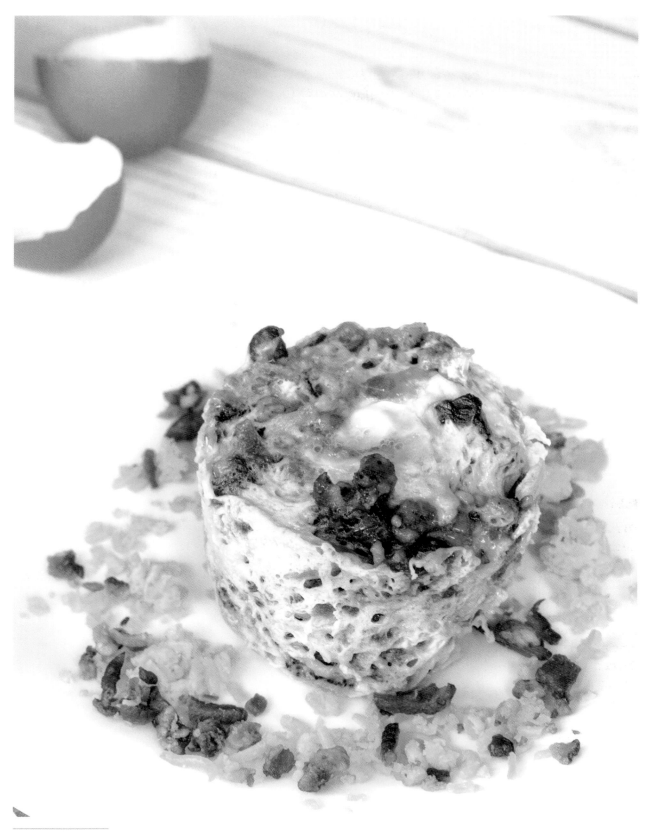

NUTRITION FACTS: Calories, fat, protein, carbs, and fiber will vary depending on the meats, veggies, and cheeses you choose.

Breakfast Sausage

While there are a lot of commercial breakfast sausages available, many contain sugars and food starches that can interfere with weight loss. One easy way to avoid those is to make your own sausage. Ground pork is the traditional choice, but the ground pork available at most grocery stores has less fat than what professional sausage makers use. As a result, the texture of homemade breakfast sausage will be slightly drier than the commercial versions you may be used to. Adding bacon fat (or any fat) will help make the texture more moist. You can adjust the seasonings to your taste.

MAKES: 1 pound (8 servings)

1 pound ground pork

2 tablespoons bacon fat, melted

1½ teaspoons ground dried sage

½ teaspoon garlic powder

½ teaspoon ground dried thyme

½ teaspoon salt

¼ teaspoon ground black pepper

¼ teaspoon red pepper flakes

1. Place all the ingredients in a bowl and use your hands to mix until well combined. Chill the sausage mixture in the refrigerator for at least 20 minutes, then shape into 8 patties.

2. Fry the patties in a skillet over medium-high heat until browned and no longer pink in the center, 12 to 15 minutes. Serve warm. Refrigerate leftovers for up to 5 days.

Substitution Suggestion:

If you avoid pork, you may use ground turkey or chicken instead.

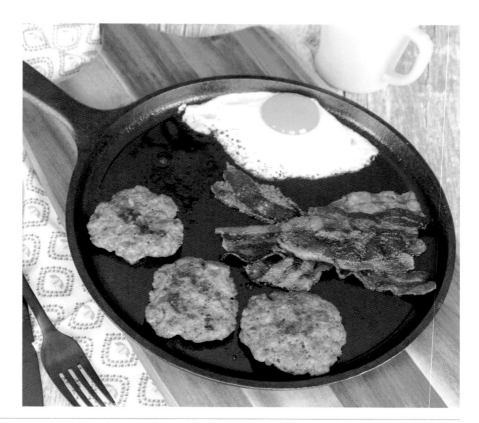

NUTRITION FACTS (PER SERVING):   Calories: 182 | Fat: 15.7g | Protein: 9.6g | Carbs: 0.5g | Fiber: 0.1g

Sausage Gravy

Perhaps even more than pancakes, I associate creamy sausage gravy with a decadent breakfast. It's rich and thick and full of fatty protein. The instant coffee in this recipe is optional, but it gives the gravy a richer, deeper flavor. Without flour, this gravy is actually very low in carbs! I love that I can eat foods like this and lose weight. While there are low-carb biscuit options, many are higher in carbs than I prefer. As you're getting started on keto, it may be better to serve this gravy over scrambled eggs or even a side of sausage.

MAKES: 6 servings

1 pound breakfast sausage, homemade (opposite) or store-bought

6 ounces cream cheese (¾ cup)

½ cup heavy cream

½ cup beef bone broth, homemade (page 187) or store-bought

1 teaspoon garlic powder

½ teaspoon onion powder

⅛ teaspoon instant coffee powder (optional)

¼ teaspoon salt

1. In a large skillet over medium heat, cook the sausage until well browned and crumbled. Reduce the heat to low, then add the cream cheese and stir until melted. Stir in the cream and broth.

2. Add the remaining ingredients and stir until the gravy comes to a simmer. Simmer for a few minutes to thicken the gravy before serving.

Carb Check:

If using store-bought sausage, be sure to check the ingredients for wheat, sugar, and food starches.

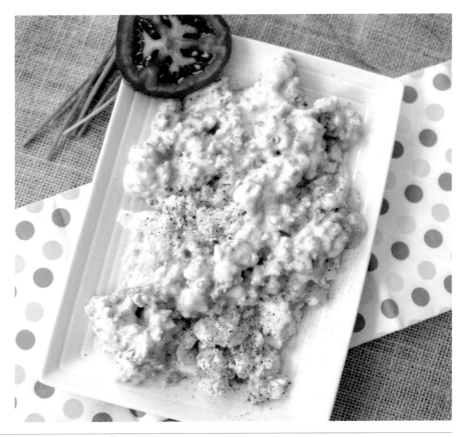

NUTRITION FACTS (PER SERVING): Calories: 380 | Fat: 35g | Protein: 15.2g | Carbs: 1.9g | Fiber: 0.2g

Breakfast Skillet Scrambles

Some people can make gorgeous omelets and flip them in the air. My omelets look as if they were flipped in the air, but often end up too well-done on the outside while remaining runny on the inside, even when I babysit them carefully and keep the heat low. A compromise that saves me time and frustration is to cook or warm the fillings first, then add the eggs to the skillet. As the eggs cook, I scramble them with the omelet fillings. Adding the cheese last melts the cheese without it getting lost in the scramble. The following are three of my favorite Breakfast Skillet Scramble combinations. While the recipes call for ghee, you can also use bacon fat.

Sausage and Goat Cheese Skillet Scramble with Spinach and Sun-Dried Tomatoes

Something about the combination of spinach and eggs just seems healthy. I also love the creamy goat cheese and the punch of flavor from the sun-dried tomatoes and sausage, which hides the egg taste a bit.

MAKES: 1 serving

1 tablespoon ghee

2 ounces breakfast sausage, homemade (page 224) or store-bought

1 ounce fresh spinach

1 teaspoon finely chopped sun-dried tomatoes

2 large eggs, beaten

2 ounces fresh (soft) goat cheese, crumbled (about ½ cup)

Dash of salt

Dash of ground black pepper

1. In a medium-sized skillet over medium heat, melt the ghee. Add the sausage and cook until browned and crumbled. Add the spinach and sun-dried tomatoes and cook until the spinach just begins to wilt.

2. Pour the beaten eggs over the mixture in the skillet. As the eggs cook, use a spatula to scramble them with the sausage, spinach, and sun-dried tomatoes. When the eggs are softly scrambled, sprinkle in the goat cheese, salt, and pepper and remove the skillet from the heat. Serve immediately.

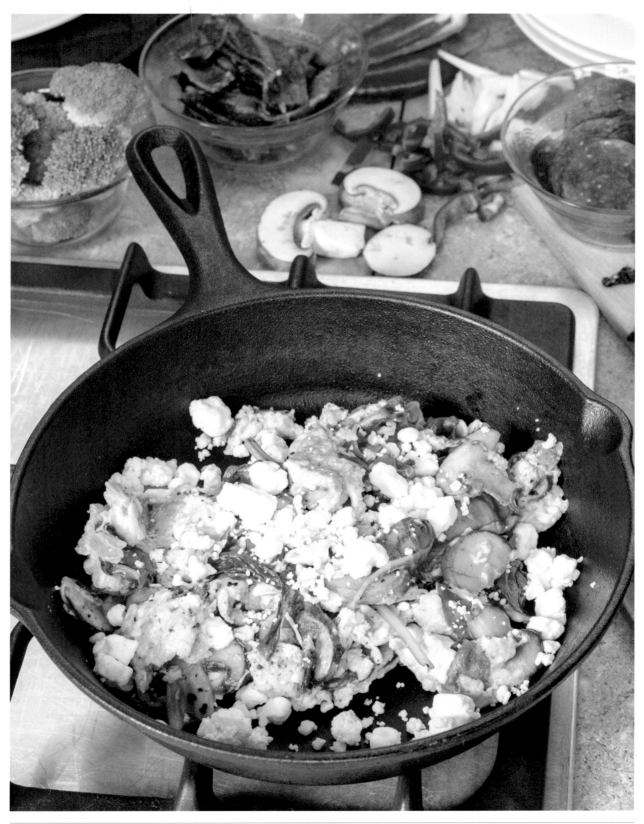

NUTRITION FACTS (PER SERVING): | Calories: 680 | Fat: 56.6g | Protein: 34g | Carbs: 2.9g | Fiber: 0.9g

Pizza Skillet Scramble

Because my family does not love eggs, I am constantly looking for ways to combine them with nontraditional breakfast foods that I know they will enjoy. I also like to use leftovers to make meals, which makes this pizza-flavored scramble an even better breakfast option.

MAKES: 1 serving

1 tablespoon ghee

2 ounces bulk Italian sausage

1 tablespoon chopped green bell peppers

1 ounce mushrooms, chopped

1 ounce pepperoni, chopped

¼ teaspoon garlic powder

¼ teaspoon onion powder

2 large eggs, beaten

Dash of salt

Dash of ground black pepper

2 ounces mozzarella cheese, shredded (about ½ cup)

1. In a medium-sized skillet over medium heat, melt the ghee. Add the sausage and cook until browned and crumbled. Add the bell peppers and mushrooms and cook until tender, about 3 minutes. Add the pepperoni and garlic and onion powders and stir to combine.

2. Pour the beaten eggs over the mixture in the skillet. As the eggs cook, use a spatula to scramble them with the sausage, bell peppers, mushrooms, and pepperoni. When the eggs are softly scrambled, season with the salt and pepper. Remove from the heat and sprinkle the mozzarella over the scramble. Serve immediately.

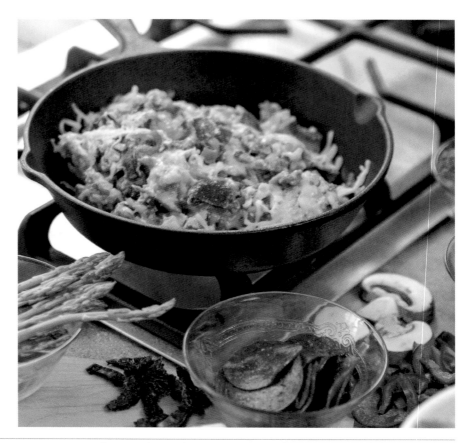

NUTRITION FACTS (PER SERVING):   Calories: 699 | Fat: 58.6g | Protein: 35.3g | Carbs: 3.6g | Fiber: 0.6g

Spring Veggie Skillet Scramble

The combination of asparagus, broccoli, and ham gives this scramble a light, springlike taste. I tend to make it when I have leftover asparagus since a little asparagus adds a lot of flavor. I also love the green onion in this dish.

MAKES: 1 serving

1 tablespoon ghee

6 asparagus spears, trimmed and cut into 2- to 3-inch pieces

¼ cup broccoli florets

1 green onion, chopped

2 ounces ham, chopped

½ teaspoon onion powder

2 large eggs, beaten

Dash of salt

Dash of ground black pepper

2 ounces sharp cheddar cheese, shredded (about ½ cup)

1. In a medium-sized skillet over medium heat, melt the ghee. Add the asparagus, broccoli, and green onion and cook until tender, 6 to 8 minutes. Stir in the ham and onion powder.

2. Pour the beaten eggs over the mixture in the skillet. As the eggs cook, use a spatula or wooden spoon to scramble them with the ham and vegetables. When the eggs are softly scrambled, season with the salt and pepper. Remove from the heat and sprinkle the cheddar cheese over the scramble. Serve immediately.

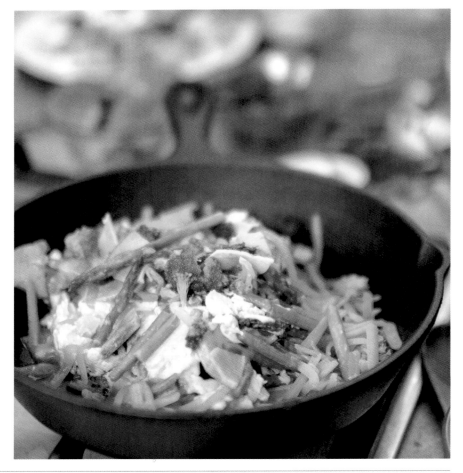

NUTRITION FACTS (PER SERVING):   Calories: 622 | Fat: 45.6g | Protein: 42g | Carbs: 7.4g | Fiber: 3g

Mexican Eggs in Purgatory

My family doesn't always enjoy eating the same thing twice, so I am constantly trying to reinvent leftovers. We aren't always lucky enough to have leftover Taco Bake, but when we do, this recipe is a great way to disguise it. The flavors of the spicy chorizo, cheese, and tomato become even more intense after the Taco Bake sits in the fridge overnight. This dish is incredibly easy to make and looks impressive. I try to serve it so that each person gets a sunny-side-up egg and gets the joy of cutting into that rich, gooey yolk. This is one of those dishes that makes you wonder why anyone would ever call keto a diet. It is excellent for brunch. The Taco Bake can easily be made ahead of time and transformed in a flash into this dish, whenever your guests are hungry.

MAKES: 4 servings

½ recipe Taco Bake (page 312)

4 large eggs

Chopped fresh cilantro, for garnish (optional)

1. Preheat the oven to 350°F.

2. Spread out the taco bake in a 9-inch oven-safe skillet. Crack the eggs, one at a time, over the taco bake, leaving some space between the eggs. Bake for 15 to 18 minutes, until the taco bake is bubbly and the egg whites are set but the yolks are still runny. Serve warm, garnished with cilantro, if desired.

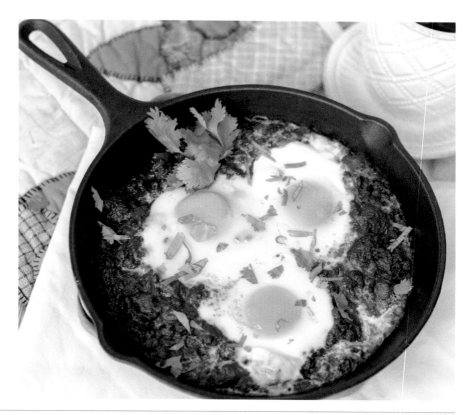

| NUTRITION FACTS (PER SERVING): | Calories: 469 | Fat: 33g | Protein: 28g | Carbs: 7.8g | Fiber: 2g |

Western Quiche

Canadian bacon, bell peppers, and onions are the stars of this humble quiche. I love biting into a pepper, although I am careful with the amount I use in this dish because peppers do add carbs. The flavors are light and simple, but this quiche packs a lot of protein and fat. It should keep hunger at bay for at least four hours.

MAKES: 6 servings

CRUST:

1 cup blanched almond flour

3 ounces Parmesan cheese, grated (about 1 cup)

1 large egg

1 teaspoon water

¼ teaspoon salt

FILLING:

½ cup cooked bacon pieces (about 8 slices)

6 ounces Canadian bacon, chopped

½ cup chopped green bell peppers

⅓ cup chopped onions

6 ounces cheddar cheese, shredded (about 1½ cups), divided

8 large eggs

½ cup heavy cream

1 teaspoon mustard powder

1 teaspoon onion powder

½ teaspoon ground dried thyme

½ teaspoon salt

⅛ teaspoon ground black pepper

1. Preheat the oven to 350°F.

2. Place the ingredients for the crust in a food processor. Pulse until a soft dough forms, then press the dough into the bottom and up the sides of a 9-inch deep-dish pie plate.

3. Distribute the bacon, Canadian bacon, bell peppers, onions, and 1 cup of the cheddar cheese evenly over the crust. Set aside.

4. In a blender, combine the eggs, cream, mustard powder, onion powder, thyme, salt, and pepper. Pour the egg mixture over the ingredients in the pie plate. Sprinkle the remaining ½ cup of cheese over the top.

5. Bake for 35 to 45 minutes, until golden brown on top and set in the center. Let cool for at least 5 minutes before serving.

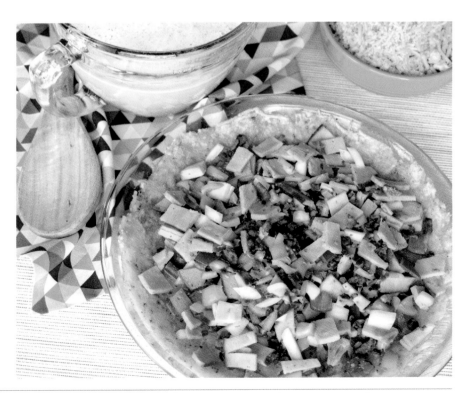

NUTRITION FACTS (PER SERVING): Calories: 338 | Fat: 24g | Protein: 24.5g | Carbs: 3.5g | Fiber: 0.5g

Frittatas

Frittatas are a staple in my house for a lot of reasons. First, the flavor combinations are limited only by your imagination and can easily be tweaked to appeal to individual preferences. In addition, frittatas can be made the night before and baked or warmed just before serving. They are also a great way to use up leftover vegetables.

Broccoli, Ham, and Cheese Frittata

This is my favorite frittata. The ham is subtle but provides some protein, while the broccoli gives the frittata a little texture and the cheese makes it creamy and rich. This dish is a complete meal and the flavors have universal appeal, so it is generally safe to serve to guests.

MAKES: **6 servings**

8 large eggs

½ cup heavy cream

1 teaspoon mustard powder

½ teaspoon salt

2 tablespoons bacon fat

1 cup chopped broccoli

⅓ cup chopped green onions

6 ounces ham, chopped

6 ounces cheddar cheese, shredded (about 1½ cups)

1. Preheat the oven to 350°F.

2. Using a whisk, mix the eggs, cream, mustard powder, and salt until well blended. Set aside.

3. Melt the bacon fat in a 10-inch oven-safe skillet over medium heat. Add the broccoli and onions and cook until the broccoli is tender and the onions are translucent, 10 to 12 minutes. Remove the skillet from the heat.

4. Add the ham to the skillet with the broccoli and onions and stir well to evenly distribute the ingredients. Sprinkle the cheese over the ham, broccoli, and onions, then pour the egg mixture over the top. Bake for 35 to 45 minutes, until browned and set. Let cool for at least 10 minutes before serving.

Time-Saver Tip:

Both this frittata and the Southwestern version on page 234 can be baked in a standard-size 12-well muffin pan to create a grab-and-go breakfast. These muffin-sized individual servings are great for portion control. Simply divide the ham and broccoli mixture evenly among the greased muffin wells, sprinkle evenly with the cheese(s), and then pour in the egg mixture, filling each well about three-quarters full. Bake the egg muffins for 15 to 18 minutes, until set in the middle and browned. Let cool in the pan for at least 5 minutes before removing. Refrigerate leftovers for up to 5 days and reheat in the microwave on low power.

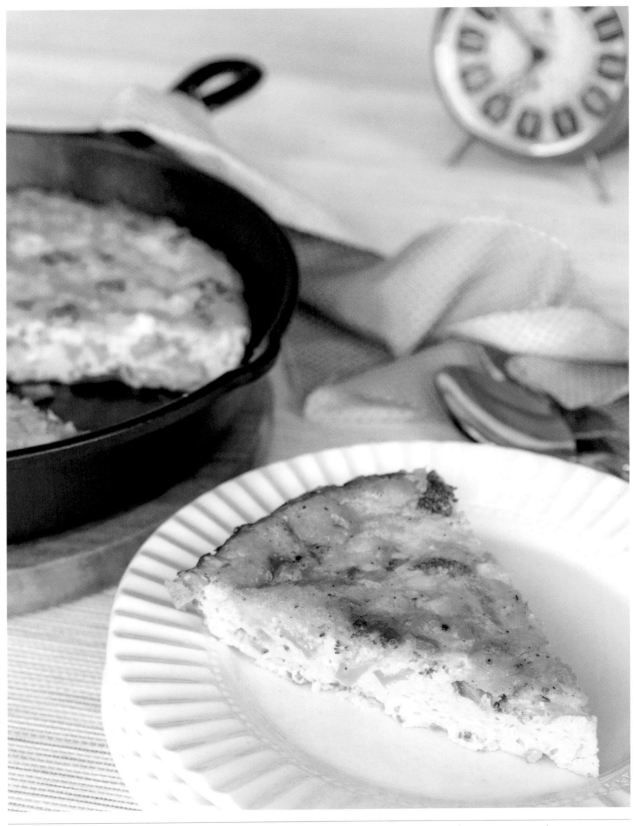

NUTRITION FACTS (PER SERVING):   Calories: 319 | Fat: 25.7g | Protein: 22.2g | Carbs: 2.9g | Fiber: 0.6g

Southwestern Frittata

My husband does not like eggs, but he really enjoys this frittata. The hearty chorizo, jalapeños, cream cheese, and shredded cheddar cheese make it a great brunch dish, especially if you're feeding a crowd that includes fellas.

MAKES: 6 servings

1 pound Mexican-style fresh (raw) chorizo, casings removed

⅓ cup chopped green bell peppers

¼ cup finely chopped onions

2 jalapeño peppers, seeded and chopped

6 ounces cheddar cheese, shredded (about 1½ cups)

4 ounces cream cheese (½ cup), cut into small cubes

8 large eggs

½ cup heavy cream

1 teaspoon mustard powder

½ teaspoon salt

⅛ teaspoon ground black pepper

FOR SERVING:

Chopped fresh cilantro

Diced avocado

Sour cream

1. Preheat the oven to 350°F. Grease a 13 by 9-inch baking dish.

2. Cook the chorizo, bell peppers, onions, and jalapeños in a large skillet over medium heat until the chorizo is browned and the vegetables are tender.

3. Spread the chorizo mixture in the greased baking dish. Top with the shredded cheese. Distribute the cubes of cream cheese evenly over the dish. Set aside.

4. Using a blender or whisk, beat the eggs, cream, mustard powder, salt, and pepper until frothy. Pour the egg mixture over the meat and cheeses. Use a fork to mix the egg mixture throughout the dish.

5. Bake for 30 to 40 minutes, until browned and set. Let cool for at least 10 minutes before serving. Serve with chopped fresh cilantro, diced avocado, and sour cream.

Time-Saver Tip:

I often make a frittata on Sunday evening while I cook dinner, then slice and refrigerate it for weekday mornings. It is nice to be able to pull a tasty low-carb breakfast from the fridge, warm it up quickly, and get everyone out the door on time!

Substitution Suggestion:

If you can't find a good chorizo, or if you don't care for chorizo, you can substitute ground pork or beef and add 2 tablespoons of Taco Seasoning (page 207) to the meat when you cook it.

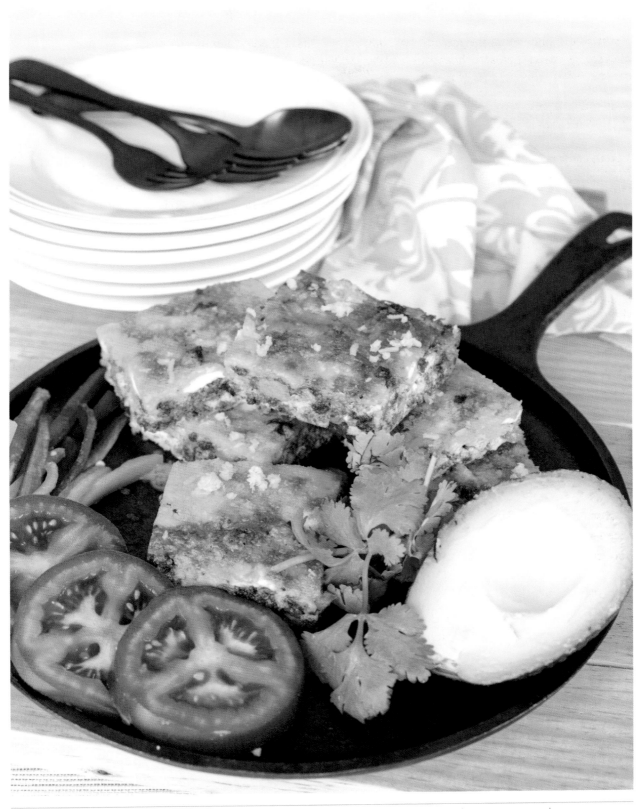

NUTRITION FACTS (PER SERVING):   Calories: 346 | Fat: 28.7g | Protein: 18.6g | Carbs: 2.9g | Fiber: 0.4g

Faux-gurt

Few people think of yogurt as an unhealthy breakfast choice. On a ketogenic diet, however, commercial yogurt is often too high in sugar and carbs. Some "plain" brands can have 12 to 15 grams of carbohydrate in a 1-cup serving! Because low-carb yogurt is hard to find, I have found a few excellent low-carb alternatives to yogurt.

The following is a list of products that behave like yogurt and make excellent substitutes when lightly sweetened and combined with a few low-carb berries, such as blackberries, raspberries, or blueberries.

Product	Serving Size	Fat	Protein	Carbohydrate
Crème fraîche	28g	11g	< 1g	< 1g
Mascarpone	28g	12g	< 1g	0
Sour cream	30g	6g	1g	1g

To make faux yogurt, or faux-gurt, you want to maximize fat and flavor while keeping carbs very low. Either of the two options described below makes a great faux-gurt. Once you add just a bit of your preferred sweetener and some berries, they make surprisingly tasty substitutes for yogurt. But if you're looking for a particularly thick faux yogurt, go for Option 1: The mascarpone gives the crème fraîche a nice texture and makes a faux-gurt that is thicker than crème fraîche or sour cream alone. Also, being higher in fat, Option 1 makes a delicious breakfast fat bomb.

MAKES: 2 servings

OPTION 1:

¾ cup crème fraîche

½ cup mascarpone

OPTION 2:

1 cup sour cream

FOR SERVING (OPTIONAL):

Keto sweetener of choice

Fresh blackberries, raspberries, or blueberries

TO MAKE OPTION 1:

Stir together the crème fraîche and mascarpone until smooth. Divide between two small bowls. This ratio of crème fraîche to mascarpone (3:2) gives you 45 grams of fat, 4 grams of protein, and fewer than 3 grams of carbohydrate per serving.

TO MAKE OPTION 2:

Divide the sour cream between two small bowls. This amount of sour cream gives you 24 grams of fat, 4 grams of protein, and 4 grams of carbohydrate.

If desired, sweeten each serving with a little keto sweetener and top with a few berries.

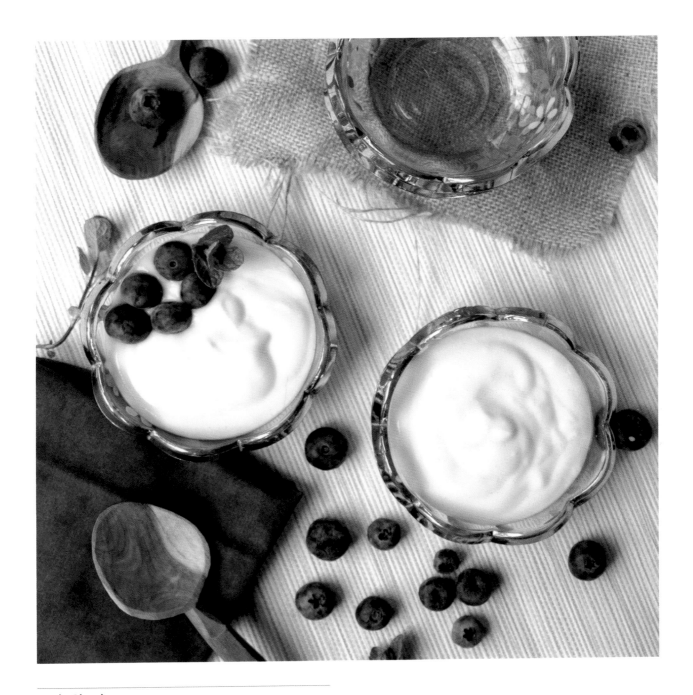

Carb Check:

Check the labels to make sure that the product you choose is full-fat and contains no sugar. Some brands of mascarpone have added sugars, and some brands of sour cream are higher in carbs than others.

NUTRITION FACTS (PER SERVING, OPTION 1):	Calories: 433	Fat: 45g	Protein: 4g	Carbs: 3g	Fiber: 0g
NUTRITION FACTS (PER SERVING, OPTION 2):	Calories: 248	Fat: 24g	Protein: 4g	Carbs: 4g	Fiber: 0g

Breakfast Pizza

Pizza for breakfast? Why not! Pick your own toppings—try traditional breakfast meats, eggs, and cheese or use your favorite pizza toppings. Using a variety of cheeses gives you a lot of options—Brie, fresh mozzarella, Gouda, Parmesan, Gruyère, and aged cheddar are all delicious. Breakfast doesn't have to be boring!

MAKES: 4 servings

1 large Sullivans' KeDough Pizza Crust (page 216), par-baked

SAUCE:

2 ounces cream cheese (¼ cup), softened, or ¼ cup tomato sauce

SUGGESTED TOPPINGS:

4 ounces cheese(s) of choice, shredded or sliced

8 ounces diced ham, chopped cooked bacon, or crumbled and cooked breakfast sausage, homemade (page 224) or store-bought

4 large eggs (see Note)

⅓ cup broccoli florets, sautéed

⅓ cup diced fresh tomatoes

¼ cup diced bell peppers, sautéed

1 green onion, thinly sliced

1. To make the par-baked pizza crust, complete Steps 1 through 4 of the pizza crust recipe.

2. Top the par-baked crust with cream cheese or tomato sauce and your favorite low-carb breakfast pizza toppings. Return the topped pizza to the oven to bake at 375°F until the toppings are browned and the cheese (if used) is melted, 6 to 8 minutes.

Note:

I either softly scramble eggs before putting them on the par-baked crust in Step 2 or crack them right onto the par-baked crust; the raw eggs will bake while the other toppings warm and the cheese melts.

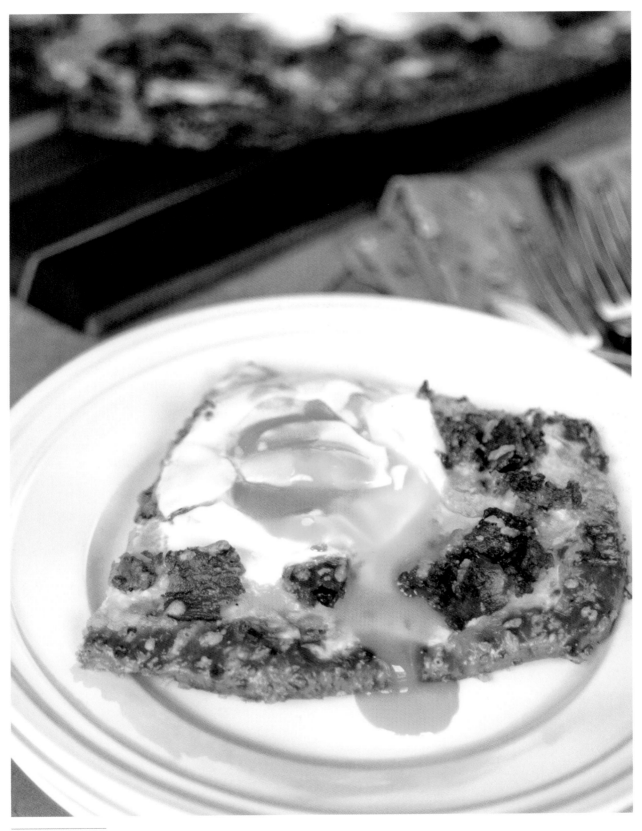

NUTRITION FACTS: Calories, fat, protein, carbs, and fiber will vary depending on the sauce and toppings you choose.

Simple
Keto Pancakes

I have to confess: the first keto pancakes I made were horrible! The recipes themselves were not the problem. In large part, it was me. I used to adore fluffy wheat-based pancakes. My children loved them, too. Making pancakes on a weekend morning was an event! Alas, while these are very good low-carb pancakes, they are no rival for the fluffy, gluten-filled version that you may be accustomed to serving. Having said that, these pancakes are a great low-carb option. Keeping them small makes them easier to turn. Use low heat and be patient while cooking them; low-carb pancakes do not cook as quickly as traditional pancakes. Before you know it, you'll be wearing a smaller robe while you stand over the stove to flip them!

MAKES: 16 small pancakes (4 per serving)

½ cup heavy cream

1 tablespoon white vinegar

⅓ cup plus 1 tablespoon unflavored whey protein isolate

⅓ cup granulated sweetener

1 teaspoon baking powder

1 teaspoon baking soda

1 teaspoon vanilla extract

Dash of ground cinnamon (optional)

2 large eggs

Ghee, for the pan

1. In a small bowl, whisk together the cream and vinegar. Set aside.

2. In another mixing bowl, whisk together the dry ingredients. Add the eggs and cream mixture to the dry ingredients and mix with a rubber spatula until the ingredients are well blended. Let the batter rest for 3 to 4 minutes.

3. Heat a large skillet or griddle over low heat and grease the pan with ghee. Ladle a scant ¼ cup of the batter into the skillet to make a small pancake, no more than 3½ to 4 inches in diameter. Cook the pancakes in batches. They are ready to flip when they are starting to brown around the edges and multiple bubbles have formed on top, 5 to 7 minutes. Take care to flip them gently and to keep the heat low. Once flipped, cook for another 2 to 4 minutes, until lightly browned on both sides.

Time-Saver Tip:

These pancakes freeze well and can be reheated in the toaster or microwave. They can also be used to make a quick breakfast sandwich. Just use less sweetener for a savory option.

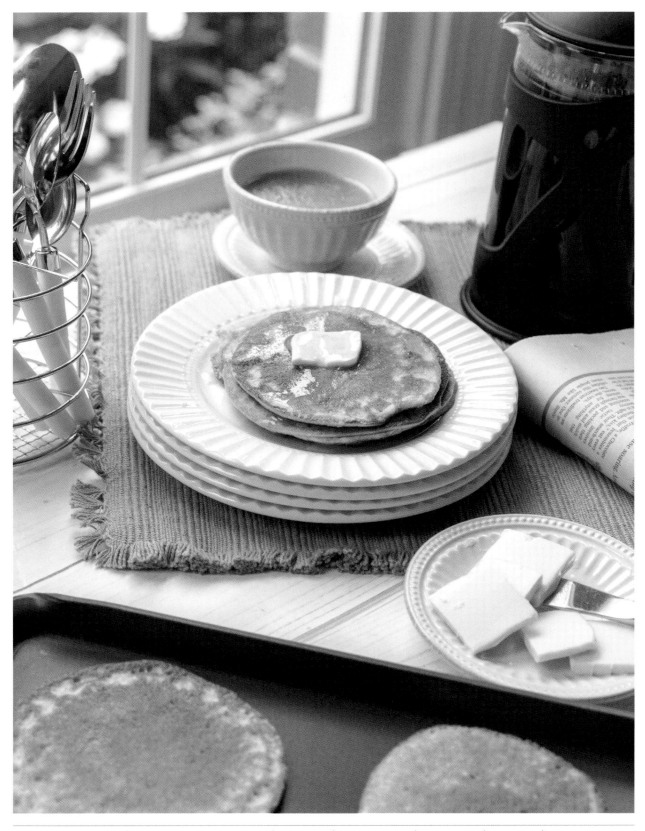

NUTRITION FACTS (PER SERVING):   Calories: 160 | Fat: 11.6g | Protein: 12.8g | Carbs: 0.8g | Fiber: 0g | Erythritol: 32g

One-Minute
French Toast

For many families, breakfast during the work week has to be fast. No one in my family really likes eggs unless the taste is masked by other ingredients, so I came up with this simple low-carb substitute for French toast that we all enjoy. The texture becomes surprisingly breadlike as it cools. If you avoid dairy, you can omit the cream cheese and substitute ghee for the butter. The texture will be softer without the cream cheese, but it's still delicious. Try topping this French toast with homemade pancake syrup (page 244).

MAKES: 2 servings

2 tablespoons unsalted butter

1 tablespoon cream cheese

2½ tablespoons unflavored whey protein isolate

1 tablespoon granulated sweetener

Dash of ground cinnamon

Dash of ground nutmeg (optional)

1 large egg, beaten

⅛ teaspoon vanilla extract

⅛ teaspoon maple extract (optional)

FOR GARNISH (OPTIONAL):

Whipped cream

A few fresh berries

1. Grease two 8-ounce microwave-safe ramekins or mugs with butter.

2. In a small microwave-safe bowl, microwave the butter and cream cheese until the butter is melted and the cream cheese is softened. Use a fork or spatula to blend.

3. Add the whey protein isolate, sweetener, cinnamon, and nutmeg, if using, and mix well. Add the egg and extracts and beat until smooth.

4. Pour the batter into the buttered ramekins or mugs and microwave for 50 to 60 seconds. The French toast should be slightly wet; it will firm up as it cools. Let sit for at least 3 minutes before serving. Garnish with some whipped cream and a few berries, if desired.

Time-Saver Tip:

Eat one serving fresh from the microwave and refrigerate the second serving for breakfast later in the week. You can reheat it in the microwave for 15 to 20 seconds or enjoy it cold.

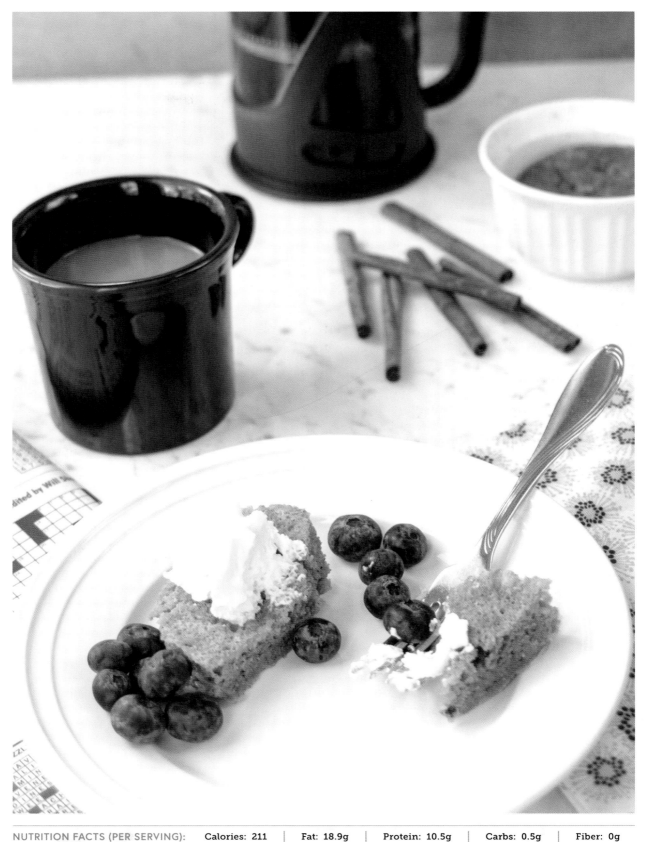

NUTRITION FACTS (PER SERVING): Calories: 211 | Fat: 18.9g | Protein: 10.5g | Carbs: 0.5g | Fiber: 0g

Simple
Pancake Syrup

I tested this recipe on a carbivore friend of my son, and he loved it! I never intended to be deceitful, but I was playing around with the proportions and had just made a batch of low-carb pancakes, and my son's friend asked to try them. I explained that they were low-carb. He grabbed a plate and fork and then exclaimed, "Wow! I didn't know you could even make real syrup!" This syrup can also be used to top a Sweet Dutch Baby (page 246) or drizzled over Faux-gurt (page 236).

OPTION

MAKES: about ¾ cup (1 tablespoon per serving)

½ cup (1 stick) unsalted butter or ghee

¼ cup water

½ cup powdered sweetener

2 teaspoons vanilla extract

1 teaspoon maple extract

¼ teaspoon salt

4 drops liquid sweetener, or to taste

1. Melt the butter in a small saucepan over low heat. Whisk in the water and powdered sweetener and simmer for 3 to 4 minutes. Stir in the extracts, salt, and liquid sweetener.

2. The syrup will thicken as it cools, and it may separate and crystallize. Be sure to whisk it well; using an immersion blender helps keep it blended. Serve warm and stir before serving.

Carb Check:

You really do want to avoid commercial syrups that are labeled "low-carb" or "sugar-free." I haven't found even one that is made with sweeteners that don't impact blood glucose and/or cause intestinal distress. Besides, making this homemade syrup is less expensive and far easier than running to the grocery store.

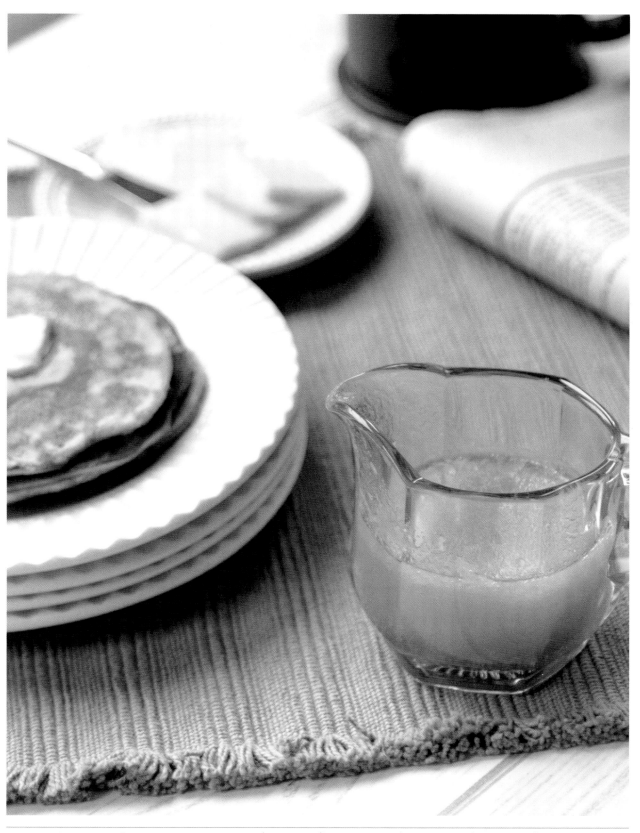

NUTRITION FACTS (PER SERVING):   **Calories: 70** | **Fat: 7.7g** | **Protein: 0.1g** | **Carbs: 0.1g** | **Fiber: 0g** | **Erythritol: 48g**

Sweet Dutch Baby
with Vanilla and Cinnamon

A Dutch baby is a little like a pancake, a little like a custard, and a whole lot of delicious! I had several friends test this recipe. A few had never heard of a Dutch baby, and the others were smitten with the high-carb versions they had enjoyed growing up. Both camps declared that my Dutch baby was a hit! Their carbivore family members asked for seconds and argued that the serving size was surely much larger than I suggested.

If you've never made a Dutch baby, the key is to melt butter in an oven-safe skillet or baking dish, pour the batter into the center of the sizzling pan so that the butter comes up over the top of the batter, and then bake that baby at high heat so that the outside browns and the inside stays somewhat custardlike. Don't be alarmed if your Dutch baby gets a lopsided, puffy top; that's exactly what it's supposed to do. It is likely to deflate as it cools. I top mine with powdered sweetener and a sprinkle of cinnamon. You can also drizzle it with Simple Pancake Syrup (page 244).

MAKES: **6 servings**

BATTER:

½ cup heavy cream, room temperature

4 large eggs, room temperature

2 ounces cream cheese (¼ cup), softened

1 teaspoon lemon juice

1 teaspoon vanilla extract

3 drops liquid sweetener

¼ cup granulated sweetener

2 tablespoons unflavored whey protein isolate

½ teaspoon baking powder

¼ teaspoon salt

3 tablespoons unsalted butter, for the pan

TOPPINGS (OPTIONAL):

Fresh berries

Ground cinnamon, for dusting

Powdered sweetener, for dusting

1. Preheat the oven to 400°F.

2. Place the ingredients for the batter in a blender and blend until creamy and foamy, about 1 minute.

3. Put the butter in a 10-inch oven-safe skillet or baking dish and place the pan in the oven. As soon as the butter begins to sizzle and brown, remove the pan from the oven. Make sure that the butter is evenly distributed throughout the pan.

4. Pour the batter into the center of the hot skillet so that the batter runs to the edges and some of the butter is pushed onto the top of the batter. Bake for 15 to 20 minutes, until the Dutch baby is puffy and dark brown. The center should be just set. The Dutch baby is likely to rise in a lopsided fashion and will deflate somewhat as it cools.

5. Serve hot from the oven, topped with a few fresh berries and a dusting of cinnamon or powdered sweetener, if desired. Leftovers can be eaten cold.

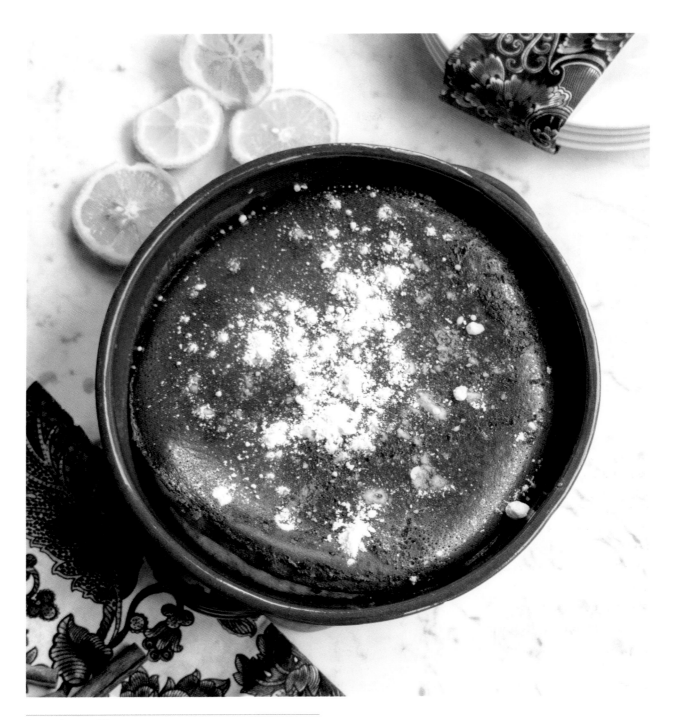

Time-Saver Tip:

This Dutch baby has an advantage over pancakes: it requires much less hands-on work because you do not have to stand by the stovetop and cook up individual pancakes. Also, no one is left waiting for more.

NUTRITION FACTS (PER SERVING): Calories: 174 | Fat: 15.8g | Protein: 7.3g | Carbs: 0.9g | Fiber: 0g | Erythritol: 22g

Savory Dutch Baby
with Bacon, Gruyère, Mushrooms, and Caramelized Onions

If you're avoiding sweeteners, then you can enjoy a savory Dutch baby. While you can use any meat, veggie, or herb combination you love, I find caramelized onions, mushrooms, and bacon hard to resist. Full of savory cheeses and rich flavors, this baby is truly delicious! Although I prefer to use Gruyère for this recipe, you can substitute any full-fat cheese. Swiss cheese is similar to Gruyère and easier to find.

MAKES: 5 servings

½ cup heavy cream, room temperature

4 large eggs, room temperature

2 ounces cream cheese (¼ cup), softened

5½ ounces Gruyère or Swiss cheese, shredded (about 1⅓ cups), divided

2 tablespoons unflavored whey protein isolate

½ teaspoon baking powder

¼ teaspoon salt

3 tablespoons unsalted butter, for the pan

½ pound bacon, chopped

½ cup sliced onions

8 ounces mushrooms, sliced

1. Preheat the oven to 400°F.

2. Make the batter: Place the heavy cream, eggs, cream cheese, ⅓ cup of the shredded cheese, whey protein isolate, baking powder, and salt in a blender and blend until creamy and foamy, about 1 minute.

3. Place the butter in a 10-inch oven-safe skillet and put the pan in the oven. As soon as the butter begins to sizzle and brown, remove the pan from the oven. Make sure that the butter is evenly distributed throughout the pan.

4. Pour the batter into the center of the hot skillet so that the batter runs to the edges and some of the butter is pushed onto the top of the batter. Bake for 15 to 18 minutes.

5. Meanwhile, prepare the savory topping: In a large skillet over medium heat, cook the bacon. When the bacon is browned, add the onions and mushrooms. Cook over low heat until the onions are caramelized, 10 to 12 minutes. Set aside.

6. Remove the Dutch baby from the oven when the top is puffy and dark brown and the center is just set. It is likely to rise in a lopsided fashion and will deflate somewhat as it cools.

7. Top the Dutch baby with the bacon, onion, and mushroom topping and the remaining 1 cup of shredded cheese. Serve immediately.

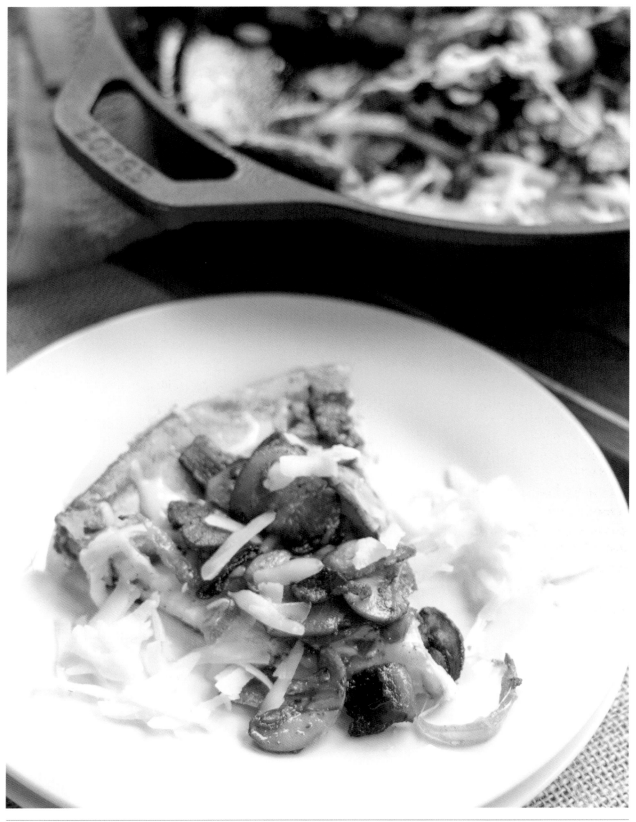

NUTRITION FACTS (PER SERVING):   Calories: 343 | Fat: 28.5g | Protein: 18.9g | Carbs: 3.8g | Fiber: 0.7g

Vanilla Coffee Creamer

One of the most frequent struggles that folks new to keto have is giving up commercial coffee creamer. After fielding nearly daily questions about what to use, I decided to create a low-carb option. Honestly, this creamer turned out even better than I imagined. It reminds me of sweetened condensed milk. It's very concentrated because it's meant for coffee, so don't go dipping your spoon into it!

OPTION

1 cup heavy cream

⅓ cup powdered sweetener

1½ tablespoons vanilla extract

6 drops liquid sweetener, or to taste

MAKES: about ¾ cup (2 tablespoons per serving)

1. In a small saucepan over low heat, bring the cream to a simmer. Add the powdered sweetener and whisk to dissolve it into the cream. Add the vanilla extract and simmer for 15 to 18 minutes, until the cream is reduced by roughly one-quarter.

2. Remove from the heat and stir in the liquid sweetener. Let the creamer cool and refrigerate the unused portion in a tightly covered container. It will keep in the refrigerator for up to 5 days.

Substitution Suggestion:

To make this creamer dairy-free, use 1 cup of coconut cream in place of the heavy cream.

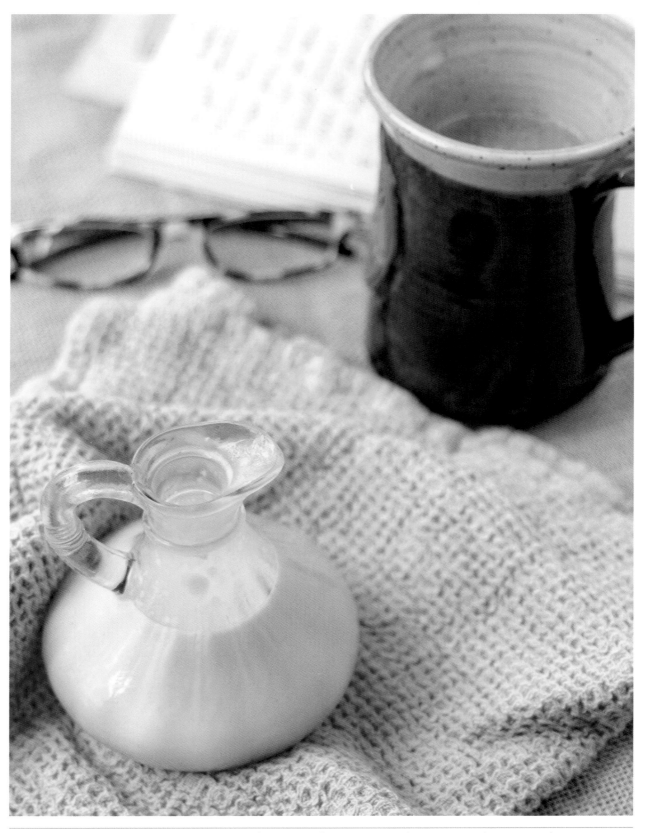

NUTRITION FACTS (PER SERVING):   **Calories:** 77 | **Fat:** 7.2g | **Protein:** 0.6g | **Carbs:** 0.9g | **Fiber:** 0g | Erythritol: 30g

Mocha Latte

Sometimes you need a little chocolate and a lotta coffee! This cold-weather treat is a sweet reminder that you can follow this eating plan, stay healthy, and never feel deprived. Because of the carb count, I don't indulge in this latte every day, but it's a nice option when I want a flavored coffee.

OPTION

MAKES: one 12-ounce serving

1½ teaspoons unsweetened cocoa powder

1 tablespoon hot water

12 ounces brewed hot coffee

3 tablespoons heavy cream or coconut cream

1 tablespoon unsalted butter or coconut oil

⅛ teaspoon vanilla extract

3 drops liquid sweetener

In a quart-sized wide-mouth jar, dissolve the cocoa powder in the tablespoon of hot water. Add the remaining ingredients and use an immersion blender to mix well. Serve hot.

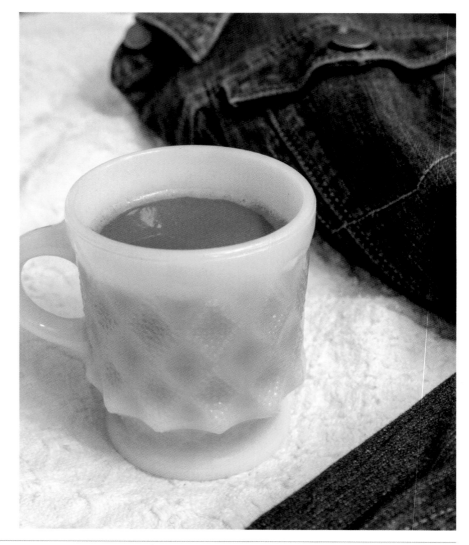

NUTRITION FACTS (PER SERVING):   Calories: 182 | Fat: 20.1g | Protein: 1.4g | Carbs: 2.1g | Fiber: 0.9g

Chai Latte

While I'm not as enamored with chai as most people seem to be, I see a great many folks enjoying the high-sugar version of chai latte. I can't let that continue to happen, so I've made a sugar-free version. Don't worry, I've run this recipe by true chai latte snobs, and all of them have given it their stamp of approval.

OPTION

12 ounces freshly brewed chai, hot

2 tablespoons heavy cream or coconut cream

1 tablespoon unsalted butter or coconut oil

¼ teaspoon maple extract

¼ teaspoon ground cardamom

¼ teaspoon ground cinnamon

⅛ teaspoon ground cloves

⅛ teaspoon ginger powder

⅛ teaspoon ground nutmeg

Liquid sweetener, to taste (optional)

MAKES: one 12-ounce serving

Using an immersion blender or other mixer that is safe for hot liquids, blend all the ingredients. Add sweetener as desired. Serve hot.

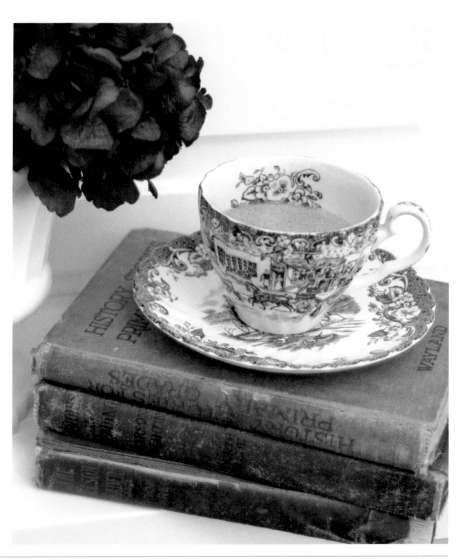

Carb Check:

In case you weren't aware, spices have carbs. Before you add an extra dash of this or scoop of that to a recipe, be sure to count *all* the carbs.

NUTRITION FACTS (PER SERVING): | Calories: 152 | Fat: 17.4g | Protein: 0.5g | Carbs: 0.9g | Fiber: 0g

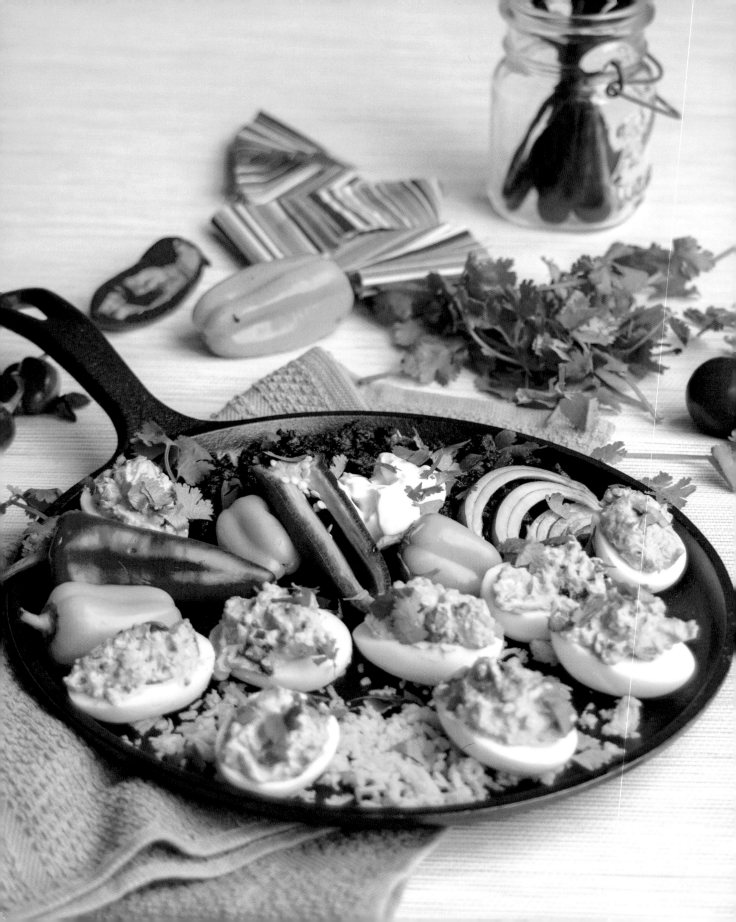

Chapter 8
Small Bites

One of the miracles of eating a ketogenic diet is finally having hunger under control. It isn't unusual to skip a meal simply because you are no longer constantly hungry. When you do eat, you will likely discover that the portions you want are far smaller. This same girl who could eat half a medium pizza now finds that one small slice of keto-friendly pizza is plenty.

This chapter is for those times when you want a smaller meal or you find yourself needing to prepare an appetizer for a party or gathering. These are simply delicious, healthful dishes that are easily shared with others or kept all to yourself. Your guests will never think of these recipes as diet food, but many will ask you for the recipes!

Cheddar Cheese Chips

Simple shredded cheese can be transformed into taco shells or chips in minutes. Use parchment paper or a silicone baking mat to make any size chips you want. You can use any semi-firm or hard cheese, such as cheddar or Parmesan, to experiment with different flavors. You can also add various seasonings or top each chip with a sliced olive or slice of jalapeño. Be sure to shred your own cheese to avoid the food starches that are almost always added to preshredded cheeses.

8 ounces cheddar cheese or other semi-firm or hard cheese of choice, shredded (about 2 cups)

MAKES: 32 chips (8 per serving)

1. Preheat the oven to 350°F. Line a rimmed baking sheet with parchment paper or a silicone baking mat.

2. Using a 1-tablespoon measuring spoon, drop 32 piles of shredded cheese onto the lined baking sheet, leaving at least ½ inch of space between piles. Bake for 8 to 10 minutes, until the cheese is melted and the edges of the chips are slightly browned. Let cool on the baking sheet before eating. Store in an airtight container in the refrigerator for up to 5 days.

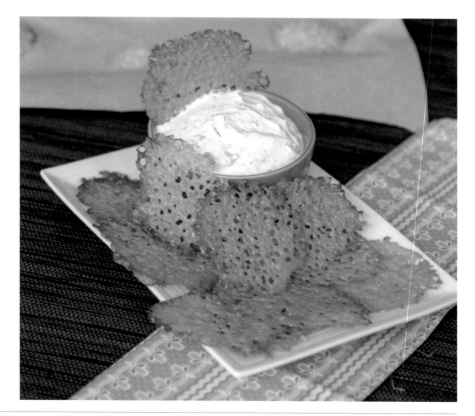

NUTRITION FACTS (PER SERVING): | Calories: 228 | Fat: 18.5g | Protein: 14g | Carbs: 0.7g | Fiber: 0g

Crispy Pepperoni Chips

Pepperoni chips are perfect for kids to enjoy in lunch boxes or with friends. They are easy enough for older kids to make on their own, and they're great for kids and adults alike to eat with a favorite dip, such as homemade Ranch Dressing (page 209).

MAKES: **24 chips (6 per serving)**

24 slices pepperoni

1. Preheat the oven to 350°F. Line a rimmed baking sheet with parchment paper or a silicone baking mat.

2. Lay the pepperoni slices in a single layer on the lined baking sheet. Bake for 6 to 9 minutes, until lightly browned. Store in an airtight container in the refrigerator for up to 4 days.

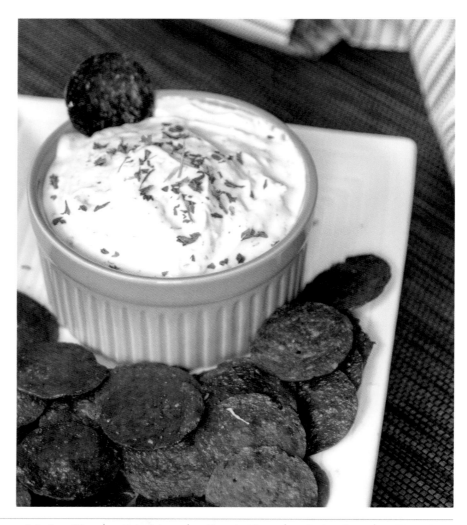

NUTRITION FACTS (PER SERVING): | Calories: 60 | Fat: 5.4g | Protein: 3g | Carbs: 0g | Fiber: 0g

BLT Boats

This is so simple that it hardly warrants being called a recipe, but it is a great keto meal when you don't have the time or energy to cook. While mayo is the standard condiment for BLTs, these boats are even better with homemade Ranch Dressing (page 209). The macros on these, once loaded with mayo or ranch, are excellent. Just limit the tomatoes, as one medium tomato packs 4.8 grams of carbs. These boats also work well on a buffet table.

MAKES: 8 meal servings or 16 appetizer servings

16 romaine lettuce leaves, washed and patted dry

32 tomato slices (about 5 medium tomatoes)

48 slices bacon (about 2½ pounds), cooked

1 cup mayonnaise, homemade (page 192) or store-bought

Salt and pepper

Lay the lettuce leaves in a single layer on a large serving platter. Top each leaf with 2 slices of tomato and 3 slices of bacon. Drizzle a tablespoon of mayonnaise over each boat. Season with salt and pepper and serve immediately.

Time-Saver Tip:

Use precooked bacon for an even faster keto meal!

Carb Check:

Don't be tempted to add an extra slice of tomato to each boat. I love tomatoes, too, but they have more carbs than other low-carb produce. Limiting yourself to two slices per boat will keep the carb count in check.

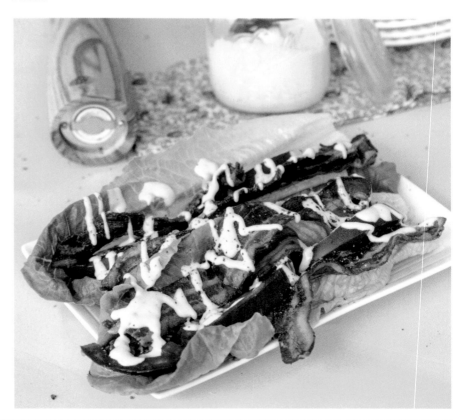

NUTRITION FACTS (PER APPETIZER SERVING):   Calories: 269 | Fat: 24.6g | Protein: 9.5g | Carbs: 2.6g | Fiber: 0.8g

Roasted Chicken Wings

Before going keto, I rarely ate chicken wings. That's nearly forty years I won't ever get back! I make up for lost time by eating these wings anytime I can. Thankfully, they are easy enough to make at least once a week. Roast the wings until the skins are crispy, then dip them in a delicious fatty dip like homemade Ranch Dressing (page 209), Parmesan Peppercorn Dressing (page 210), or the classic combination of Blue Cheese Dressing (page 213) and celery sticks.

MAKES: **4 meal servings or 12 appetizer servings**

2 pounds chicken wings and/or drumettes

2 tablespoons bacon fat, melted

1 tablespoon salt

2 teaspoons garlic powder

¼ teaspoon ground black pepper

1 teaspoon red pepper flakes (optional)

1. Pat the chicken wings dry with a paper towel to remove as much moisture as possible and place the wings in a large bowl. Add the melted bacon fat, salt, and spices. Mix until all the wings are well coated. Place in the refrigerator to marinate for at least an hour or up to overnight.

2. When you are ready to cook the wings, preheat the oven to 425°F. Place the wings on a rimmed baking sheet and roast for 30 to 45 minutes, until the skin is crispy and the juices run clear. Serve hot.

Substitution Suggestion:

Chicken legs and bone-in, skin-on chicken thighs also work well in this recipe. Just be sure to leave the skin on and cook the chicken to an internal temperature of 165°F.

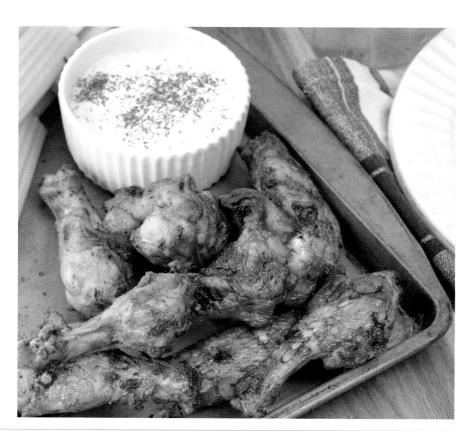

NUTRITION FACTS (PER APPETIZER SERVING): Calories: **189** | Fat: **14.3g** | Protein: **13.7g** | Carbs: **0.4g** | Fiber: **0.1g**

Pork Rind Nachos

Who doesn't love a pile of spicy, meaty nachos loaded with cheese? You can keep these simple with pork rinds, taco meat, and shredded cheese or kick it up a notch with homemade queso. These nachos are excellent served with sour cream, guacamole, or diced avocado; salsa fresca or chopped fresh tomatoes; and chopped jalapeños for heat.

MAKES: 4 meal servings or 8 appetizer servings

1 pound ground beef (93% lean)

2 tablespoons Taco Seasoning (page 207)

3 ounces pork rinds

1 recipe Chile con Queso (page 200) (optional)

1 jalapeño pepper, seeded and chopped (optional)

2 tablespoons chopped fresh cilantro (optional)

FOR SERVING (OPTIONAL):

Sour cream

Guacamole (page 205) or diced avocado

Simple Salsa Fresca (page 206) or chopped tomatoes

1. Brown the ground beef in a large skillet over medium heat, stirring often to crumble the meat as it cooks. Add the taco seasoning and mix well. Set aside.

2. Layer the pork rinds on a plate or serving platter, then top them with the seasoned ground beef. If desired, top the platter with the queso, chopped jalapeño, and/or cilantro. Serve warm with your choice of sour cream, guacamole or diced avocado, and salsa fresca or chopped tomatoes.

Carb Check:

Though you can use a commercial taco seasoning, many brands have added sugars and/or food starches. Whenever possible, I avoid commercial spice blends and use my homemade mixes instead. Also, remember that avocados and tomatoes are low-carb but not carb-free. Use them sparingly, especially if you are including both of them in your nachos.

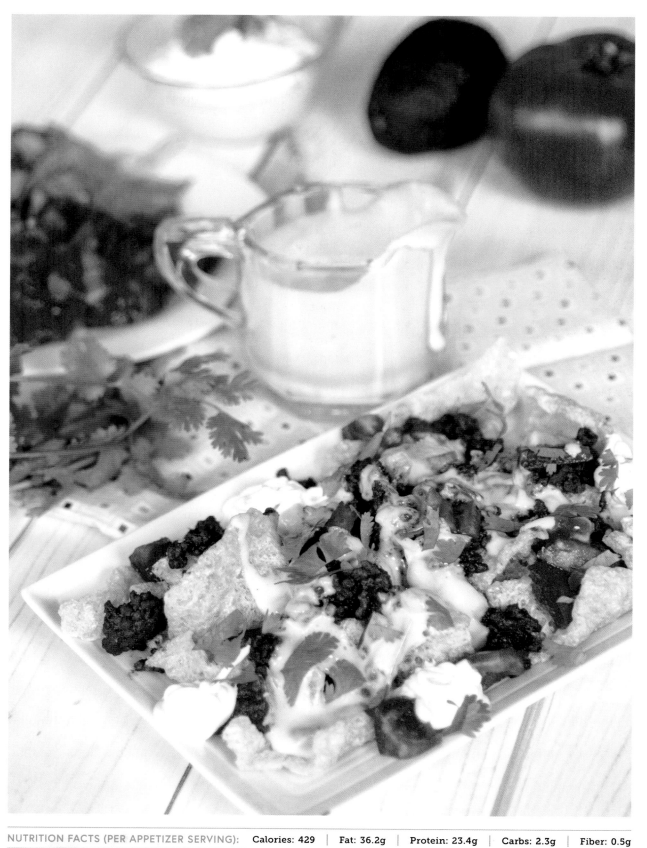

NUTRITION FACTS (PER APPETIZER SERVING):   **Calories: 429** | **Fat: 36.2g** | **Protein: 23.4g** | **Carbs: 2.3g** | **Fiber: 0.5g**

Swedish Meatballs
in Keto Gravy

These are my favorite meatballs ever! I love their texture, and I love the gravy that goes with them. While this standout needs no side dish, it is really good served with Cabbage Noodles (page 342), Cauli Rice (page 343), or Creamy Cauli Mash (page 344).

MAKES: **42 meatballs (6 per serving)**

MEATBALLS:

1 pound ground beef (93% lean)

1 pound ground pork

1½ ounces Parmesan cheese, grated (about ½ cup)

½ cup pork dust (ground pork rinds)

2 large eggs

2 tablespoons dried minced onions

2 tablespoons dried parsley

1 teaspoon salt

1 teaspoon garlic powder

GRAVY:

2 cups beef bone broth, homemade (page 187) or store-bought

¼ cup (½ stick) salted butter

¼ cup dried minced onions

1 teaspoon salt

½ teaspoon ground black pepper

¼ teaspoon Worcestershire sauce

⅛ teaspoon instant coffee powder

½ cup sour cream

1. Preheat the oven to 375°F.

2. Make the meatballs: In a large bowl, mix all the meatball ingredients with your hands until thoroughly combined. Shape the meat mixture into 1½-inch balls. Place the meatballs on a rimmed baking sheet in a single layer, spaced about ½ inch apart. Bake for 12 to 14 minutes, until the meatballs are browned and cooked through.

3. Meanwhile, make the gravy: In a 2-quart saucepan over medium heat, bring the broth, butter, onions, salt, pepper, Worcestershire sauce, and coffee powder to a simmer. Continue to simmer for 15 to 20 minutes, until the gravy has thickened. Reduce the heat to low and stir in the sour cream.

4. Add the cooked meatballs to the gravy and simmer over low heat for 5 to 10 more minutes. Serve hot.

Substitution Suggestion:

If you avoid pork, you can use all ground beef or a combination of ground beef and ground lamb or chicken instead. There is no good substitute for pork rinds, so just omit those. While the texture of the meatballs will be different, they should still hold together well without the pork rinds. As with any recipe, making these substitutions will alter the nutritional information, so please calculate it yourself based on the changes you make.

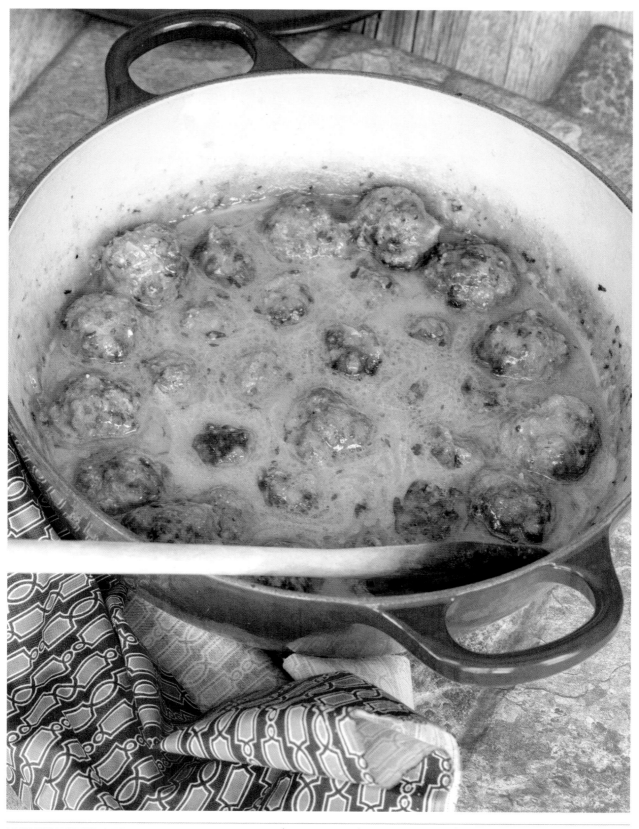

Classic Deviled Eggs

My mother used to make these deviled eggs for Easter. While they are very simple, my children like them, and this recipe uses ingredients that are nearly always stocked in my kitchen, and probably in yours, too.

MAKES: 12 deviled egg halves (3 per serving)

6 hard-boiled eggs, peeled and halved lengthwise

¼ cup mayonnaise, homemade (page 192) or store-bought

1½ teaspoons prepared yellow mustard

½ teaspoon white vinegar

Dash of salt

Dash of ground black pepper

Paprika, for garnish

1. Remove the yolks from the hard-boiled eggs and place them in a small mixing bowl; set the whites aside on a plate or small platter.

2. Use a fork to crumble the egg yolks. Add the mayonnaise, mustard, vinegar, salt, and pepper to the yolks and mix until creamy.

3. Using a spoon or piping bag, fill the egg white halves with the yolk mixture. Sprinkle with paprika just before serving.

Time-Saver Tip:

Buy hard-boiled eggs in the refrigerated section of the grocery store to save the time and hassle of boiling and peeling them yourself.

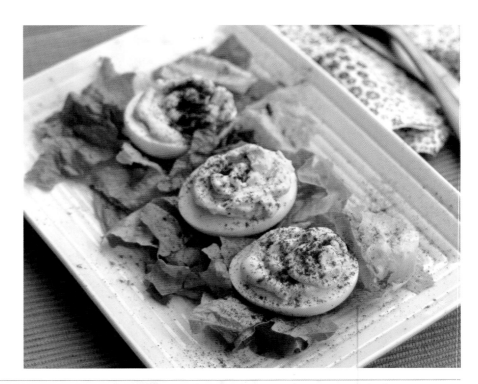

NUTRITION FACTS (PER SERVING): Calories: 234 | Fat: 21.3g | Protein: 9.6g | Carbs: 0.6g | Fiber: 0g

Buffalo Chicken
Deviled Eggs

When your husband doesn't like deviled eggs but he does like Buffalo chicken dip, you invent recipes like this! The filling is substantial and is generally well received on a buffet table. You can also chop the egg whites and serve this as an egg salad or use the filling to stuff celery sticks. Some folks like to add a little hot sauce, such as Tabasco, which can easily be served on the side.

MAKES: 12 deviled egg halves (3 per serving)

6 hard-boiled eggs, peeled and halved lengthwise

⅓ cup mayonnaise, homemade (page 192) or store-bought

2 ounces cream cheese (¼ cup), softened

2 tablespoons Buffalo wing sauce

3 ounces cooked chicken, chopped

1 ounce cheddar cheese, shredded (about ¼ cup)

2 tablespoons finely chopped celery, plus extra for garnish

2 tablespoons crumbled blue cheese, plus extra for garnish

1. Remove the yolks from the hard-boiled eggs and place them in a small mixing bowl; set the whites aside on a plate or small platter.

2. Use a fork to crumble the egg yolks. Add the mayonnaise, cream cheese, and wing sauce to the yolks and mix until creamy. Add the remaining ingredients and stir to make a creamy filling.

3. Using a spoon, stuff the filling into the egg white halves. Garnish the filled egg halves with additional blue cheese and/or finely chopped celery, if desired.

Carb Check:

Check the ingredient list before buying a bottle of Buffalo wing sauce. Some products contain added sugar.

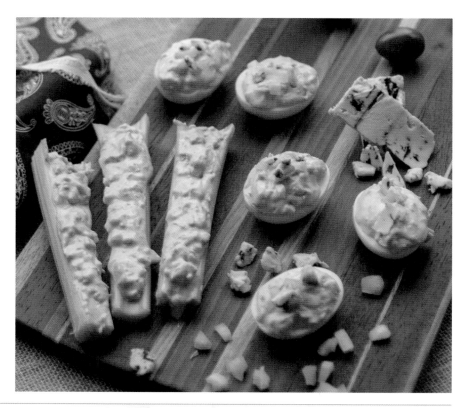

NUTRITION FACTS (PER SERVING): | Calories: 438 | Fat: 38.4g | Protein: 19.8g | Carbs: 1.5g | Fiber: 0g

Ham and Cheese
Deviled Eggs

This deviled egg recipe is probably my favorite. It reminds me of the deviled ham that I enjoyed as a child. It has fresh springlike flavors and works well for brunch or an Easter buffet table. Like the other deviled egg recipes in this book, you can also chop the egg whites and serve this dish as an egg salad.

MAKES: 12 deviled egg halves (3 per serving)

6 hard-boiled eggs, peeled and halved lengthwise

⅓ cup mayonnaise, homemade (page 192) or store-bought

2 tablespoons cream cheese, softened

2 teaspoons Ranch Seasoning (page 208)

2 ounces ham, finely chopped

1 ounce cheddar cheese, shredded (about ¼ cup)

1½ tablespoons finely chopped celery

1½ tablespoons finely chopped green onions

Sliced green onion tops, for garnish (optional)

1. Remove the yolks from the hard-boiled eggs and place them in a small mixing bowl; set the whites aside on a plate or small platter.

2. Use a fork to crumble the egg yolks. Add the mayonnaise, cream cheese, and ranch seasoning to the yolks and mix until creamy. Then add the ham, cheddar cheese, celery, and green onions and stir until everything is well combined.

3. Using a spoon, stuff the filling into the egg white halves. Serve with a garnish of green onion tops, if desired.

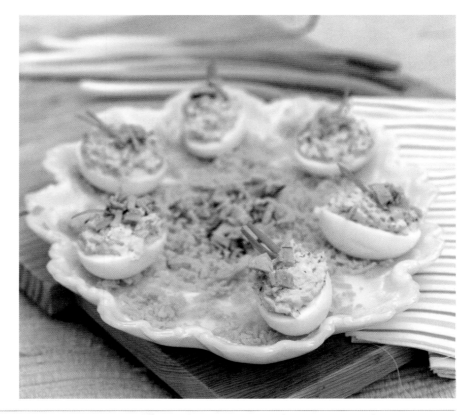

NUTRITION FACTS (PER SERVING): | Calories: 354 | Fat: 31.5g | Protein: 15g | Carbs: 2.1g | Fiber: 0.3g

Southwestern
Deviled Eggs

A favorite of the fellas, these spicy deviled eggs are hearty enough to make an easy meal or become a buffet favorite. This dish is especially popular with football fans and can be served with fresh avocado and chopped tomatoes as well as a dollop of guacamole (page 205) or salsa fresca (page 206). You can also kick up the flavor by using pepper Jack cheese instead of cheddar.

MAKES: 12 deviled egg halves (3 per serving)

6 hard-boiled eggs, peeled and halved lengthwise

⅓ cup mayonnaise, homemade (page 192) or store-bought

⅓ cup sour cream

2 teaspoons Taco Seasoning (page 207)

4 ounces Mexican-style fresh (raw) chorizo (casings removed), browned and crumbled

1⅓ ounces cheddar cheese, shredded (about ⅓ cup)

2 tablespoons seeded and finely chopped jalapeño peppers

2 tablespoons finely chopped onions

Fresh cilantro leaves or smoked paprika, for garnish

1. Remove the yolks from the hard-boiled eggs and place them in a small mixing bowl; set the whites aside on a plate or small platter.

2. Use a fork to crumble the egg yolks. Add the mayonnaise, sour cream, and taco seasoning to the yolks and mix until creamy. Then add the browned chorizo, cheddar cheese, jalapeños, and onions and stir until everything is well combined.

3. Using a spoon, stuff the filling into the egg white halves. Serve with a garnish of cilantro leaves or smoked paprika.

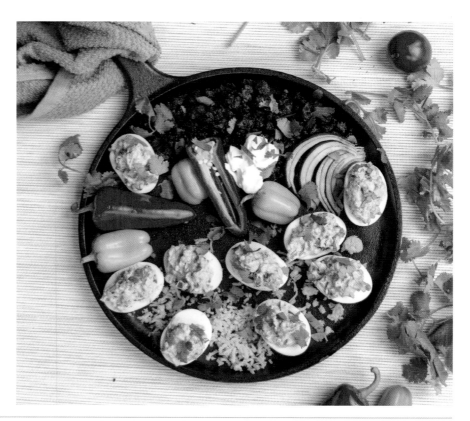

Substitution Suggestion:

Use ground pork or ground beef instead of chorizo.

NUTRITION FACTS (PER SERVING): | Calories: 411 | Fat: 40.2g | Protein: 17.4g | Carbs: 2.7g | Fiber: 0.6g

Antipasti Platter

An antipasti platter serves up the best of Italy. Who needs pasta when you have fresh mozzarella, basil, tomatoes, and fabulous fatty meats like pepperoni, prosciutto, salami, and soppressata? This platter is a frequent meal for my daughter and me. We tuck fresh basil among the layered mozzarella and tomato slices and drizzle it all with balsamic vinegar and olive oil. Delizioso!

OPTION

4 ounces pepperoni, sliced

4 ounces prosciutto, sliced

4 ounces salami, sliced

4 ounces soppressata, sliced

1 pound fresh mozzarella cheese, sliced

3 large tomatoes, sliced

16 to 20 fresh basil leaves

1½ tablespoons balsamic vinegar

1 tablespoon olive oil

Salt and pepper

MAKES: **4 meal servings or 8 appetizer servings**

Arrange the meats on one half of a large serving platter. On the other half of the platter, layer the mozzarella slices, tomato slices, and basil leaves. Drizzle the balsamic vinegar and olive oil over the mozzarella and tomato slices, then sprinkle them with salt and pepper. Serve immediately.

Carb Check:

Check the label before buying a bottle of balsamic vinegar. The sugar content varies greatly by brand. Ideally, you want a brand with no more than 2 grams of carbs per tablespoon.

Substitution Suggestion:

To make this platter dairy-free, omit the mozzarella.

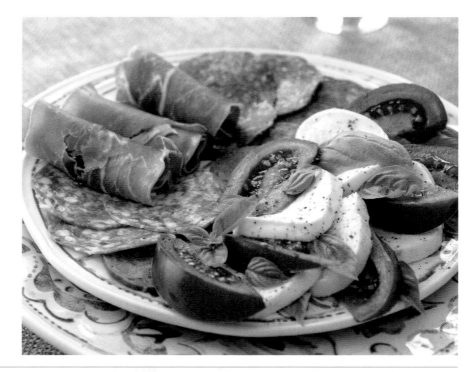

NUTRITION FACTS (PER APPETIZER SERVING):   Calories: 382 | Fat: 13.4g | Protein: 25g | Carbs: 3.1g | Fiber: 0.6g

Baked Spinach Bites

Before going keto, I had a favorite spinach ball recipe that I once made for a vegetarian friend. This recipe was inspired by that high-carb version that included a lot of breadcrumbs. This recipe uses pork dust instead of breadcrumbs, but the pork dust can easily be omitted. These bites are delicious when served with homemade Ranch Dressing (page 209), Parmesan Peppercorn Dressing (page 210), or Marinara Sauce (page 203).

MAKES: 15 bites (3 per serving)

8 ounces frozen spinach, thawed and drained

1½ ounces Parmesan cheese, grated (about ½ cup)

2 ounces fresh (soft) goat cheese, crumbled (about ½ cup)

⅓ cup cooked chopped bacon (5 to 6 slices)

¼ cup pork dust (ground pork rinds) (optional)

1 large egg, beaten

1 tablespoon dried minced onions

2 teaspoons finely chopped sun-dried tomatoes (optional)

1. Preheat the oven to 375°F. Line a rimmed baking sheet with parchment paper.

2. In a large bowl, mix together all the ingredients with a rubber spatula until well combined. Shape the mixture into fifteen 1-inch balls and place in a single layer on the lined baking sheet.

3. Bake the spinach bites for 10 to 12 minutes, until lightly browned. Serve warm or cold.

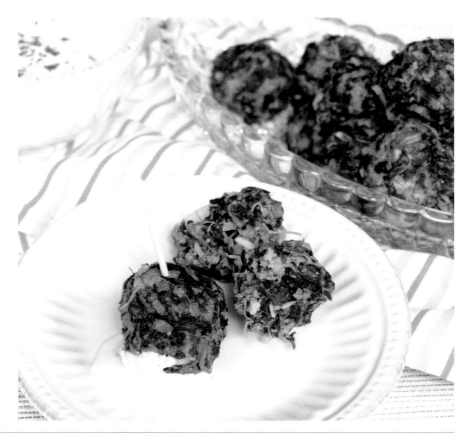

NUTRITION FACTS (PER SERVING): | Calories: 207 | Fat: 14.7g | Protein: 14.1g | Carbs: 3.3g | Fiber: 1.2g

Crab-Stuffed Mushrooms

These yummy bites top my list of party foods to make and share. I prefer to use crab claw meat because it is less expensive and more flavorful than other grades of crabmeat. You can use white mushrooms, too, but I prefer the consistent size and meaty flavor of baby bellas. You might want to scoop out more mushroom than usual to make more room for the tasty filling! Be careful to not overfill the mushrooms or the filling will run out.

You can convert this dish to a filling meal by dividing the filling among four large portobello mushroom caps, which will need 15 to 20 more minutes to bake.

MAKES: **about 20 stuffed mushrooms (2 per serving)**

1½ pounds baby bellas or white mushrooms (about 20), cleaned and stemmed

4 ounces cream cheese (½ cup), softened

2 tablespoons mayonnaise, homemade (page 192) or store-bought

1½ ounces Parmesan cheese, grated (about ½ cup)

2 green onions, chopped

2 teaspoons lemon juice

1 tablespoon dried parsley

1 teaspoon garlic powder

½ teaspoon mustard powder

½ teaspoon salt

¼ teaspoon onion powder

Dash of ground white pepper

8 ounces crabmeat, flaked and cartilage removed

Chopped fresh parsley and/ or sliced green onions, for garnish (optional)

1. Preheat the oven to 350°F. Line a rimmed baking sheet with parchment paper.

2. Arrange the mushroom caps in a single layer on the lined baking sheet.

3. Make the filling: In a large bowl, mix the cream cheese and mayonnaise until smooth. Add the Parmesan cheese, green onions, lemon juice, parsley, garlic powder, mustard powder, salt, onion powder, and pepper and stir to combine. Add the crabmeat and combine with the cream cheese mixture.

4. Fill each mushroom cap with a small mound of the filling. Bake for 15 to 20 minutes, until the filling is hot and lightly browned and the mushrooms are tender. Garnish with chopped parsley and/or sliced green onions before serving, if desired. These are best served warm.

VARIATION: **Hot Crab Dip**

To save lots of time, skip the mushrooms. You end up with a party dip that's very popular in the mid-Atlantic and Southern coastal states. Simply spread the filling mixture in an 8-inch square baking dish and bake in a preheated 350°F oven until bubbling and lightly browned, 25 to 30 minutes. Serve with pork rinds, Cheddar Cheese Chips (page 256), sliced fresh veggies, or spoons for dipping!

Substitution Suggestion:

If you are allergic to shellfish or using crabmeat feels like a splurge, you can use a different meat, such as cooked chicken, Italian sausage, or ground beef. If you prefer shrimp, you can use cooked and chopped shrimp instead of or in addition to crabmeat.

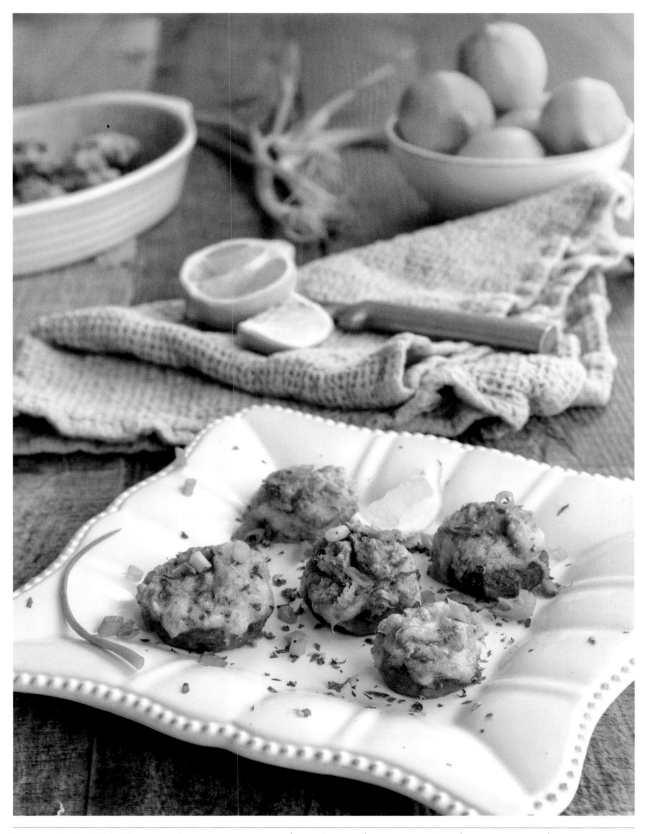

NUTRITION FACTS (PER SERVING):　　Calories: 124　|　Fat: 9g　|　Protein: 9g　|　Carbs: 3g　|　Fiber: 0.8g

Shrimp Cocktail

Shrimp is a special treat for my family, as we live just far enough from the coast to make fresh shrimp expensive. When I find a good sale, we enjoy shrimp cocktail served with cocktail sauce and/or tartar sauce. Cocktail sauce is more traditional, but tartar sauce has a higher fat content. If you don't serve this with tartar sauce, be sure to add a fatty side or offer melted butter for dipping, as shrimp is naturally low in fat. You can also serve the shrimp cocktail alongside a small salad topped with bacon and drizzled with a fatty dressing.

MAKES: 4 meal servings or 8 appetizer servings

1½ quarts water

1 lemon, sliced

12 whole black peppercorns

2 bay leaves

2 tablespoons dried parsley

2 pounds large shrimp, peeled and deveined (leave tails on)

1 large lemon, quartered, for serving

½ cup Cocktail Sauce (page 198) or Tartar Sauce (page 197), for serving

Carb Check:

Commercial cocktail sauces are typically high in sugar, so be sure to use homemade. Watch your portions.

1. In a large pot, bring the water, lemon slices, peppercorns, bay leaves, and parsley to a boil. Lower the heat and simmer rapidly for 15 to 20 minutes.

2. Add the shrimp and continue to simmer, stirring occasionally, until the shrimp curl and turn pink, 3 to 4 minutes. Do not overcook.

3. Drain the shrimp and rinse with cold water. Refrigerate for 1 to 2 hours or until cold. Serve with lemon quarters and cocktail sauce or tartar sauce for dipping.

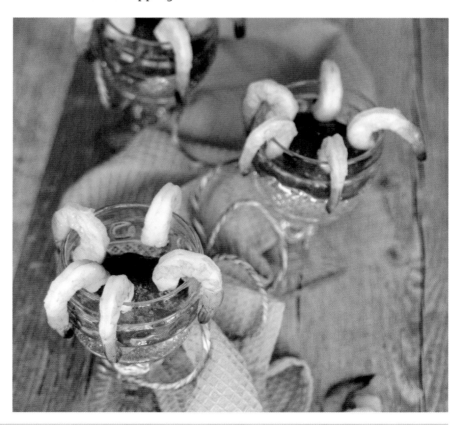

NUTRITION FACTS (PER APPETIZER SERVING):   Calories: 97 | Fat: 0.6g | Protein: 22.6g | Carbs: 0.2g | Fiber: 0.1g

Smoked Salmon Cucumber Bites

Grace and I love these cucumber bites. We eat them whenever we have smoked salmon on hand. We also enjoy these as a breakfast treat with slices of hard-boiled egg! These bites come together quickly and look as impressive as they taste, so they are great for serving to guests.

MAKES: 24 cucumber bites (4 per serving)

1 seedless cucumber, about 8 inches long

4 ounces cream cheese (½ cup), softened

2 tablespoons mayonnaise, homemade (page 192) or store-bought

1 tablespoon dried dill weed

1 teaspoon lemon juice

½ teaspoon salt

8 ounces cold-smoked salmon, such as Nova lox, sliced into 24 small pieces

Fresh dill sprigs, for garnish

1. Slice the cucumber crosswise into 24 rounds, about ¼ inch thick. Lay the cucumber slices on a serving plate in a single layer.

2. In a small bowl, mix the cream cheese, mayonnaise, dill, lemon juice, and salt until well combined. Top each cucumber slice with a teaspoon of the cream cheese mixture.

3. Place one piece of smoked salmon on each cucumber slice, on top of the cream cheese mixture. Serve the bites chilled, garnished with fresh dill.

Substitution Suggestion:

If you aren't a fan of smoked salmon, this recipe is also good with small pieces of cooked shrimp or chicken.

Carb Check:

I left the peel on the cucumber for a nice green color in the photo, but peeling the cucumber reduces the carb count of these tasty bites.

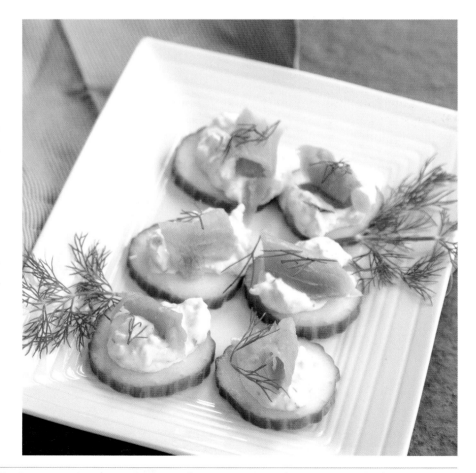

NUTRITION FACTS (PER SERVING): Calories: 156 | Fat: 13.2g | Protein: 8g | Carbs: 1.6g | Fiber: 0.4g

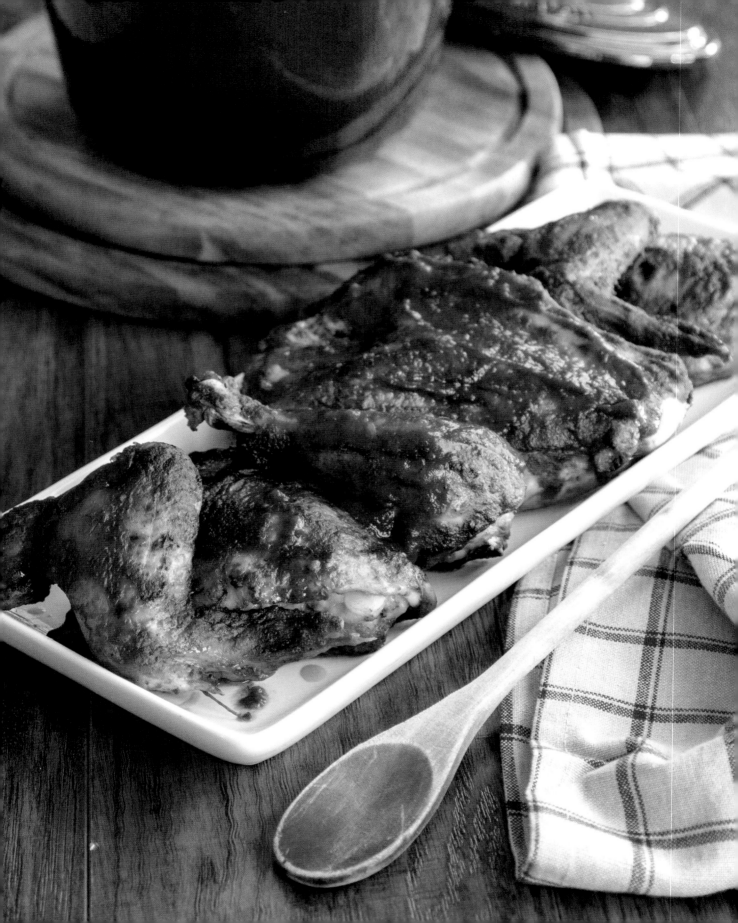

Chapter 9

Mains

This chapter contains main dishes organized by type of protein: beef, pork, poultry, and seafood. The idea is to simplify meal planning and to enable you to create menus based on grocery store sales or food preferences. Some of my favorites are those that I call "one-pot wonders," or recipes that are meals in themselves without the need for sides, which means that you don't have to dirty a lot of dishes.

If you are just getting started on a ketogenic lifestyle and perhaps are just getting used to cooking, you will find some very simple recipes to get you going. I've included different recipes for everyday cuts of meat and easy-to-find low-carb vegetables so that you won't have a lot of ingredients to buy or anything to special order.

Burgers—Six Ways

A burger recipe? Yes. I'm giving you a basic burger recipe for two reasons. First, I was once talking with a friend about starting a ketogenic lifestyle. I shared with her that ground beef is on sale for $2.99 a pound every Tuesday, and I stock up once a month. She gave me a curious look and asked, "What do I do with raw ground beef? I've never cooked it before!" She was young, but it was a clear reminder that many people are not accustomed to cooking with fresh meats and vegetables. If you're one of those people, this recipe is for you. Second, my grandmother had a few tricks up her sleeve when it came to making moist and juicy burgers, and this is my chance to share those tricks with you. I've adapted her recipe because she always added a slice or two of white bread.

We won't do that, but adding a little vinegar and heavy cream gives these burgers a great texture. I don't know why or how it works, but it does! Lastly, these burgers will convince you that, while having a bun may be convenient, the flavor is not in the bun! If you think about it, all the best flavors are tucked inside the bun. Cook up a batch of these burgers, grab a knife and fork, and you will see what I mean.

While my simple take on my grandmother's burgers is delicious on its own, the toppings are what really make a burger special. You can take this basic recipe and use it to make dozens of different meals. I have never tired of eating burgers. See below for some of my favorite topping combinations.

Basic Fatty Burgers

MAKES: 4 burgers (1 per serving)

1 pound ground beef (80% lean)

1½ tablespoons heavy cream

1 teaspoon apple cider vinegar

1 teaspoon salt

½ teaspoon ground black pepper

Condiments and/or toppings of choice (see sidebar, opposite, for ideas)

1. Place all the ingredients in a large mixing bowl and, using your hands, mix until thoroughly combined. Divide the mixture into fourths and shape each portion into a patty about 1 inch thick and 4 inches in diameter.

2. Fry the patties in a skillet over medium-high heat. For safety, the meat should reach a minimum internal temperature of 160°F. The burgers are usually done when the juices run clear or when you can cut into the center and see only a little pink. I tend to cook burgers well-done, which takes 4 to 6 minutes per side.

3. Top the burgers with the condiments and/or toppings of your choice and eat with a knife and fork.

Time-Saver Tip:

Make a double or triple batch of burgers and fry them all up at once. After they cool, freeze them in freezer-safe containers. Whether you eat them for breakfast, lunch, or a quick dinner, they are easy to warm in a skillet, in the microwave, or in the oven. Whether you are cooking for one, two, or six people, you can warm as many or as few burgers as you need!

BURGER CONDIMENTS AND TOPPINGS

Here is a list of my family's go-to toppings when we're looking to add a little excitement to basic burgers.

Blue Cheese Dressing (page 213)

Classic BBQ Sauce (page 195)

Ketchup, homemade (page 190) or store-bought

Mayonnaise, homemade (page 192) or store-bought

Mustard

Parmesan Peppercorn Dressing (page 210)

Lettuce

Skillet Mushrooms (page 349)

Sliced avocado

Sliced green onions

Sliced jalapeños

Sliced red onions

Sliced tomatoes

Southern Table Pickles (page 365)

Cheese: blue cheese, Brie, cheddar, Muenster, pepper Jack, Swiss

Crispy bacon slices

VARIATION: Egg-Topped Burgers (aka Kristie's Favorite)

I could eat this burger every day of the week, and it is my favorite breakfast! Complete Steps 1 and 2 for the basic burgers (opposite), then top each burger with an egg fried sunny side up, 4 slices of cooked bacon, and 2 ounces of sliced cheese. Serve with lettuce and tomato and a heaping spoonful or two of mayonnaise. Break the egg yolk and let all that rich, fatty goodness drip into the beef patty. Use the bacon, beef, and cheese to sop up the yolk.

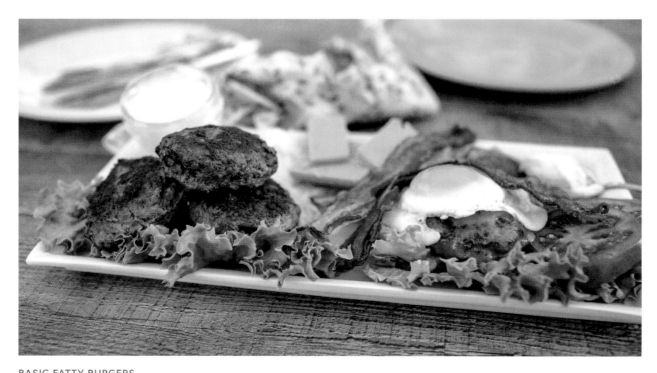

BASIC FATTY BURGERS

| NUTRITION FACTS (PER BURGER): | Calories: 285 | Fat: 22.7g | Protein: 19.2g | Carbs: 0.1g | Fiber: 0g |

EGG-TOPPED BURGERS (AKA KRISTIE'S FAVORITE)

| NUTRITION FACTS (PER BURGER): | Calories: 761 | Fat: 59.4g | Protein: 51.5g | Carbs: 1.6g | Fiber: 0g |

A classic! Complete Steps 1 and 2 for the basic burgers on page 276, then top each burger with 2 ounces of sliced Swiss cheese, 4 slices of cooked bacon, and ¼ recipe of Skillet Mushrooms (page 349). A drop or two of Worcestershire sauce is really good with this burger. Serve with mayonnaise. *Tip:* Have the mushrooms made ahead of time.

Carb Check:

Keep an eye on the amount of onions you use. Because they are so yummy, they are easy to overeat.

VARIATION: **The Westerner**

Slowly caramelize 1 cup of sliced onions with 1 tablespoon of bacon fat in a skillet over medium-low heat. Don't turn them often so that they brown and soften. The onions will need 15 to 20 minutes to become caramelized. (*Note:* This quantity of onions is for 4 burgers; adjust the amount as needed for the number of burgers you're making.) While the onions are caramelizing, complete Steps 1 and 2 for the basic burgers on page 276, then top each burger with 2 ounces of cheddar cheese, 6 slices of cooked bacon, 2 tablespoons of caramelized onions, and 2 tablespoons of Classic BBQ Sauce (page 195).

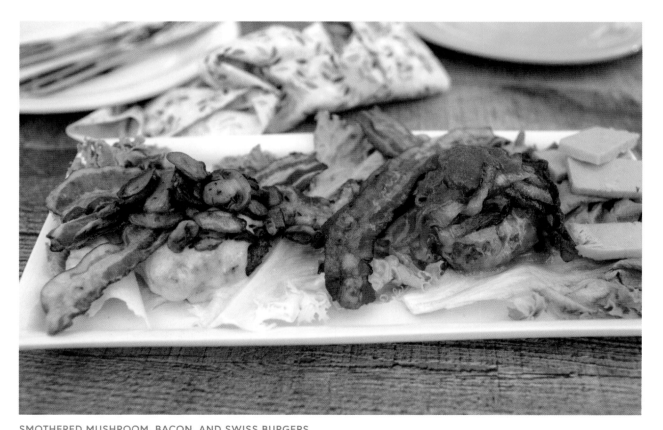

SMOTHERED MUSHROOM, BACON, AND SWISS BURGERS

NUTRITION FACTS (PER BURGER):	Calories: 711	Fat: 55.7g	Protein: 48.9g	Carbs: 5.5g	Fiber: 0.7g

THE WESTERNER

NUTRITION FACTS (PER BURGER):	Calories: 797	Fat: 62.5g	Protein: 51.1g	Carbs: 4.5g	Fiber: 0.7g

VARIATION: **Bacon and Blue Burgers**

I tend to make this version when I have leftover blue cheese dressing, but if you don't have any on hand, you can use crumbled blue cheese instead. This is one of my favorite lunches, and it keeps me full until dinner. Complete Steps 1 and 2 for the basic burgers on page 276, then top each burger with 2 tablespoons of Blue Cheese Dressing (page 213) or 2 ounces of crumbled blue cheese, 4 slices of cooked bacon, 2 lettuce leaves, and 2 slices of tomato.

VARIATION: **The Husband's Favorite**

Anytime I make a meal with spicy cheese and fresh jalapeños, my husband is pleased. Add bacon and he thinks it is even better! Complete Steps 1 and 2 for the basic burgers on page 276, then top each burger with 2 ounces of sliced Monterey Jack cheese, 1 sliced jalapeño pepper, 6 slices of cooked bacon, 2 lettuce leaves, and one-third of an avocado, sliced. Serve with mayonnaise and mustard.

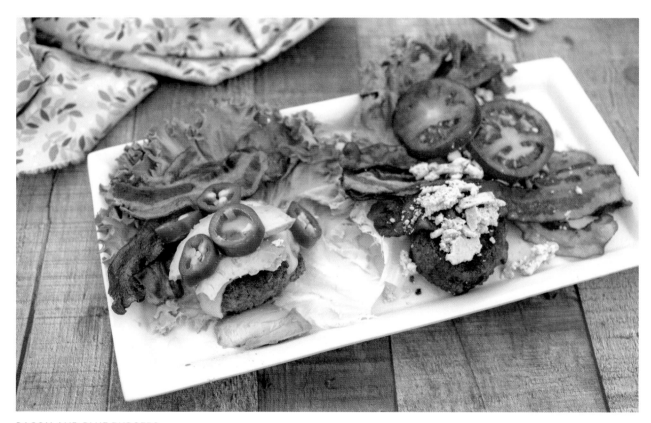

BACON AND BLUE BURGERS

| NUTRITION FACTS (PER BURGER): | Calories: 569 | Fat: 44.7g | Protein: 37.6g | Carbs: 2.7g | Fiber: 0.4g |

THE HUSBAND'S FAVORITE

| NUTRITION FACTS (PER BURGER): | Calories: 850 | Fat: 68.8g | Protein: 51.7g | Carbs: 6.4g | Fiber: 3.7g |

Open-Faced
Taco for Two

This is an easy meal to make on a weeknight when schedules vary or when family members have varying food preferences. The toppings are easy to customize. For example, Grace and I like to top our tacos with chopped olives, which neither David nor Jonathan would touch, while David piles his taco with fresh jalapeños, which would be way too spicy for me. These tacos are also excellent with homemade guacamole (page 205) and salsa fresca (page 206).

MAKES: 2 servings

½ pound ground beef
(80% lean)

2 tablespoons minced
onions

1 tablespoon Taco Seasoning
(page 207)

5 ounces cheddar cheese,
shredded (about 1¼ cups),
divided

1 cup shredded lettuce

1 small tomato, chopped

**ADDITIONAL TOPPINGS
(OPTIONAL):**

2 tablespoons sour cream

1 jalapeño pepper, seeded
and chopped

½ avocado, diced

1. Brown the ground beef and onions in a medium nonstick skillet over medium heat, stirring often to crumble the meat as it cooks. When the beef is browned, drain the fat and add the taco seasoning. Mix well. Transfer the seasoned meat to a bowl and set aside.

2. Return the skillet to the stovetop over medium heat. Sprinkle ¾ cup of the cheese into the skillet, spreading it out in a thin layer. The cheese will melt and form a solid layer. Let the cheese brown for 4 to 6 minutes, then remove from the heat. Let cool in the pan for 3 to 5 minutes before turning the cheese shell onto a cutting board. Top the shell with the seasoned meat, remaining ½ cup of cheese, lettuce, and tomato, then cut in half. Serve with additional toppings as desired.

VARIATION: Tacos for a Crowd

For a party or large gathering, double or triple the recipe. Instead of making two or three large open-faced tacos, make several small cheese shells and serve the fillings and toppings individually. Guests can create their own open-faced tacos according to their preferences.

Time-Saver Tip:

Keep batches of browned and taco-seasoned ground beef in the freezer to make this quick meal even faster to prepare and easier to clean up afterward.

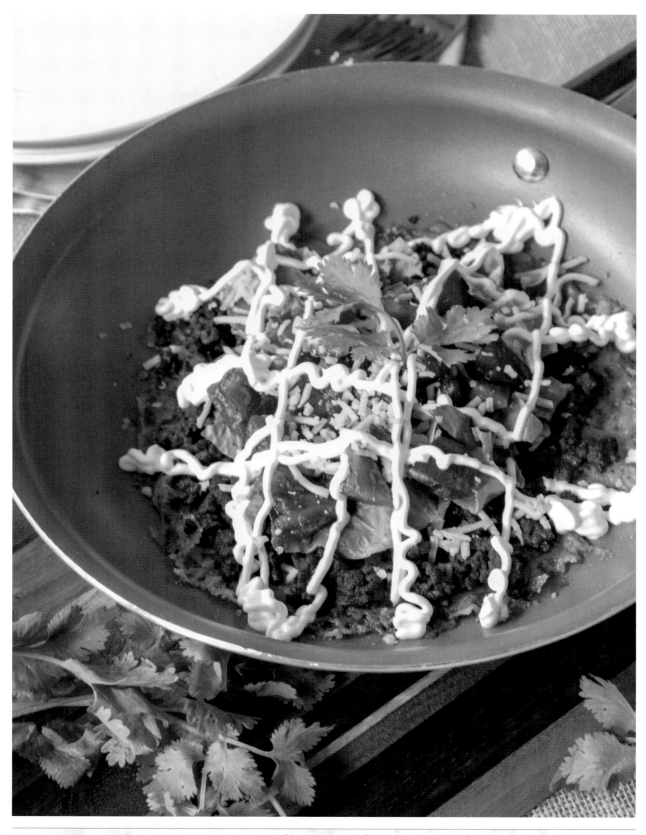

NUTRITION FACTS (PER SERVING):　　Calories: 459　|　Fat: 29.2g　|　Protein: 42.3g　|　Carbs: 5.5g　|　Fiber: 1.9g

Meatloaf

My kids love meatloaf. My husband loves meatloaf. I have never really been a fan, but this is one of two meatloaves that I make often and my whole family enjoys, including me. It is especially good served with Ranch Cauli Mash with Bacon (page 345), but it goes well with all sorts of side dishes. Other favorites are Skillet Mushrooms (page 349), Creamed Brussels Sprouts (page 361), and Bacon-Wrapped Asparagus (page 362). Grace likes it with low-carb ketchup (page 190) or Classic BBQ Sauce (page 195). I use leaner ground beef so that the meatloaf doesn't shrink as much during cooking.

MAKES: 8 servings

1 pound ground beef (93% lean)

1 pound ground pork

1 large egg, beaten

½ cup pork dust (ground pork rinds)

2 tablespoons dried minced onions

2 teaspoons Italian seasoning

2 teaspoons Worcestershire sauce

1 teaspoon white vinegar

1 teaspoon garlic powder

1 teaspoon ground dried thyme

1 teaspoon salt

½ teaspoon ground black pepper

1. Preheat the oven to 375°F.

2. Place all the ingredients in a large mixing bowl and, using your hands, mix thoroughly. Fill a 9 by 5-inch loaf pan with the meat mixture. Smooth out the top or shape it into a dome.

3. Bake the meatloaf for 60 to 70 minutes, until it is dark brown with no pink in the middle and the juices run clear when sliced. If using a meat thermometer, the internal temperature should register at least 165°F.

Time-Saver Tip:

I often bake the meatloaf in two smaller loaf pans instead of one large one so that it bakes faster and dinner gets on the table sooner.

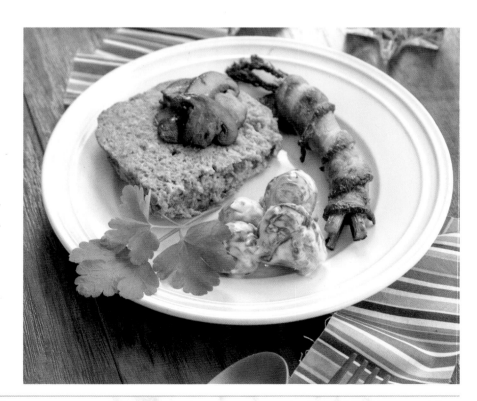

NUTRITION FACTS (PER SERVING):   Calories: 302 | Fat: 28.4g | Protein: 19.3g | Carbs: 2.2g | Fiber: 0.3g

Big Mac Salad

I was never really a fan of McDonald's legendary burger, the Big Mac, but my whole family is enamored with this simple salad. In fact, my husband, who was not keen to try this recipe, asked when I would be making it again. The key seems to be the pickles. Salty, sour sliced pickles are, without a doubt, what make this recipe work. Trust me on this one, even if you don't care for pickles.

OPTION

MAKES: 4 servings

1 pound ground beef (93% lean)

1 tablespoon Worcestershire sauce

1 tablespoon dried minced onions

1 teaspoon garlic powder

2 cups shredded lettuce

4 ounces cheddar cheese, shredded (about 1 cup)

1 medium tomato, chopped

1 tablespoon chopped onions, or ¼ small red onion, sliced

12 dill pickle slices

1 cup Thousand Island Dressing (page 211)

1 tablespoon toasted sesame seeds

1. Brown the ground beef in a large skillet over medium-high heat, stirring often to crumble the meat as it cooks. Add the Worcestershire sauce, dried minced onions, and garlic powder and stir until well combined. Remove from the heat and set aside.

2. Prepare the salad: Divide the lettuce equally among 4 plates or bowls. Top the lettuce with the prepared ground beef, cheese, tomato, onions, and pickles. Drizzle each salad with ¼ cup of the Thousand Island dressing and sprinkle with sesame seeds. Serve immediately.

Substitution Suggestion:

To make this salad dairy-free, omit the cheese.

Time-Saver Tip:

Make the beef ahead of time and reheat it just before serving the salad. The seasoned beef can also be frozen for later use.

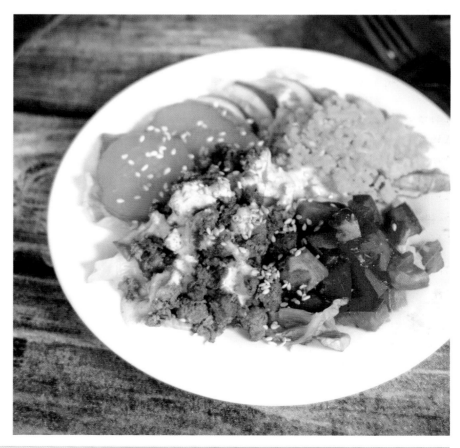

NUTRITION FACTS (PER SERVING): | Calories: 346 | Fat: 35.4g | Protein: 27.3g | Carbs: 5.7g | Fiber: 1.4g

Kristie's Crack Slaw

In case you are dubious about the addictive nature of this recipe, I will tell you about my middle schooler sharing it with her friends. Apparently, her lunch became so popular that I was instructed to include two servings of slaw in separate containers so that she had one to eat and one to share. I also was asked to send copies of the recipe to her teachers, who had sampled the slaw as well. As a final bit of proof, Grace once had a friend over, and I gave the girls the option to pick a restaurant for dinner. Instead of a restaurant, Grace's friend asked me to make my crack slaw. Just make it!

MAKES: 6 servings

2 pounds ground beef (80% lean)

1½ tablespoons minced fresh ginger

1 tablespoon dried minced onions

1 teaspoon garlic powder

½ teaspoon salt

¼ cup coconut aminos

4 cups shredded green cabbage

1 teaspoon red pepper flakes (optional)

3 drops liquid sweetener (optional)

1 tablespoon toasted sesame oil

1. Brown the ground beef in a large skillet over medium-high heat, stirring often to crumble the meat as it cooks. Add the ginger, dried onions, garlic powder, and salt and mix thoroughly. Pour in the coconut aminos.

2. Add the cabbage and cook until tender, 8 to 10 minutes. Add the red pepper flakes and sweetener, if using. Just before serving, drizzle the toasted sesame oil over the dish and toss to coat the beef and cabbage.

Time-Saver Tip:

Use preshredded cabbage to save time and reduce cleanup.

Substitution Suggestion:

While coconut aminos is the better option, you can use tamari instead. Tamari is much saltier than coconut aminos, so if you make this substitution, omit the ½ teaspoon of salt from the recipe.

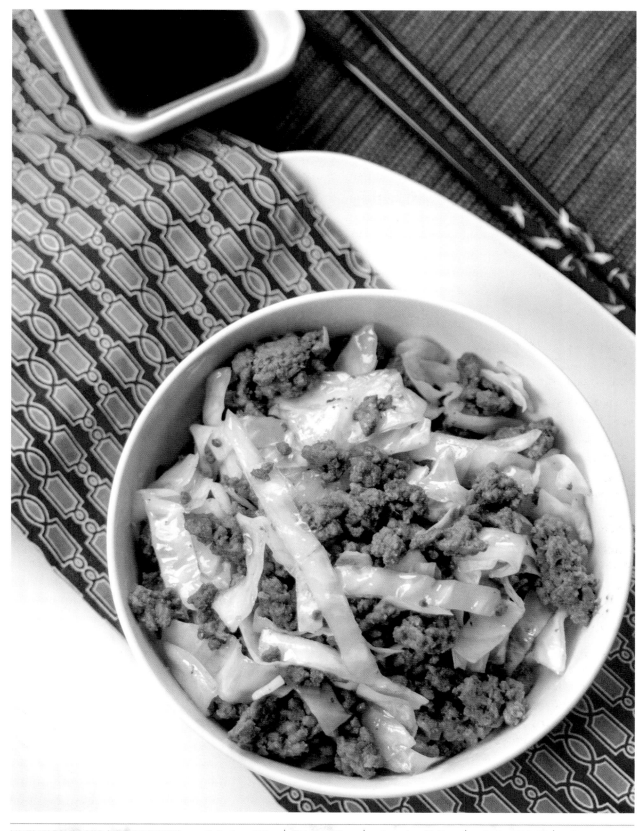

NUTRITION FACTS (PER SERVING):   Calories: 410 | Fat: 31.3g | Protein: 26.3g | Carbs: 5.2g | Fiber: 1.4g

Noodle-less Lasagna

Consider this truth: in a traditional lasagna, the noodles provide texture and structure for the layers of filling, but very little flavor. The rich taste we love comes from the meat sauce and cheeses. This keto-friendly lasagna packs all the flavors of a traditional lasagna but uses long strips of zucchini instead of high-carb noodles. Don't worry about getting the slices perfect; you will cover them with meat sauce and cheeses. Both of my kids are fans of this recipe, except that I have to peel the green skin from the zucchini for my picky son. Once, when I was in a hurry, I didn't, and I got the dreaded question, "Hey, Mom, what's this green stuff in my lasagna?" Take the time to trim off the green stuff if you have a picky eater at your table.

MAKES: 6 servings

2 medium zucchini

1 pound ground beef (93% lean)

8 ounces bulk Italian sausage

⅓ cup chopped onions

1 teaspoon minced garlic

2 teaspoons Italian seasoning

1 recipe Marinara Sauce (page 203)

1 cup ricotta cheese

8 ounces mozzarella cheese, shredded (about 2 cups)

1 ounce Parmesan cheese, grated (about ⅓ cup), plus extra for garnish

1. Preheat the oven to 375°F.

2. Using a sharp knife, thinly slice the zucchini lengthwise into broad, planklike slices similar to lasagna noodles. Lay the slices in a single layer on a paper towel to dry. Set aside.

3. In a large skillet, brown the ground beef and sausage with the onions, garlic, and Italian seasoning over medium heat, stirring often to crumble the meat as it cooks. When the meat is browned, add the marinara sauce and stir to combine. Set the meat sauce aside.

4. Layer the ingredients in a 13 by 9-inch or similar-sized baking dish. Start with 1 cup of the meat sauce to just cover the bottom of the dish. Then make a layer using half of the zucchini noodles. Top the zucchini layer with half of the ricotta and half of the mozzarella. Cover the cheeses with 1½ cups of the meat sauce. Repeat these layers, ending with the remaining meat sauce.

5. Sprinkle the Parmesan cheese over the top of the lasagna and bake until bubbly and browned, 40 to 50 minutes. Sprinkle the baked lasagna with more Parmesan and let cool for at least 10 minutes before serving.

Substitution Suggestions:

Cabbage Noodles (page 342) make an excellent substitution for the zucchini noodles. Slices of cooked bacon can also serve as noodles, as can slices of deli turkey or shaved roast beef.

Time-Saver Tip:

Leftovers are excellent for portioning into freezer-safe containers and freezing for later consumption.

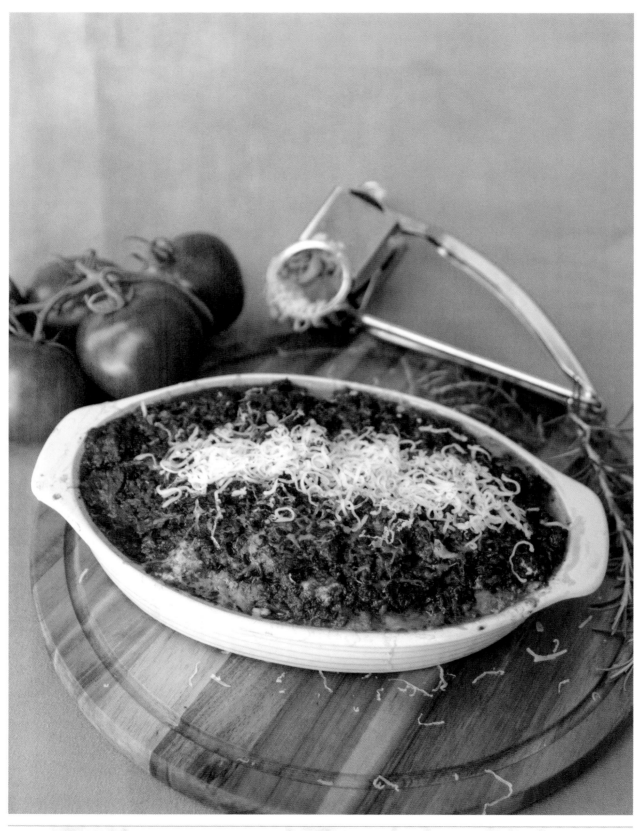

NUTRITION FACTS (PER SERVING): Calories: 567 | Fat: 49.7g | Protein: 36.5g | Carbs: 8.2g | Fiber: 2.3g

20-Minute
Skillet Dinner

I love cheap, easy, and quick meals, especially on weeknights when my family has had a busy day and we still have homework or other evening obligations. This recipe was a plan B. I had planned to make taco salad but discovered at the last minute that I didn't have any romaine lettuce on hand. The family still expected dinner, so I made up this dish! It ended up tasting like a low-carb version of Hamburger Helper. It's just as easy to make as the boxed kind but is more flavorful and much healthier. In my version, cauliflower replaces high-carb pasta and heavy cream and cream cheese up the fat content. I knew I had a winner when my daughter said, "Hey, you made a healthy Hamburger Helper!" The recipe has since become a part of our monthly meal rotation.

MAKES: 4 servings

1 pound ground beef
(80% lean)

1 tablespoon bacon fat

1 cup finely chopped
cauliflower florets

2 teaspoons Jane's Crazy
Mixed-Up Salt

⅓ cup water

4 ounces cream cheese
(½ cup)

2 tablespoons unsalted
butter

1 teaspoon onion powder

⅓ cup heavy cream

2 ounces cheddar cheese,
shredded (about ½ cup), plus
extra for garnish if desired

1. Brown the ground beef in a large skillet with a lid over medium-high heat, stirring often to crumble the meat as it cooks.

2. Add the bacon fat, chopped cauliflower, and seasoning salt and cook over medium heat, stirring occasionally. When the cauliflower is just beginning to soften, add the water and cover the skillet with the lid. Cook for 5 to 7 minutes, until the cauliflower is tender.

3. Remove the lid and reduce the heat to low. Add the cream cheese, butter, and onion powder and stir until melted. Add the heavy cream and stir until smooth and creamy. Remove from the heat, stir in the cheddar cheese, and serve immediately. Garnish with additional shredded cheddar, if desired.

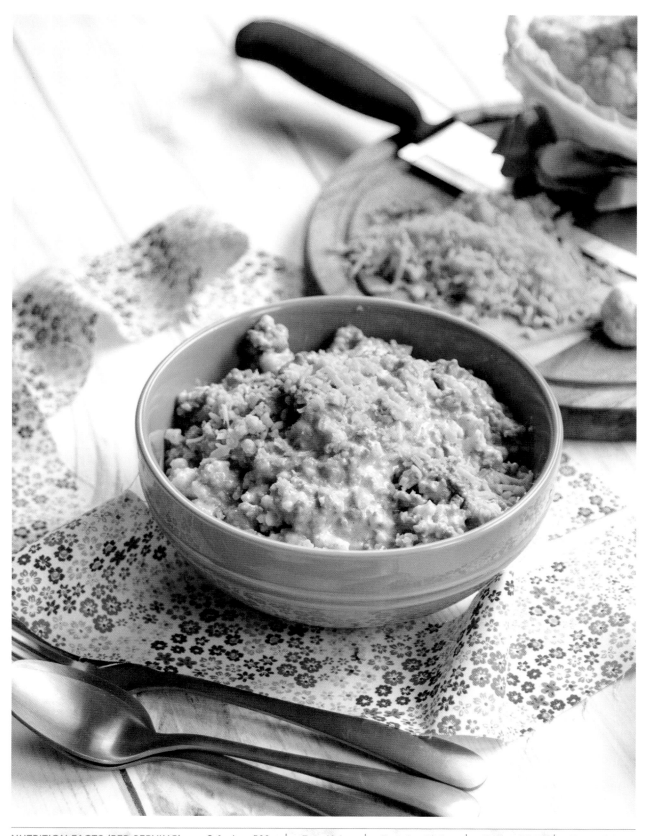

NUTRITION FACTS (PER SERVING):   Calories: 502 | Fat: 49.1g | Protein: 25.3g | Carbs: 2.8g | Fiber: 0.6g

Three-Meat Chili

This very-low-carb chili recipe yields eight generous servings. It uses 3 pounds of meat, which ensures that it is hearty and filling. One of the reasons I add so much meat is that chili can be high in carbs. Between the tomatoes and the seasonings, which include some of the highest-carb spices out there, traditional chili is not really low-carb. Using various cuts of meat provides different textures. The bite-sized pork and steak lend a texture similar to beans, which are out of the question on a ketogenic diet. With those varying textures, you won't miss those little carb bombs. Like most chili recipes, this chili tastes best a day or two after it's made. We like to top ours with a dollop of sour cream and/or some shredded cheese just before serving.

OPTION

MAKES: 8 servings

1 tablespoon bacon fat

1 pound beef round steak, cut into bite-sized pieces

1 pound ground beef (93% lean)

1 pound cubed pork steak or ground pork

2 tablespoons dried minced onions, or ½ cup chopped fresh onions

2 teaspoons minced garlic

2 teaspoons salt

3 tablespoons chili powder

2 teaspoons ground cumin

2 teaspoons paprika

1 teaspoon onion powder

1½ cups strained tomatoes

2 cups beef bone broth, homemade (page 187) or store-bought

1 cup water

½ cup (1 stick) unsalted butter or ghee

1. Heat the bacon fat in a 6-quart or larger saucepan over medium-high heat. Brown the meats one at a time, stirring often to crumble the meat as it cooks, then return all the browned meats to the saucepan. Add the onions, garlic, salt, and spices and stir to coat the meats with the seasonings.

2. Add the tomatoes, broth, water, and butter. Lower the heat and simmer, uncovered, for 35 to 45 minutes, until the meats are tender and the chili has thickened.

Time-Saver Tip:

Freeze individual portions for quick meals on busy days.

Substitution Suggestion:

You can use any combination of boneless cuts of beef, pork, or chicken that you prefer, as long as the total amount of meat is 3 pounds. Choose types and cuts of meat that cook at about the same rate, and keep in mind that tougher cuts of beef or pork will require a longer cooking time.

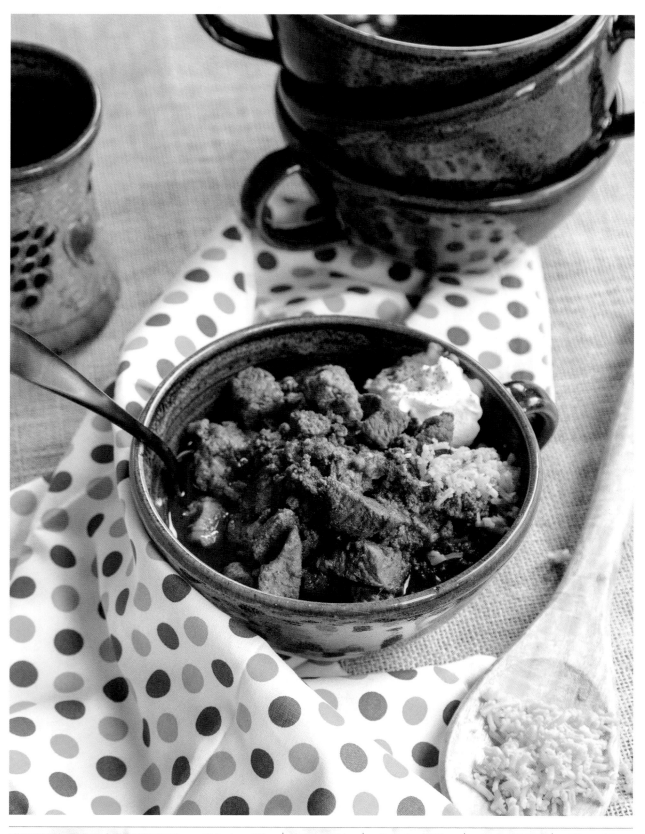

NUTRITION FACTS (PER SERVING):   Calories: 415 | Fat: 32.6g | Protein: 25.8g | Carbs: 5.9g | Fiber: 2.1g

Asian-Style
Beef and Broccoli

This recipe is a favorite, and I can assure you that one of the reasons my family enjoys it so much is an ingredient they don't like. Promise to keep my secret? Not one of us is a fan of oysters, yet oyster sauce is the key ingredient to making an extraordinarily rich beef and broccoli. Before you rush to the store, let me tell you that you don't want to buy a bottle of oyster sauce. Simply buy a can of oysters and strain the brine for a homemade oyster sauce without the added sugars commonly found in commercial brands. Another game-changer in this recipe is sesame oil. Pouring it over the dish just before serving keeps your taste buds chasing the flavor and the fat. This classic dish is delicious paired with Cauli Rice (page 343).

MAKES: 8 servings

1 tablespoon coconut oil or bacon fat

2 pounds beef round steak, cut into strips

2 cloves garlic, minced

2 tablespoons minced fresh ginger

1 teaspoon salt (omit if using tamari)

¼ cup beef bone broth, homemade (page 187) or store-bought

¼ cup Chinese rice wine or dry sherry (optional)

¼ cup coconut aminos or tamari

3 tablespoons oyster brine from 1 (8-ounce) can whole oysters packed in water

2 cups broccoli florets

2 teaspoons toasted sesame oil

1. Heat the coconut oil in a large skillet with a lid over high heat. When the oil is hot, add the steak, garlic, ginger, and salt and stir-fry for 8 to 12 minutes, until the beef is browned on all sides.

2. Add the broth, rice wine (if using), coconut aminos, and oyster brine and reduce the heat to medium-low. Once at a simmer, cover the skillet and simmer over low heat for 12 to 15 minutes, until the beef is tender.

3. Add the broccoli and cook, uncovered, over medium-low heat for 12 to 15 more minutes, stirring frequently. When the broccoli is tender, remove the pan from the heat and pour in the sesame oil. Stir to distribute the oil, then serve.

Note:

My recipe for Moo Goo Gai Pan (page 330) also uses this keto-friendly oyster sauce substitution, in case you end up with leftover brine. You can discard the oysters or set them aside to fry, using a "breading" made up of equal parts pork dust and Parmesan cheese.

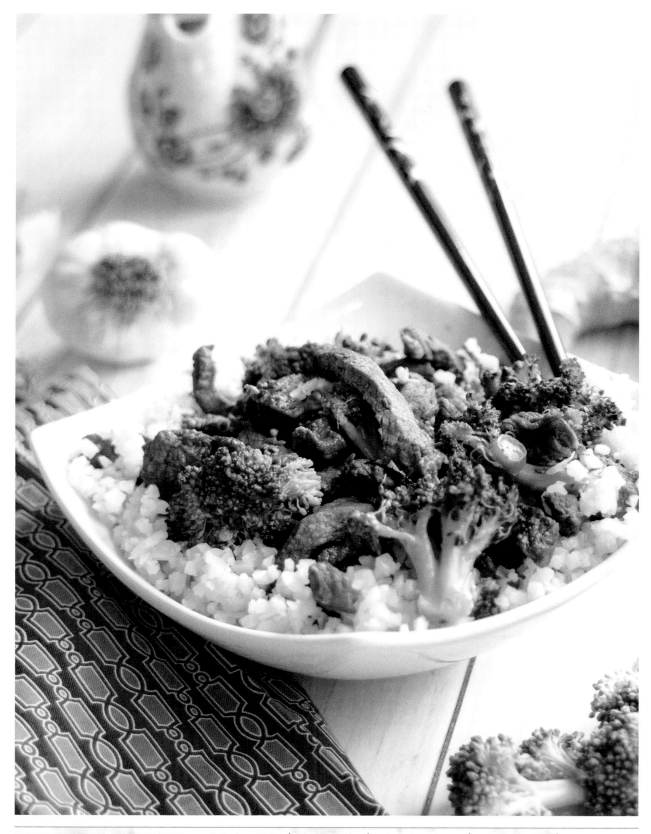

NUTRITION FACTS (PER SERVING): Calories: 264 | Fat: 16.7g | Protein: 24.5g | Carbs: 3.6g | Fiber: 0.8g

Savory
Pepper Steak

While I generally make meals to feed my family of four, I often make an extra-large batch of this steak dish. It's that good! Plus, the leftovers, if there are any, taste even better a day or two later. We enjoy this dish on its own or with Cauli Rice (page 343). You can also serve it over Cabbage Noodles (page 342), but the peppers and onions in this dish are already fairly high in carbohydrates, so I see no good reason to add even more carbs.

MAKES: 8 servings

1 tablespoon coconut oil or bacon fat

2 pounds round steak, cut into 3-inch long by ¼- to ½-inch-thick strips

2 cloves garlic, minced

1 teaspoon salt

1 medium onion, sliced

8 ounces mushrooms, sliced

2 stalks celery, chopped

1 cup beef bone broth, homemade (page 187) or store-bought

2 medium-sized bell peppers (any color), cut into strips

¼ cup coconut aminos or tamari

1. Heat the coconut oil in a large skillet over high heat. When hot, add the steak, garlic, and salt and brown the steak for 8 to 10 minutes, stirring frequently.

2. When the steak is browned, add the onion, mushrooms, and celery and continue cooking for 8 to 10 minutes, until the vegetables are tender.

3. Add the broth and reduce the heat to low. Simmer, covered, for 10 to 15 minutes, until the meat is tender. Remove the lid and continue to simmer for 4 to 6 minutes, until the sauce has thickened.

4. Increase the heat to medium. Add the bell peppers and coconut aminos and cook for 6 to 7 minutes, until the peppers are tender but not soft.

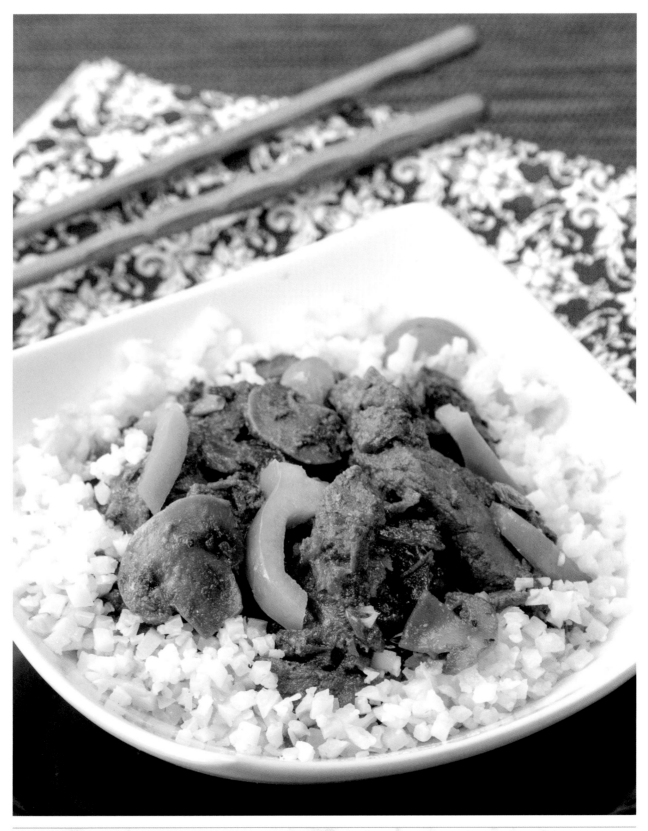

NUTRITION FACTS (PER SERVING):   **Calories: 264** | **Fat: 15.5g** | **Protein: 25.9g** | **Carbs: 5.2g** | **Fiber: 1.3g**

Mississippi Roast

Dinner doesn't get easier than this three-ingredient beef roast, especially if you have the ranch seasoning prepared in advance. While a popular version of this dish is prevalent online, that version uses packaged ranch dressing powder that includes food starches and other undesirable ingredients. My homemade ranch seasoning is a much healthier option.

My family loves Creamy Cauli Mash (page 344) as a side dish with this roast. I get bonus points if I make the gravy to go with it! You can also serve it with Herb-Roasted Radishes (page 347), as shown here—or, to save time, add the radishes to the slow cooker so that they cook right along with the meat.

MAKES: **8 servings**

1 (4- to 5-pound) boneless beef chuck roast

3 tablespoons Ranch Seasoning (page 208)

½ cup (1 stick) salted butter

GRAVY (OPTIONAL):

Reserved cooking liquid from the slow cooker

2 ounces cream cheese (¼ cup)

¼ cup heavy cream

Salt and pepper

1. Rinse the beef roast in cold water and place in a 4-quart or larger slow cooker. Sprinkle half of the ranch seasoning over the roast. Turn the roast over and sprinkle the other side with the remaining seasoning. Place the butter on top of the roast. (You can leave it whole or cut it into chunks.)

2. Cook the roast on high for 5 to 6 hours or on low for 8 to 9 hours, until it is quite tender and easy to slice or shred. Reserve the liquid in the slow cooker to serve as an "au jus" with the roast, or use it to make a rich pan gravy.

3. If making a pan gravy, strain the remaining cooking liquid into a saucepan and place over medium heat. Simmer until the liquid is reduced by one-third to one-half. Add the cream cheese and stir until melted. Add the heavy cream and simmer for 4 to 5 minutes, until the gravy has thickened. Season with salt and pepper to taste and serve with the roast.

Carb Check:

Please take the time to make homemade ranch seasoning. It is easy to prepare and less expensive and more flavorful than commercial brands.

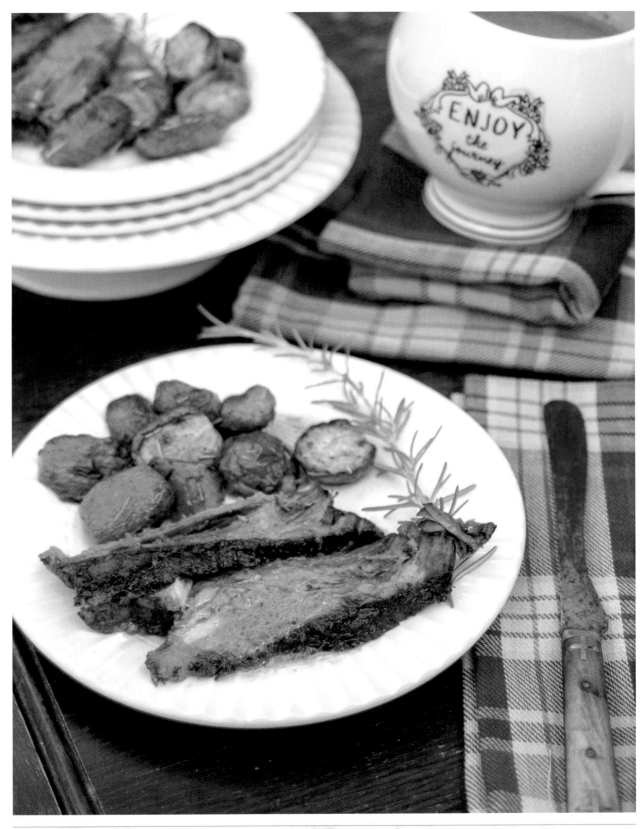

NUTRITION FACTS (PER SERVING):   Calories: 783 | Fat: 65.8g | Protein: 43.7g | Carbs: 1.1g | Fiber: 0.2g

Dry-Rubbed
Beef Ribs

Beef ribs are a hearty meat for grilling or smoking, and my whole family enjoys them. Maybe it's because ribs are best cooked low and slow, but cooking them is like a ritual at our house. The anticipation builds with each step in the process, and when that big plate of ribs and all the sides are set on the table, it's time to dig in! We serve them up with plenty of Unsweetened Iced Tea (page 218) and traditional sides liked Baked Cauliflower Mac and Cheese (page 368), Homecoming Broccoli Salad (page 350), and Cucumber, Tomato, and Feta Salad (page 356). Ribs are messy finger food at its finest. If you don't leave the table wearing a little sauce or with grease stains on your clothes, then you probably aren't eating them right!

My husband smokes the ribs in a ceramic smoker, but you can follow this same process using your oven. Don't let the lengthy steps deter you from trying this recipe. These ribs are well worth the wait!

MAKES: **4 servings**

DAVID'S DRY RUB FOR BEEF RIBS:

2 tablespoons ground black pepper

1 tablespoon onion powder

1 tablespoon salt

2 teaspoons chili powder

2 teaspoons garlic powder

2 teaspoons mustard powder

1 teaspoon instant coffee powder

½ teaspoon cayenne pepper (optional)

6 pounds beef back ribs

⅓ cup prepared yellow mustard

1 recipe Classic BBQ Sauce (page 195)

1. Put the ingredients for the dry rub in a small bowl and stir until well combined. Set aside.

2. Prepare the ribs: Use a sharp knife to remove the membrane covering the back of the rack of ribs. The ribs will remain intact. After removing the membrane, place the ribs on a baking sheet. Use your hands or the back of a spoon to spread a thin layer of the mustard all over the surface of the ribs, then coat the ribs on all sides with the dry rub. Cover and refrigerate for at least an hour or up to overnight.

3. If using a smoker, preheat the smoker to 300°F. When the smoker has reached temperature, place the ribs in a single layer on the rack. Smoke for 2 hours. Remove the ribs from the smoker, cover in the BBQ sauce, and wrap tightly in foil. Return the ribs to the smoker and smoke at 250°F for 1 hour. Remove the ribs from the smoker and discard the foil. Return the ribs to the smoker for 1 more hour. The ribs should reach a minimum internal temperature of 160°F when a meat thermometer is inserted into the thickest part of the rack; however, the ribs are the most tender when they reach 190°F to 200°F. You can also test for doneness by inserting a toothpick into the meat between the bones.

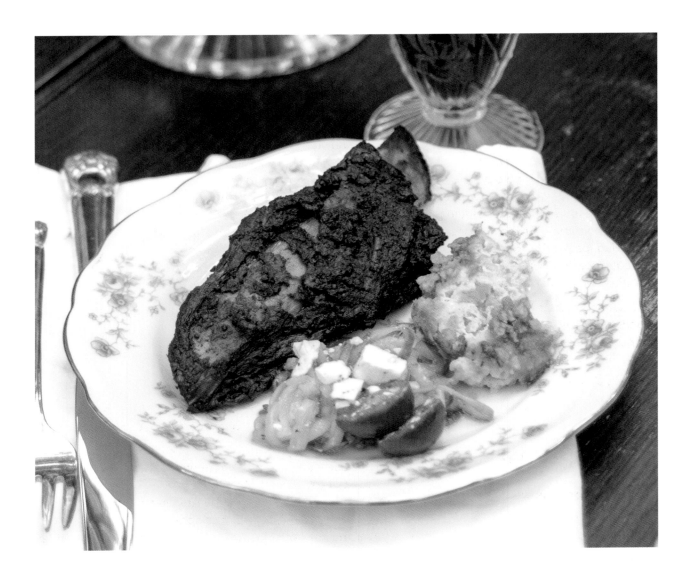

If using the oven, preheat the oven to 300°F. Set a wire rack inside a rimmed baking sheet. Set the ribs on top of the rack and bake for 2 hours. Remove the ribs from the oven, cover in the BBQ sauce, and wrap tightly in foil. Return the ribs to the oven, reduce the temperature to 250°F, and bake for 1 hour. Remove the ribs from the oven and discard the foil. Return the ribs to the oven for 1 more hour. The ribs should reach a minimum internal temperature of 160°F when a meat thermometer is inserted into the thickest part of the rack; however, the ribs are the most tender when they reach 190°F to 200°F. You can also test for doneness by inserting a toothpick into the meat between the bones.

4. Serve the ribs immediately or wrap in foil to rest at room temperature until you are ready to serve them.

Note:

The protein per serving for this recipe is higher than I would typically consume in one meal. I would eat a smaller portion and balance the meal with fatty sides so that the total number of fat grams in the meal would be equal to or greater than the total number of protein grams.

NUTRITION FACTS (PER SERVING): Calories: 768 | Fat: 59.4g | Protein: 54.4g | Carbs: 6.8g | Fiber: 2.7g

Bolognese

Although I make Bolognese an average of three times per month, if you asked my children if they like Bolognese, they would likely answer, "We've never had it!" They know this as "spaghetti sauce," and I'm guessing you probably do, too. Bolognese is the proper name for this meat sauce, but we rarely call it that; we just call it "a good dinner"! Another bonus is that it is inexpensive and fast. You can serve it over Zoodles (page 340), Cabbage Noodles (page 342), glucomannan noodles (such as Miracle Noodles), or a scoop of full-fat ricotta cheese. We often eat it from a bowl just as we would eat stew.

MAKES: 4 servings

½ **pound ground beef (93% lean)**

½ **pound ground pork**

2 (8-ounce) cans tomato sauce

1 cup beef bone broth, homemade (page 187) or store-bought

1 tablespoon Italian seasoning

2 teaspoons garlic powder

2 bay leaves

1 teaspoon salt

1. Brown the ground beef and pork in a large skillet with a lid over medium heat, stirring often to crumble the meat as it cooks. When the meat is browned, add the tomato sauce, broth, and seasonings. Reduce the heat and simmer for about 15 minutes, until the sauce has thickened.

2. Cover and simmer for another 10 to 15 minutes, until the meat is tender and the flavor of the sauce has intensified. Remove and discard the bay leaves before serving.

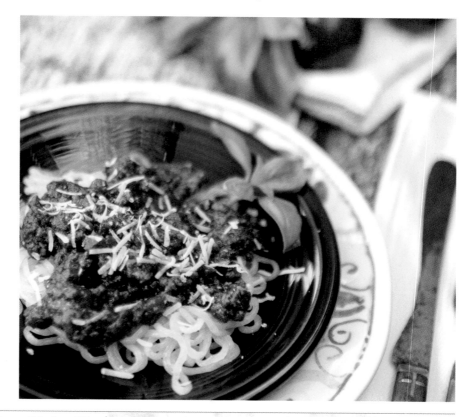

NUTRITION FACTS (PER SERVING):   Calories: 279 | Fat: 15.8g | Protein: 24.9g | Carbs: 7.2g | Fiber: 1.3g

No-Vodka
Vodka Sauce

This recipe breaks tradition in two ways: one) it contains no vodka, and two) it includes meat. Perhaps Vodka Sauce is not the right name for it, but I love the heavy cream that is a typical part of vodka sauce, and I wanted to make a keto version. Whatever you call it, this sauce is excellent served over Cabbage Noodles (page 342) or glucomannan noodles (such as Miracle Noodles).

MAKES: 4 servings

½ pound ground beef (93% lean)

½ pound ground pork

1 tablespoon minced garlic

2 (8-ounce) cans tomato sauce

½ cup beef bone broth, homemade (page 187) or store-bought

2 tablespoons unsalted butter

2 teaspoons dried basil

1 teaspoon onion powder

½ teaspoon salt

Pinch of red pepper flakes (optional)

1 cup heavy cream

Grated Parmesan cheese, for garnish

1. Brown the ground beef and pork with the garlic in a large skillet over medium-high heat, stirring often to crumble the meat as it cooks. When the meat is browned, add the tomato sauce, broth, butter, and seasonings. Reduce the heat and simmer for 10 to 15 minutes, until the sauce has thickened.

2. Stir in the cream, lower the heat, and simmer gently for about 5 minutes. Serve topped with a generous sprinkle of grated Parmesan.

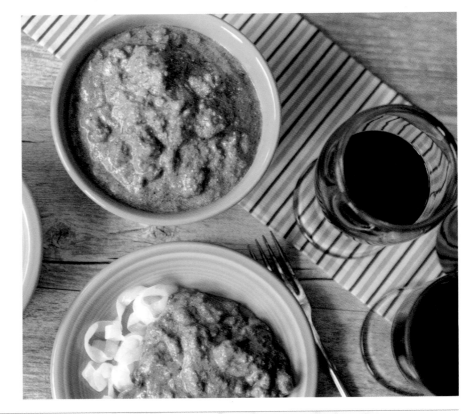

NUTRITION FACTS (PER SERVING):   Calories: 427 | Fat: 31.9g | Protein: 24.8g | Carbs: 8.6g | Fiber: 1.4g

Taco Soup

During a period of short-term success on Weight Watchers, I lived on taco soup. I made a huge batch every Sunday and ate it throughout the week ad nauseam. When I discovered how well a ketogenic diet works for me, I swore I would never eat that soup again. To be truthful, this really isn't that soup. This is a healthier, more flavorful version with satiating fat, so it is easy to enjoy.

MAKES: 6 servings

1 pound Mexican-style fresh (raw) chorizo, casings removed

1 pound ground beef (93% lean)

⅓ cup chopped green bell peppers

⅓ cup chopped onions

1 jalapeño pepper, seeded and chopped

2 tablespoons Taco Seasoning (page 207)

2 cups beef bone broth, homemade (page 187) or store-bought

1 (8-ounce) can tomato sauce

1 cup chopped zucchini

FOR SERVING (OPTIONAL):

Sour cream

Shredded cheddar cheese

Sliced avocado

Fresh cilantro leaves

1. Brown the chorizo and ground beef in a 6-quart saucepan over medium-high heat, stirring often to crumble the meat as it cooks. Add the bell peppers, onions, jalapeño, and taco seasoning and cook until the vegetables are tender and slightly browned, 8 to 10 minutes.

2. Add the broth, tomato sauce, and zucchini and stir to combine. Simmer, uncovered, over low heat for 20 to 25 minutes, until the zucchini is tender. Serve the soup topped with a dollop of sour cream, some shredded cheese, a slice of avocado, and/or some cilantro leaves, if desired.

Time-Saver Tip:

Use browned and seasoned taco meat that you have already prepped and frozen to create this meal in less than half an hour.

Substitution Suggestion:

If you can't find an acceptable brand of chorizo or you prefer not to use pork, you can make an equally delicious all-beef taco soup. Simply replace the chorizo with an additional pound of ground beef and increase the taco seasoning to 3 tablespoons.

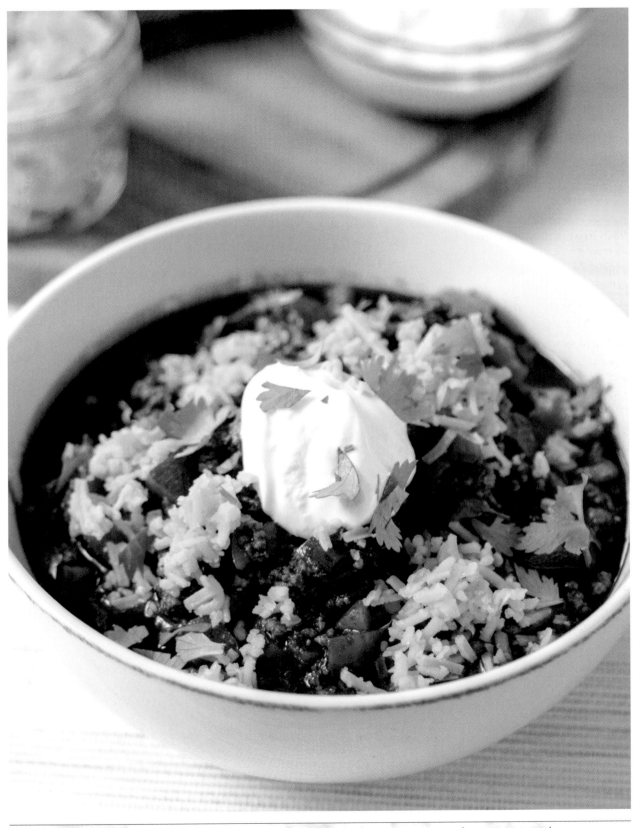

NUTRITION FACTS (PER SERVING):   Calories: 350 | Fat: 26.1g | Protein: 23.8g | Carbs: 5.4g | Fiber: 2.2g

Simple Pulled Pork

Pulled pork is on the menu at least once a month at my house. The cut of meat used is inexpensive, making pulled pork a great choice for feeding a crowd. You can use either pork butt or pork shoulder. While the two cuts are similar, pork butt tends to have more marbling and shreds more easily. Because both cuts have quite a bit of gristle and sinew, they need to be cooked at a lower temperature for a longer period than a more tender cut like tenderloin. A slow cooker is perfect if you don't have a smoker or you don't want to heat up the oven for several hours. This recipe includes directions for both the oven (which are similar to the directions for using a smoker) and a slow cooker.

I serve this pulled pork with the classic tomato-based BBQ sauce on page 195 as well as the eastern Carolina–style vinegar-based sauce on page 194 and the mayonnaise-based white BBQ sauce on page 196.

MAKES: ten to twelve 4-ounce servings

2 tablespoons smoked paprika

1 tablespoon garlic powder

1 tablespoon onion powder

1 tablespoon salt

2 teaspoons ground black pepper

1 (4- to 5-pound) boneless pork butt or pork shoulder

½ cup prepared yellow mustard (omit if using a slow cooker)

OVEN OR SMOKER METHOD:

1. Preheat the oven or smoker to 275°F. Mix together the dry seasonings in a small bowl and set aside.

2. Coat every surface of the pork with the mustard, then sprinkle with the seasoning mixture to coat.

3. If using the oven, place the prepared pork in a roasting pan. If using a smoker, place it directly on the rack. Be sure to place it fatty side up so that the fat and juices run into the meat as it cooks. Roast or smoke the pork for 3½ to 4 hours, until the internal temperature reaches 165°F. Wrap the meat in foil and let rest for 20 to 30 minutes before shredding, chopping, or slicing and serving. Reserve the pan drippings to serve with the pork, if desired.

Time-Saver Tip:

Because the yield of this recipe is high, I frequently freeze the meat without BBQ sauce. To reheat, put the frozen meat in a large skillet with ¼ cup of water. Cover the skillet with a lid and set over medium heat until the pulled pork is warmed through.

SLOW COOKER METHOD:

Mix together the dry seasonings in a small bowl. Place the pork in a 6-quart or larger slow cooker and sprinkle with the seasoning mixture to coat. Cook on low for 10 to 12 hours, until the internal temperature of the pork reaches 165°F. Remove the meat from the slow cooker and shred, chop, or slice and serve.

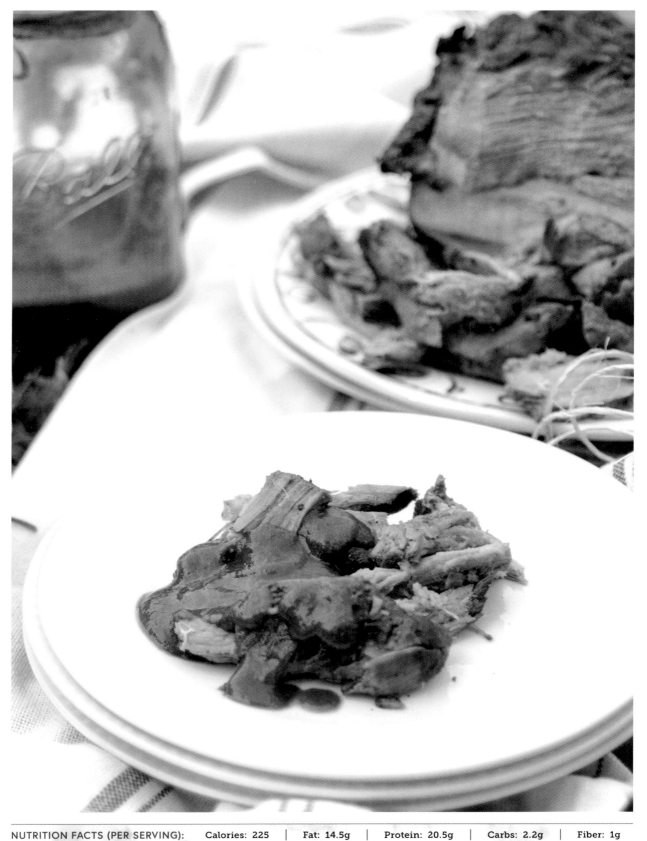

NUTRITION FACTS (PER SERVING):   Calories: 225 | Fat: 14.5g | Protein: 20.5g | Carbs: 2.2g | Fiber: 1g

Slow Cooker
Tender Baby Back Ribs

While beef ribs are delicious, I'm actually fonder of pork baby back ribs because they are foolproof to prepare: no matter how I make them, they turn out very tender nearly every single time. Here I've given you a super easy method for making ribs in a slow cooker. If you want to smoke or roast them, and I suggest that you do for classic smoked ribs with a deeper flavor, please follow the method used to make the beef ribs on page 298. Note: While people swear by boiling pork ribs before roasting or smoking them, I prefer them smoked or roasted without being boiled first.

MAKES: 4 servings

2 racks pork baby back ribs

DAVID'S DRY RUB FOR PORK:

1 tablespoon onion powder

1 tablespoon salt

1 tablespoon ground black pepper

2 teaspoons garlic powder

2 teaspoons mustard powder

2 teaspoons smoked paprika

1 teaspoon ground coffee

1 recipe Classic BBQ Sauce (page 195)

1. Rinse the ribs and pat them dry. Combine the ingredients for the dry rub in a small bowl.

2. Cover the ribs with the dry rub and place in a 6-quart or larger slow cooker, laying them on their sides if possible. Cook on low for 8 to 9 hours, until the meat is tender and begins to pull away from the bones.

3. Near the end of the slow-cooking time, preheat the oven to 400°F.

4. Remove the ribs from the slow cooker and place on a rimmed baking sheet in a single layer. Cover with the BBQ sauce and roast for 15 to 20 minutes, until the sauce has thickened and darkened slightly.

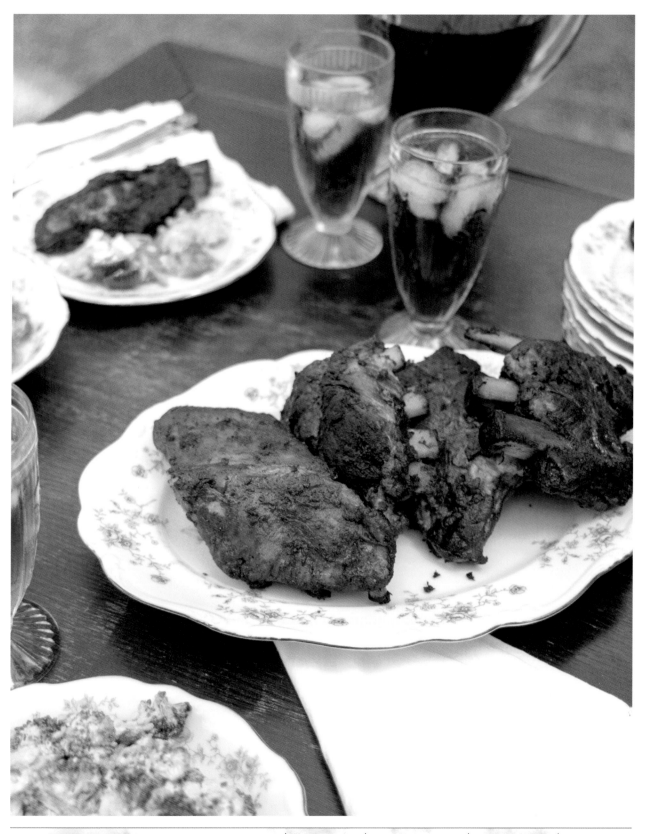

NUTRITION FACTS (PER SERVING): Calories: 544 | Fat: 37.1g | Protein: 42.1g | Carbs: 5.8g | Fiber: 2g

Pork Chops
with Pan Gravy

Once upon a time, a three-year-old Grace asked, "Mama, what is this?" while pointing to the chopped-up meat on her plate. "That's called pork chop," I explained. "Well, them pork chops is hard," she replied. She was right. Them pork chops was hard. And dry. Since then, I have learned to cook pork chops in ways that keep them moist and fatty. This recipe does that and creates a pan gravy to serve over the pork, just in case.

MAKES: **4 servings**

1 tablespoon bacon fat

1 pound boneless pork chops (about ½ inch thick), untrimmed

2 teaspoons Jane's Crazy Mixed-Up Salt

2 green onions, chopped

½ cup chicken or beef bone broth, homemade (pages 186 and 187) or store-bought

1. In a large skillet with a lid, melt the bacon fat over medium-high heat. Season the pork chops on both sides with the seasoning salt and place in the hot skillet in a single layer. Brown the chops on both sides, 5 to 7 minutes per side.

2. Reduce the heat to low. Cover the skillet with a lid and cook for 8 to 10 minutes, then turn the pork chops and cook, covered, for another 5 to 7 minutes, until tender. Remove the lid and cook, uncovered, for 3 to 5 more minutes, until the pan juices have simmered down. Remove the chops from the skillet.

3. Increase the heat to medium and add the green onions and broth. Use a spatula to scrape up the pan drippings and mix them with the broth. Simmer for 8 to 10 minutes, until the liquid is reduced. Return the pork chops to the pan and simmer for 2 to 3 minutes to rewarm. Serve warm with the pan gravy ladled over the chops.

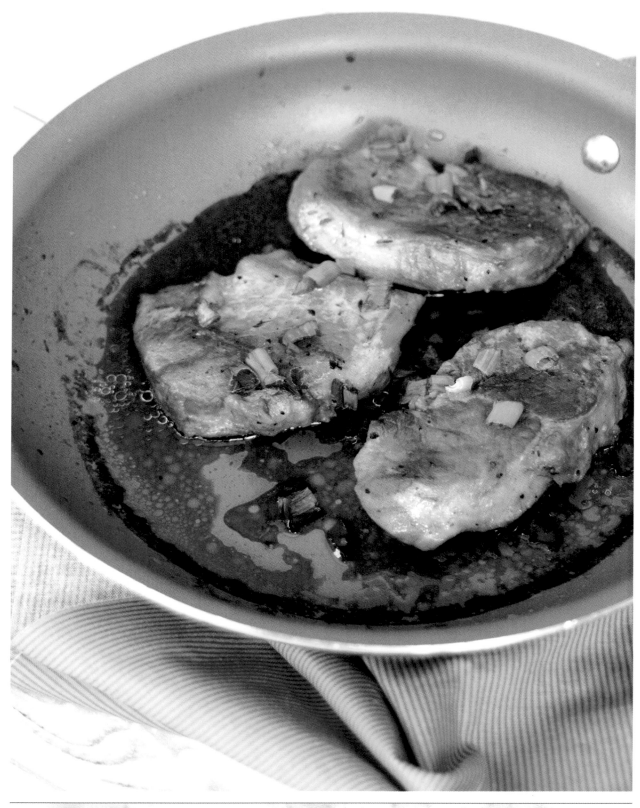

NUTRITION FACTS (PER SERVING):   Calories: 319 | Fat: 12.5g | Protein: 48.3g | Carbs: 0.3g | Fiber: 0.1g

Simple
Roasted Pork Tenderloin

Pork tenderloin is reliably moist and tender and relatively quick to cook. Find tenderloins on sale and you can make a simple but impressive meal for your family and friends. I either roast them, as described below, or smoke them in a smoker. If you're fortunate enough to own a smoker, then grab some Applewood chips and make this recipe in the smoker. I have tried nearly every seasoning combination imaginable and have found that the best flavor comes from a simple mix of salt and pepper, especially if you grill or smoke the meat.

Because tenderloin is so lean, I usually serve it with a fatty side like Cauliflower au Gratin (page 346) or Homecoming Broccoli Salad (page 350). In the summer, it is nice with a cold salad like my Cucumber, Tomato, and Feta Salad (page 356). You can also keep it simple and pair it with a steamed vegetable smothered in Simple Cheese Sauce (page 199).

MAKES: 6 servings

1½ pounds pork tenderloin

2 tablespoons bacon fat, salted butter, or ghee, melted

1 teaspoon salt

¼ teaspoon ground black pepper

1. Preheat the oven to 375°F.

2. Pat the pork dry. Rub the meat with the melted bacon fat and season with the salt and pepper. Place the pork in a baking dish.

3. Roast the pork for 30 to 45 minutes, until the internal temperature reaches a minimum of 145°F. (I prefer it cooked to 160°F.) The roast should be dark on the outside, and the juices should run clear when the meat is sliced.

4. Let the pork rest for at least 10 minutes before slicing and serving so that the meat remains moist. Pour the pan drippings over the sliced pork.

Time-Saver Tip:

For an even quicker meal, you can cut the tenderloin into 1- to 1½-inch-thick slices and pan-fry them. The leftovers freeze well and can be pulled from the freezer and quickly reheated in a skillet or in the oven. If warming in the oven, wrap the meat in foil.

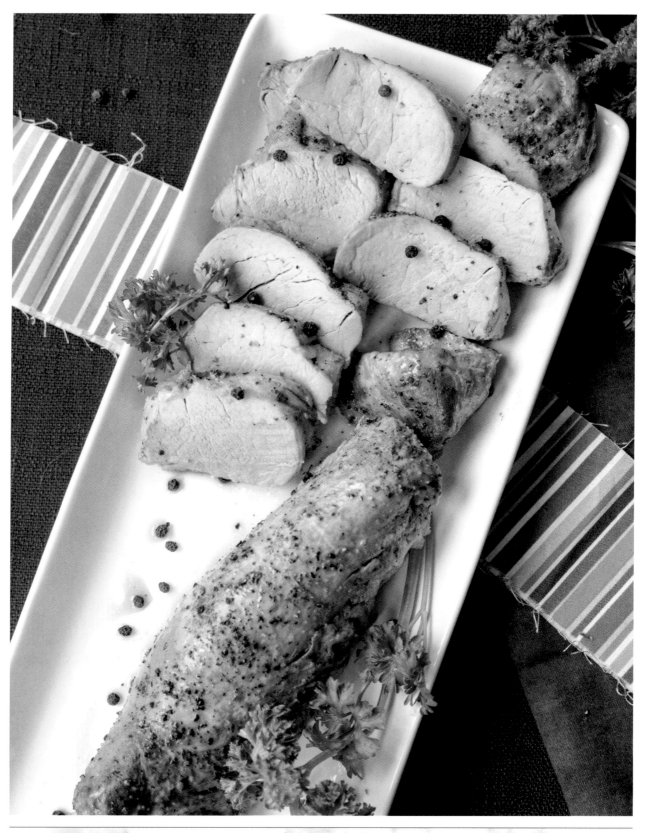

NUTRITION FACTS (PER SERVING):   Calories: 163 | Fat: 8.2g | Protein: 20.8g | Carbs: 0g | Fiber: 0g

Taco Bake

This is my favorite dish to take to a potluck or any large gathering where appetizers are served. It uses both ground beef and chorizo for a thick, diplike dish. I serve it with sliced avocado, salsa fresca (page 206) or diced tomatoes, sour cream, and/or fresh cilantro. For carbivores, I often provide tortilla chips, but a keto-adapted diner needs only a spoon. Your guests will never know how simple or how healthy this dish is! If you're lucky enough to have leftovers, you can use them to make a hearty breakfast with eggs (see page 230).

MAKES: 8 servings

1¼ pounds ground beef (80% lean)

1 pound Mexican-style fresh (raw) chorizo, casings removed

1 cup chopped onions

1 cup chopped green bell peppers

1 (14-ounce) can crushed tomatoes

1 (3.5-ounce) can green chilies

1 teaspoon chopped garlic

2 teaspoons chili powder

1 teaspoon ground cumin

½ teaspoon salt

3 ounces cream cheese (6 tablespoons)

12 ounces cheddar cheese, shredded (about 3 cups)

1. Preheat the oven to 375°F.

2. Brown the ground beef and chorizo in a 10-inch oven-safe skillet over medium heat, stirring often to crumble the meat as it cooks. Add the onions and bell peppers and cook until tender.

3. Add the tomatoes, chilies, garlic, seasonings, and cream cheese and mix well. Sprinkle the shredded cheddar cheese over the top of the dish. Bake for about 20 minutes, until hot and bubbly. Serve immediately.

Substitution Suggestion:

If you can't find an acceptable chorizo, you can substitute ground pork or use an additional pound of ground beef to make this an all-beef taco bake.

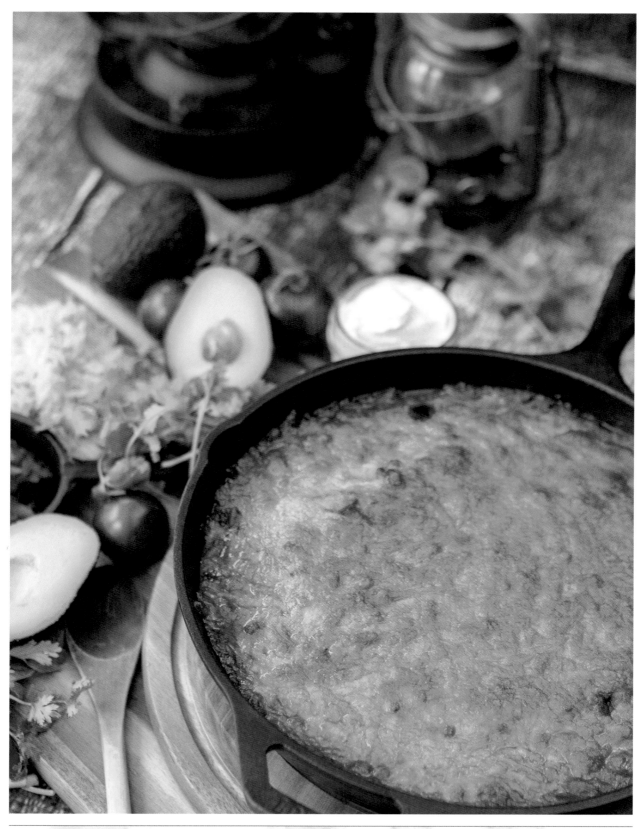

NUTRITION FACTS (PER SERVING):   Calories: 390 | Fat: 28.3g | Protein: 22.2g | Carbs: 7.9g | Fiber: 2g

Skillet Pizza

When Mom has nothing up her sleeve or isn't home for dinner, this is what my family eats. Each of the ingredients is a staple in my house, so a skillet pizza is nearly always a viable option. I also find it to be a great way to use up leftover sausage or veggies. This recipe is a great choice when only one person is eating or when people's tastes vary, and the kids can make it for themselves. Once you've tried this recipe, you'll wonder, "Why didn't I think of that?" Waiting for the pizza to cool before serving is the hardest part!

MAKES: 1 serving

3 ounces mozzarella cheese, shredded (about ¾ cup), divided

2 ounces bulk Italian sausage or other sausage of choice, cooked

2 ounces pepperoni slices

2 tablespoons chopped green bell peppers

½ teaspoon Italian seasoning

2 tablespoons tomato sauce, for serving

1. Heat a 7-inch nonstick skillet over medium heat. Sprinkle ½ cup of the cheese into the skillet. Once the cheese has melted into a thin, solid layer, reduce the heat to low and top the melted cheese with the sausage, pepperoni, and bell peppers. Cook for 3 to 4 minutes, until the toppings are warmed.

2. Top the pizza with the remaining cheese and sprinkle the Italian seasoning over the cheese. The pizza is done when the cheese on top is melted and the cheese "crust" is browned around the edges and set. Let cool for 8 to 10 minutes before serving.

3. Transfer the pizza to a plate and use a pizza cutter to cut it into slices. Serve with the tomato sauce for dipping.

Substitution Suggestion:

Nearly any pizza topping will work in this recipe. I often use cooked bacon, cooked mushrooms, and sliced black olives. You can also get creative and use leftover BBQ Chicken (page 327) to make a BBQ Chicken Skillet Pizza.

Time-Saver Tip:

Chop up leftover cooked sausage and store it with chopped veggies to make this skillet pizza come together even faster.

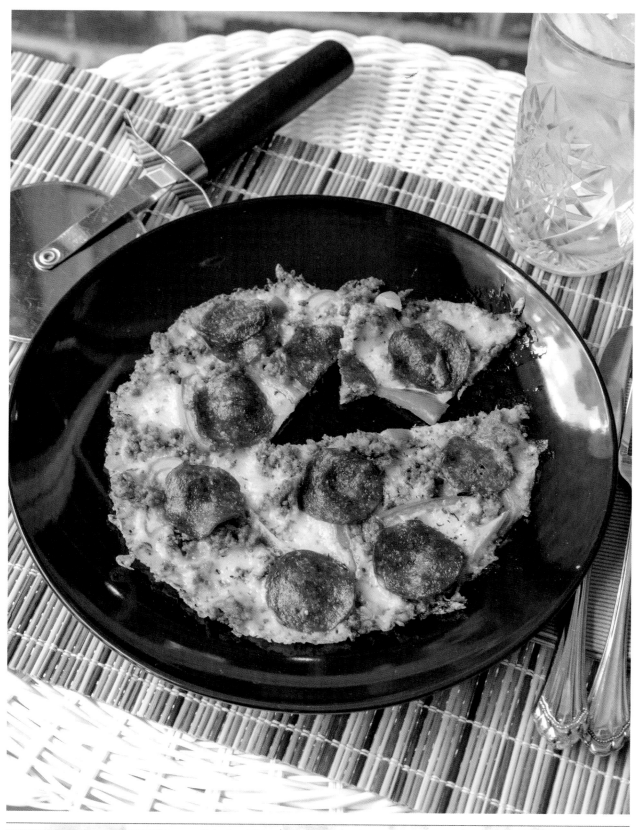

NUTRITION FACTS (PER PIZZA):   Calories: 724 | Fat: 58.4g | Protein: 40.6g | Carbs: 5.1g | Fiber: 1.5g

Whole Roasted Chicken

Buying a whole chicken is often less expensive than buying chicken pieces. I often roast a chicken when I want to have leftover meat or need bones for making broth (see pages 186 and 187). Roasted chicken is one of the easiest meals you can make, but if you'd like to make it even more effortless, you can toss the seasoned chicken into a slow cooker (see the variation below).

MAKES: 4 servings

1 (4- to 5-pound) whole chicken

1 tablespoon bacon fat, melted

1 teaspoon ground cumin

1 teaspoon Italian seasoning

1 teaspoon salt

½ teaspoon garlic powder

1. Preheat the oven to 375°F.

2. Remove the neck, gizzards, heart, and liver from the chicken cavity. Place the chicken in a roasting pan and coat with the melted bacon fat. Sprinkle the cumin, Italian seasoning, salt, and garlic powder over the chicken.

3. Roast, breast side down, for 1 hour 20 minutes to 1 hour 40 minutes, until the skin is golden brown and the juices run clear when the chicken is sliced. The chicken should register a minimum internal temperature of 165°F. Let it rest, uncovered, for at least 10 minutes before serving.

VARIATION: Slow Cooker Roasted Chicken

Instead of roasting the chicken in the oven, you can cook the chicken in a 6-quart or larger slow cooker on low for 8 to 10 hours. Although the cooking time is longer than when roasting, you can prepare the chicken ahead of time and then turn on the slow cooker in the morning so that a delicious dinner is waiting for you in the evening.

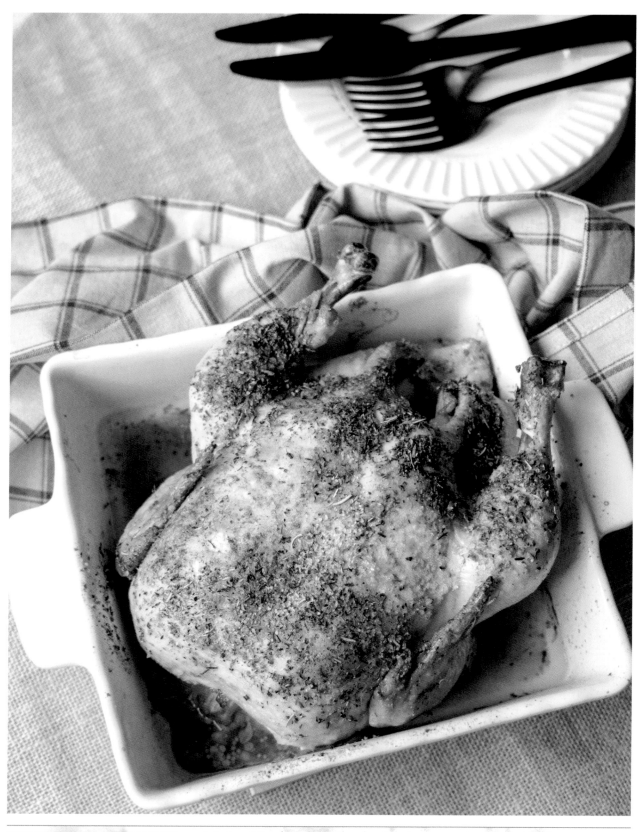

NUTRITION FACTS (PER SERVING): Calories: 275 | Fat: 42.6g | Protein: 10.3g | Carbs: 1g | Fiber: 0.4g

Pickle-Brined
Chicken Tenders

These tenders get eaten for breakfast, packed in school lunches, or devoured at dinner. While I typically save them for the kids to enjoy, when I do get a tender or two for myself, I like to dip them in homemade ranch dressing, Parmesan peppercorn dressing, classic BBQ sauce, or white BBQ sauce. I like to think of this recipe as a healthier version of frozen chicken tenders made with processed meats and fillers, and a great alternative to fast food. Someday I just might make enough of them to freeze them myself!

MAKES: 6 servings

2 pounds boneless, skinless chicken breasts, cut lengthwise into strips about 1½ inches wide

1½ cups dill pickle juice

1 cup pork dust (ground pork rinds)

1½ ounces Parmesan cheese, grated (about ½ cup)

1 tablespoon unflavored whey protein isolate

2 large eggs

1 cup Ranch Dressing (page 209), Parmesan Peppercorn Dressing (page 210), Classic BBQ Sauce (page 195), and/or White BBQ Sauce (page 196), for serving

1. Place the chicken strips and pickle juice in a 1-gallon freezer bag, seal, and refrigerate for at least 4 hours or up to overnight. After the chicken has brined in the pickle juice, drain the chicken and discard the juice. Set the chicken aside.

2. Preheat the oven to 375°F. Line a rimmed baking sheet with parchment paper.

3. Make the breading: In a small bowl, mix the pork dust, Parmesan cheese, and whey protein isolate until well combined. Set the breading aside.

4. In another bowl, beat the eggs until frothy.

5. Dip the brined chicken strips in the beaten egg and then coat with the breading. Place the breaded chicken tenders on the lined baking sheet in a single layer. Bake for 18 to 25 minutes, until the tenders are browned and the juices run clear when the chicken is cut. Serve with the dipping sauce(s) of your choice.

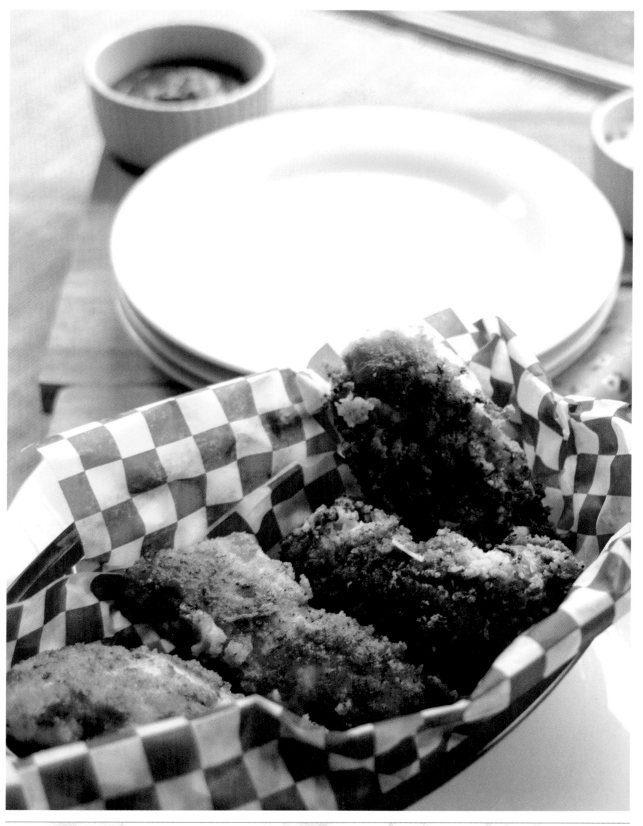

NUTRITION FACTS (PER SERVING):   Calories: 312 | Fat: 11.7g | Protein: 48.4g | Carbs: 1g | Fiber: 0g

Parmesan-Crusted
Roasted Chicken Thighs

I spent decades snubbing chicken thighs and selecting chicken breasts trimmed of all fat and skin. I was wrong. Not only are chicken thighs generally a great bargain, but they are also covered with delicious skin and have a great fat content. Fat equals flavor, so this dish is really tasty.

Chicken thighs are easy to cook in a variety of ways, but they are best when baked at high heat so that the skin crisps up to perfection. My son doesn't like the crispy skin and gives it to me, which makes me love him even more. Seriously, if you haven't tried roasted chicken thighs, you're in for a treat. They are delicious served with Roasted Mixed Veggies (page 360) and Cauli Rice (page 343).

MAKES: **4 servings**

2 pounds bone-in, skin-on chicken thighs

1 teaspoon salt

¼ teaspoon ground black pepper

½ cup mayonnaise, homemade (page 192) or store-bought

1 tablespoon dried parsley

3 ounces Parmesan cheese, grated (about 1 cup)

Chopped fresh parsley, for garnish (optional)

1. Preheat the oven to 400°F.

2. Pat the chicken dry and place the thighs in a 13 by 9-inch baking dish in a single layer. Sprinkle the thighs on all sides with the salt and pepper, then coat them all over with the mayonnaise. Turn the thighs skin side up in the dish, then sprinkle the parsley and cheese over the tops.

3. Roast the chicken for 30 to 40 minutes, until the skin is dark brown and crispy and the juices run clear when the chicken is cut. It should reach an internal temperature of at least 165°F. Garnish with chopped parsley, if desired.

Substitution Suggestion:

Any piece of chicken, pork, or fish will work nicely when roasted this way. Be sure to adjust the roasting time as needed for the cut of meat you are using.

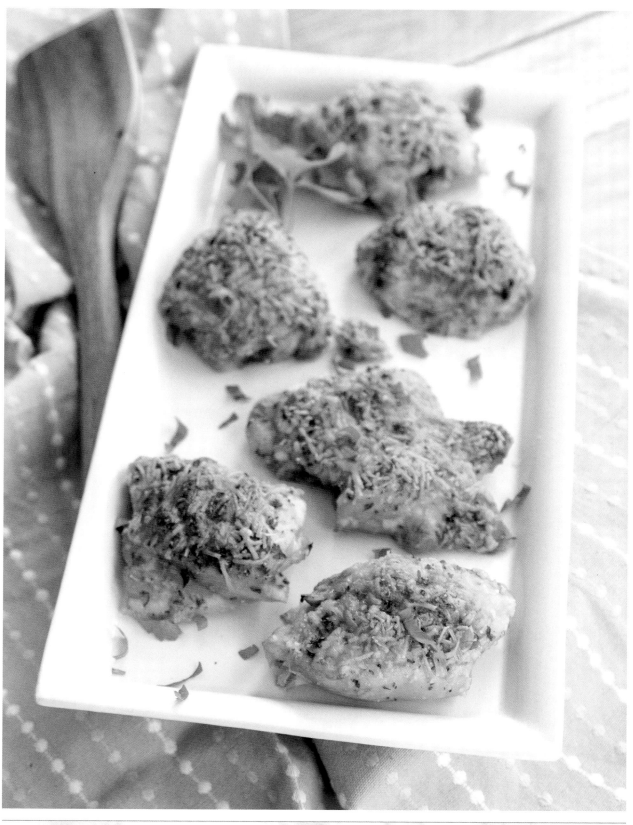

NUTRITION FACTS (PER SERVING):   Calories: 685 | Fat: 64.4g | Protein: 47g | Carbs: 1.5g | Fiber: 0.1g

Chicken Philly Cheesesteak
Casserole

When I first made this casserole, my husband and daughter looked at it, looked at each other, and then looked at me. Grace asked, "What's Plan B? Can we go get burgers?" I insisted that they try it. Not only was it a hit, but they argued over who would get the leftovers for lunch the next day!

MAKES: 6 servings

1 tablespoon ghee or bacon fat

2 pounds boneless, skinless chicken breasts or thighs, cubed

1 cup sliced green bell peppers

1 cup sliced onions

8 ounces mushrooms, sliced

2 cloves garlic, minced, divided

2 teaspoons Italian seasoning, divided

½ teaspoon salt

½ teaspoon ground black pepper

8 ounces cheddar cheese, shredded (about 2 cups)

1 (8-ounce) package cream cheese, softened

½ cup mayonnaise, homemade (page 192) or store-bought

2 tablespoons Worcestershire sauce

12 ounces provolone cheese slices

1. Preheat the oven to 375°F.

2. Melt the ghee in a large skillet over medium-high heat. When hot, add the chicken and cook until browned.

3. Add the bell peppers, onions, mushrooms, half of the garlic, 1 teaspoon of the Italian seasoning, and the salt and pepper. Continue cooking until the vegetables are just tender but not soft. Remove from the heat and set aside.

4. In a large bowl, mix together the cheddar cheese, cream cheese, mayonnaise, Worcestershire sauce, remaining minced garlic, and remaining teaspoon of Italian seasoning. Add the chicken and vegetable mixture and stir to combine.

5. Spoon the mixture into a 13 by 9-inch baking dish and top with the provolone cheese. Bake for 25 to 35 minutes, until bubbly and slightly browned.

Time-Saver Tip:

You can put this casserole together up to one day in advance and bake it just before serving.

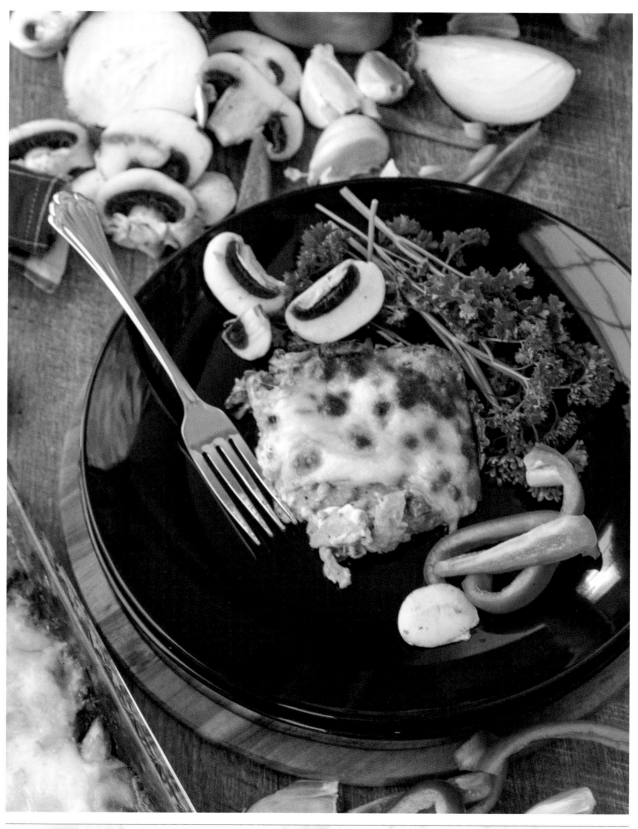

NUTRITION FACTS (PER SERVING):　　Calories: 855　|　Fat: 65g　|　Protein: 43g　|　Carbs: 7.4g　|　Fiber: 1.2g

Broccoli Cheddar Ranch
Chicken Soup

Broccoli soup is a classic comfort food, but it isn't an ideal meal for a very-low-carb diet because it contains little protein. The traditional ingredients of broccoli, onion, and a flour-thickened soup base pack a lot of carbs! My version uses chicken, bacon, cheese, and cream to kick up the protein and fat and uses my homemade ranch seasoning to boost the flavor. Grab a bowl, a spoon, and a blanket, because this is comfort food gone keto.

MAKES: 6 servings

2 tablespoons ghee or bacon fat

1½ pounds boneless, skinless chicken breasts, cut into bite-sized pieces

1 small onion, chopped

3 tablespoons Ranch Seasoning (page 208)

1½ cups chicken bone broth, homemade (page 186) or store-bought

2 cups chopped broccoli

4 ounces cream cheese (½ cup)

½ cup heavy cream

⅓ cup cooked chopped bacon (5 to 6 slices), plus extra for garnish if desired

8 ounces cheddar cheese, shredded (about 2 cups), plus extra for garnish if desired

1. In a heavy 2-quart saucepan over medium-high heat, melt the ghee. When hot, add the chicken and onion and cook until the chicken is browned on all sides. When the chicken is browned, sprinkle the ranch seasoning over the chicken and onions.

2. Add the broth and broccoli to the saucepan and cook at a low boil until the broccoli is just tender, 10 to 12 minutes.

3. When the broccoli is tender, reduce the heat to low and stir in the cream cheese and heavy cream. Continue stirring until the cream cheese is melted. Keep the heat low so that the cream cheese does not break or separate.

4. Remove from the heat and stir in the bacon and cheddar cheese. Serve immediately. Garnish with additional bacon or cheddar cheese, if desired.

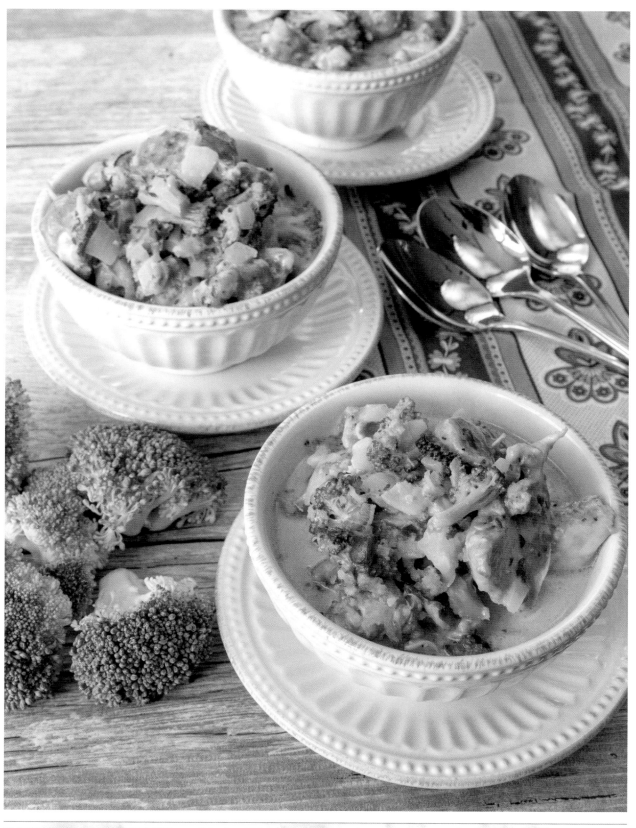

NUTRITION FACTS (PER SERVING): | Calories: 530 | Fat: 34.5g | Protein: 48.2g | Carbs: 5.8g | Fiber: 1.3g

Lemon Mushroom Chicken

This dish is easy enough to make on a weeknight but is impressive enough for company. I like to use a mix of chicken breasts and thighs for this recipe. The sauce in which the chicken bakes is particularly yummy over Cauli Rice (page 343) or asparagus.

MAKES: 6 servings

¼ cup (½ stick) unsalted butter

2½ pounds boneless, skinless chicken breasts and/or thighs, cut into 3-inch pieces

¼ cup chicken bone broth, homemade (page 186) or store-bought

3 tablespoons lemon juice

1 pound mushrooms, sliced

3 green onions, chopped

2 tablespoons grated lemon zest

2 tablespoons dried parsley

2 teaspoons salt

1 teaspoon ground black pepper

2 cups sour cream

Sliced green onions, for garnish (optional)

1. Preheat the oven to 325°F.

2. Melt the butter in a large skillet over medium-high heat. Add the chicken and cook until browned on both sides. When the chicken is browned, transfer to a 13 by 9-inch baking dish.

3. To the same skillet, add the broth and lemon juice. Scrape the bottom of the skillet to incorporate the pan juices into the broth and juice. Simmer over low heat for 2 to 3 minutes. Add the mushrooms, green onions, lemon zest, parsley, salt, and pepper to the skillet and stir well. Remove from the heat and stir in the sour cream. Pour the mixture over the chicken in the baking dish.

4. Bake, uncovered, for 1 hour. Let cool for 10 minutes before serving. Garnish with sliced green onions, if desired.

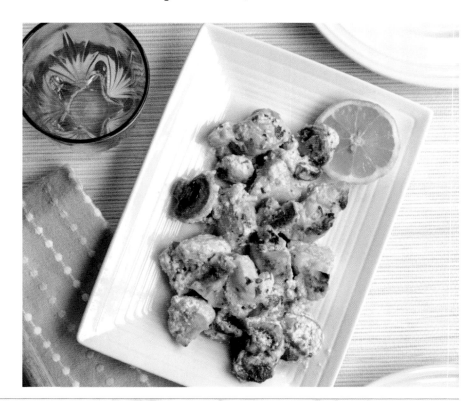

NUTRITION FACTS (PER SERVING):　　Calories: 336　|　Fat: 25.4g　|　Protein: 22.2g　|　Carbs: 5.4g　|　Fiber: 0.9g

BBQ Chicken

This recipe uses a classic tomato-based BBQ sauce. While the directions call for baking the chicken, you can also grill or smoke it, which are two of my favorite ways to prepare chicken. Because my husband does all the outdoor cooking, I can put him in charge of the meat while I prepare the sides.

MAKES: 4 servings

1 (4- to 5-pound) chicken, cut into 8 pieces

1 teaspoon salt

½ teaspoon ground black pepper

2 recipes Classic BBQ Sauce (page 195), divided

Time-Saver Tip:

Instead of roasting the pieces from an entire chicken, which include the large breast pieces, choose smaller pieces such as legs, wings, or bone-in, skin-on thighs. The smaller pieces will cook in just 25 to 35 minutes. Dark meat is also fattier and more tender than white meat.

Note:

The protein per serving for this recipe is higher than I would typically consume in one meal. I would eat a smaller portion and balance the meal with fatty sides so that the total fat in the meal would be equal to or greater than the total protein.

1. Preheat the oven to 400°F.

2. Pat the chicken pieces dry with paper towels to remove as much moisture as possible. Sprinkle the salt and pepper over each piece. Coat the pieces well with half of the BBQ sauce and place in a 13 by 9-inch baking dish. Reserve the rest of the BBQ sauce to serve at the table.

3. Bake the chicken for 40 to 55 minutes, until the thickest pieces reach an internal temperature of at least 165°F. Serve the chicken with the remaining BBQ sauce.

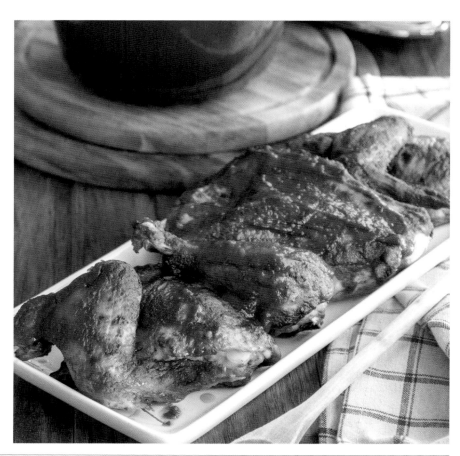

NUTRITION FACTS (PER SERVING):   Calories: 315 | Fat: 16.8g | Protein: 52.6g | Carbs: 4g | Fiber: 1.2g

Chicken Salad

More often than not, I make a double batch of this delicious chicken salad on my Sunday prep day and eat it for lunch throughout the work week. The flavors intensify in the fridge overnight as the cucumber, onion, and dill mingle. The toasted almonds are optional, but they add a nice crunch.

MAKES: 2 servings

12 ounces cooked chicken, chopped

⅓ cup mayonnaise, homemade (page 192) or store-bought

¼ cup peeled and diced cucumbers

2 tablespoons diced celery

1 tablespoon finely chopped onions

2 teaspoons lemon juice

2 teaspoons dried dill weed

¼ teaspoon salt

Dash of ground black pepper

1½ tablespoons toasted sliced almonds (optional)

Thoroughly combine all the ingredients in a small mixing bowl. Refrigerate for at least 2 hours before serving. Leftovers will keep in the fridge for up to 5 days.

Time-Saver Tip:

When making this salad, I often use canned chicken for convenience and to save time. If using canned chicken, be sure to drain the chicken well before using it to make this salad.

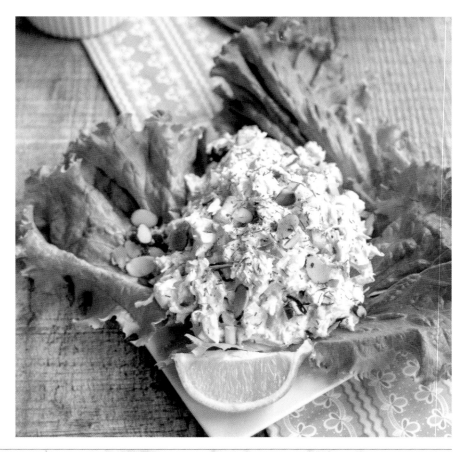

Note:

The protein per serving for this recipe is higher than I would typically consume in one meal. I would eat a smaller portion and balance the meal with fatty sides so that the total number of fat grams in the meal would be equal to or greater than the total number of protein grams.

NUTRITION FACTS (PER SERVING): | Calories: 643 | Fat: 51g | Protein: 51g | Carbs: 1.9g | Fiber: 0.4g

Shredded Mexican Chicken

My family isn't always thrilled about eating leftovers, so I created this recipe when I was heading out of town and explaining to my husband what he and the children could eat for dinner. "We've had a lot of chicken lately" was all he said. I interpreted that to mean that the meal I'd planned would end up in the back of the fridge because he and the kids had gone out to eat instead. With nothing to lose, I grabbed the slow cooker, tossed in some "different" flavorings that we hadn't eaten recently, and hoped for the best. If they didn't like it, I wouldn't be there to hear them complain! When I called from several time zones away, I was greeted with "What did you put in the chicken? That was good!" I hurried off the phone and jotted down exactly what I'd thrown into the slow cooker that morning. This has since become one of our staple meals.

MAKES: 6 servings

2 pounds boneless, skinless chicken thighs

2 tablespoons Taco Seasoning (page 207)

1 (8-ounce) can tomato sauce

½ cup (1 stick) salted butter

FOR SERVING (OPTIONAL):

Sliced jalapeño peppers

Sliced red onions

Chopped tomatoes

Diced avocado

Shredded cheese

Sour cream

1. Place the chicken thighs in a 4-quart or larger slow cooker and sprinkle each thigh with the taco seasoning. Pour the tomato sauce over the seasoned chicken and top with the butter. Cook on low for 8 to 10 hours, until the chicken is tender.

2. Shred the chicken with a fork and mix it with the liquid in the slow cooker. If desired, serve the shredded chicken with sliced jalapeños, sliced onions, chopped tomatoes, diced avocado, shredded cheese, and/or sour cream.

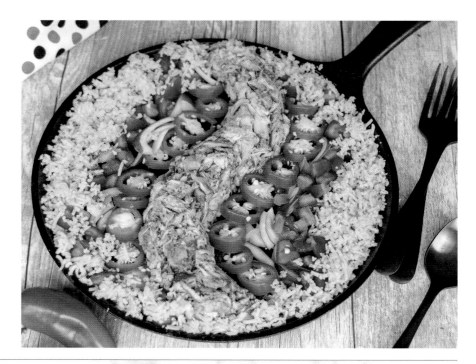

| NUTRITION FACTS (PER SERVING): | Calories: 311 | Fat: 21.9g | Protein: 26.1g | Carbs: 1g | Fiber: 0.6g |

Moo Goo Gai Pan

The flavor of this dish is subtle, although it does intensify in the leftovers, which is why I like to make a large batch. The "traditional" version includes a white sauce that is thickened with cornstarch. Here I've tried to capture the taste and consistency of that original sauce without using cornstarch. The vegetables used in American versions vary widely, but mushrooms are always a base. I've chosen to include vegetables that are very low in carbs but contribute great flavor and texture. If you have never used bok choy before, this Chinese cabbage is worth some experimentation. It lends an authentic flavor without packing many carbs. We tend to serve this dish over a small portion of Cauli Rice (page 343).

MAKES: 8 servings

¼ cup unseasoned rice wine vinegar

1 teaspoon salt

2 pounds boneless, skinless chicken pieces (white and dark meat), sliced

2 tablespoons coconut oil

2 tablespoons peeled and minced fresh ginger

1 tablespoon minced garlic

1 teaspoon salt (omit if using tamari)

½ cup chicken bone broth, homemade (page 186) or store-bought

¼ cup coconut aminos or tamari

¼ cup Chinese rice wine or dry sherry

2 tablespoons oyster brine from 1 (8-ounce) can oysters packed in water (see Note)

1 medium onion, sliced

1 pound white mushrooms, sliced

1½ cups chopped bok choy

24 stalks asparagus, trimmed and cut into 3-inch pieces

1 cup bean sprouts

1. Marinate the chicken: Put the vinegar and salt in a zip-top plastic bag. Add the chicken and place in the refrigerator to marinate for at least 2 hours or up to overnight.

2. When you are ready to cook the chicken, melt the coconut oil in a large skillet or wok over high heat. Remove the chicken from the marinade; discard the marinade. Place the chicken, ginger, garlic, and salt in the skillet or wok and stir-fry for 10 to 12 minutes, until the chicken is browned.

3. Add the broth, coconut aminos, rice wine, and oyster brine and simmer over medium heat for 12 to 15 minutes, until the chicken is tender and the sauce is reduced.

4. Add the onion and mushrooms and cook until tender, 8 to 10 minutes. Add the bok choy and asparagus and cook for 5 to 8 more minutes, until just tender. Toss in the bean sprouts and cook for 2 to 3 minutes, until warmed. Remove from the heat and serve.

Note:

You will have leftover oyster brine after making this recipe. You can use the remainder to make Asian-Style Beef and Broccoli (page 292).

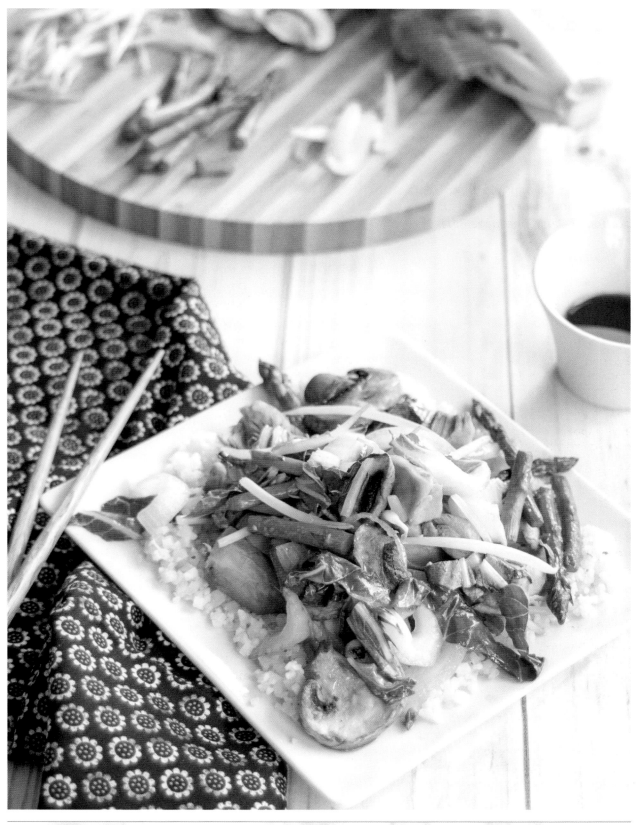

Skinny Chicken Fried "Rice"

This easy skillet dish cooks up quickly and leaves you with only one pan to wash. I giggle about calling it "skinny" because I took that name from a low-fat version that I used to make when there was nothing skinny about me but a dream! This high-fat, low-carb version is truly a *skinny recipe.*

MAKES: 8 servings

2 tablespoons coconut oil

2 pounds boneless, skinless chicken thighs, cut into bite-sized pieces

2 teaspoons garlic powder

1 teaspoon onion powder

1 teaspoon salt (omit if using tamari)

¼ cup coconut aminos or tamari

2 green onions, chopped

1 small green bell pepper, chopped

1 stalk celery, chopped

2 large eggs

2 cups Cauli Rice (page 343)

½ cup bean sprouts

1 tablespoon toasted sesame oil or unsalted butter

1. Melt the coconut oil in a large skillet or wok over medium-high heat. Add the chicken, garlic powder, onion powder, and salt and stir-fry until the chicken is browned, 12 to 16 minutes.

2. Reduce the heat to medium-low and add the coconut aminos. Simmer for 4 to 6 minutes, until the pan juices have reduced. Add the green onions, bell pepper, and celery and cook until just tender, 6 to 8 minutes.

3. Crack the eggs into the skillet and cook, stirring, so that they scramble into the other ingredients. Add the cauli rice and bean sprouts and stir until everything is thoroughly combined and hot. Remove from the heat, drizzle the toasted sesame oil over the skillet, and serve.

Carb Check:

Make sure to limit the cauli rice to ¼ cup per person. The carbohydrates in cauliflower can add up quickly!

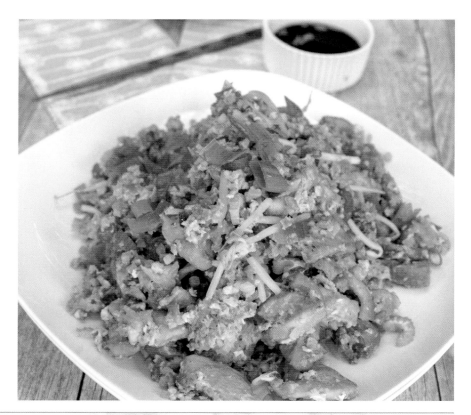

NUTRITION FACTS (PER SERVING): | **Calories: 224** | **Fat: 12.9g** | **Protein: 22.1g** | **Carbs: 4.7g** | **Fiber: 1.3g**

Chicken Broccoli Alfredo

While this dish is delicious when it's made with freshly grilled chicken, I often use reheated leftover grilled or roasted chicken (see page 316) for convenience. The chicken is cut into strips so that it absorbs more of the rich Alfredo sauce. This dish is good enough for company but simple enough for a weeknight family dinner.

MAKES: 4 servings

2 cups steamed broccoli, drained well

1 tablespoon unsalted butter, melted

½ teaspoon salt

1 pound boneless, skinless chicken breasts, grilled or roasted and sliced

1 recipe Creamy Alfredo Sauce (page 204), hot

In a large mixing bowl, toss the steamed broccoli with the melted butter and salt. Add the chicken slices and Alfredo sauce and toss to coat. Serve immediately.

Substitution Suggestion:

Use Cabbage Noodles (page 342) instead of steamed broccoli.

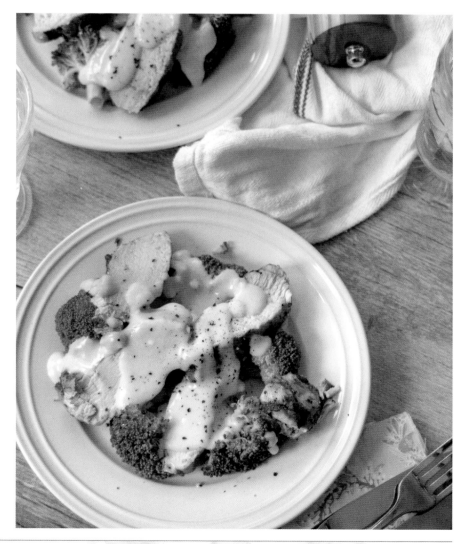

NUTRITION FACTS (PER SERVING):   Calories: 326 | Fat: 20.7g | Protein: 35g | Carbs: 3.3g | Fiber: 1.2g

Baked Salmon
with Creamy Dill Sauce

Fresh wild-caught salmon is an excellent source of omega-3 fatty acids. While Grace and I really enjoy it, David and Jonathan don't prefer it, so I don't make it often. When I do serve salmon, preparing it this way is easy. I use just enough of the sauce to cover the fish before baking and reserve the rest to serve on the side at the table.

MAKES: **4 servings**

1 (1½-pound) wild-caught salmon fillet, cleaned, skin and pinbones removed

CREAMY DILL SAUCE:

½ cup mayonnaise, homemade (page 192) or store-bought

½ cup sour cream

2 tablespoons finely chopped onions

1½ tablespoons dried dill weed

2 teaspoons lemon juice

½ teaspoon Dijon mustard

¼ teaspoon minced garlic

FOR GARNISH (OPTIONAL):

Fresh dill sprigs

1. Preheat the oven to 350°F. Line a rimmed baking sheet with parchment paper.

2. Pat the salmon dry and place it on the lined baking sheet. Set aside.

3. Put the ingredients for the sauce in a small bowl and mix until well combined. Use one-third to one-half of the sauce to coat the top of the salmon. Reserve the remaining sauce to serve at the table.

4. Bake the salmon for 30 to 40 minutes, until it flakes easily with a fork. Transfer the fillet to a serving platter and garnish with fresh dill, if desired. Serve with the remaining sauce.

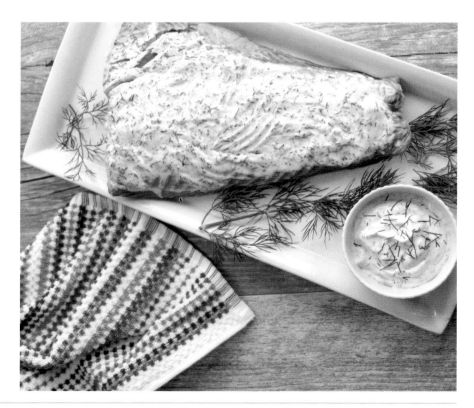

Substitution Suggestion:

You can use nearly any type of fish in this recipe. Adjust the baking time for thinner fillets or more delicate fish.

NUTRITION FACTS (PER SERVING): | Calories: **433** | Fat: **39.3g** | Protein: **18.2g** | Carbs: **2.3g** | Fiber: **0.3g**

Lemon Pepper Flounder

The flounder that I grew up eating was coated in flour and fried in vegetable oil, and I loved it! At the time, I had no idea how unhealthy it was. Until I started following keto, I didn't know that I could enjoy flounder that wasn't breaded and deep-fried. This is one of my new favorite ways to eat it, especially with tartar sauce and coleslaw on the side. Because flounder is naturally low in fat, be sure to serve it with fatty sides. You also want to coat the flounder well with butter and cover it with lemon slices so that it doesn't dry out.

OPTION

MAKES: **4 servings**

1½ pounds flounder fillets, pinbones removed

2 tablespoons unsalted butter or ghee, softened

2 teaspoons ground black pepper

1 teaspoon dried parsley

½ teaspoon salt

2 lemons, sliced

1. Preheat the oven to 350°F. Line a rimmed baking sheet with parchment paper.

2. Place the flounder on the lined baking sheet. Coat the fillets liberally with the softened butter. Sprinkle the pepper, parsley, and salt over the buttered fillets. Place the lemon slices on top.

3. Bake the flounder for 7 to 15 minutes, until it flakes easily with a fork. The baking time will vary depending on the size and thickness of the fillets. Do not overbake.

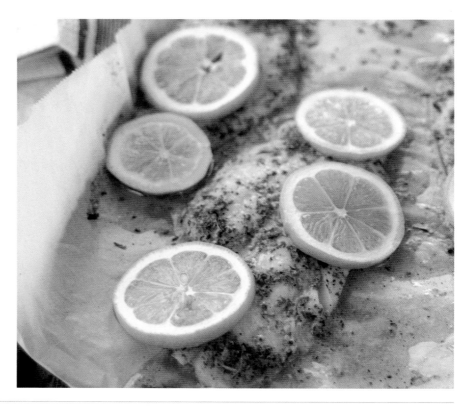

NUTRITION FACTS (PER SERVING): | Calories: **119** | Fat: **7.6g** | Protein: **10.8g** | Carbs: **1g** | Fiber: **0.6g**

Sautéed Lemon Garlic Shrimp

This dish makes me wonder why I ever ate shrimp that was coated in flour and deep-fried. This shrimp has flavor! It is unbelievably simple and fast to prepare, too. Sautéed shrimp can easily be a quick weeknight meal.

OPTION

MAKES: 2 servings

1 pound large shrimp, peeled and deveined

2 tablespoons unsalted butter or ghee

2 teaspoons minced garlic

1½ teaspoons dried parsley

¼ teaspoon salt

½ teaspoon red pepper flakes (optional)

Lemon wedges, for serving

1. Pat the shrimp dry. Combine the butter, garlic, and parsley in a large skillet over medium-high heat. When the butter is hot, add the shrimp and toss to coat. Sauté until bright pink on both sides, 4 to 6 minutes. Do not overcook or the shrimp will be tough.

2. Sprinkle the shrimp with the salt and red pepper flakes, if using, and serve with the pan juices and lemon wedges.

Time-Saver Tip:

If you buy shrimp that are already peeled and deveined, this dish comes together in less than 15 minutes from start to finish.

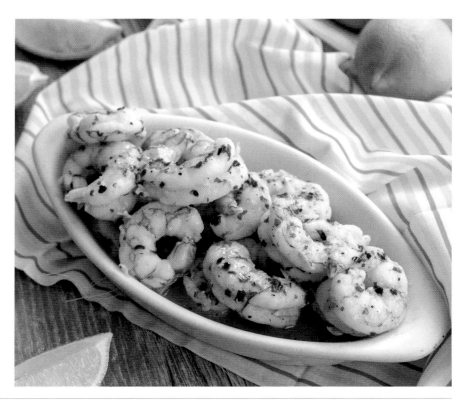

NUTRITION FACTS (PER SERVING): | Calories: 297 | Fat: 12.6g | Protein: 45.4g | Carbs: 1.1g | Fiber: 0.2g

Tuna Salad

Canned tuna isn't my first choice of protein, but it is cheap and keeps for a long time. I always have some on hand for emergencies when we lose power or when I haven't prepared lunches for myself ahead of time. This tuna salad has a light taste. Note that I use tuna packed in water and then add olive oil to the salad. Often, manufacturers pack their tuna in undesirable oils. I can avoid those by adding my own fat instead.

MAKES: 2 servings

1 (12-ounce) can tuna (packed in water), drained and flaked

⅓ cup mayonnaise, homemade (page 192) or store-bought

¼ cup chopped tomatoes

1 green onion, sliced

1 tablespoon lemon juice

1 tablespoon olive oil

Dash of salt

Dash of ground black pepper

⅓ cup diced avocado (about one-quarter of a large Hass avocado)

Combine all the ingredients in a small mixing bowl, folding in the avocado last. Chill in the refrigerator for at least 20 minutes before serving.

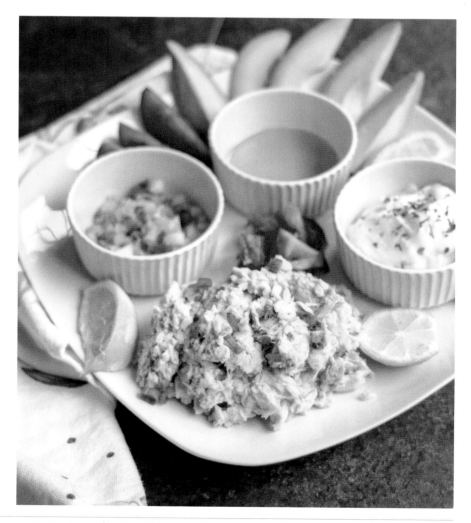

NUTRITION FACTS (PER SERVING): Calories: 658 | Fat: 53.2g | Protein: 41.3g | Carbs: 3.8g | Fiber: 2.1g

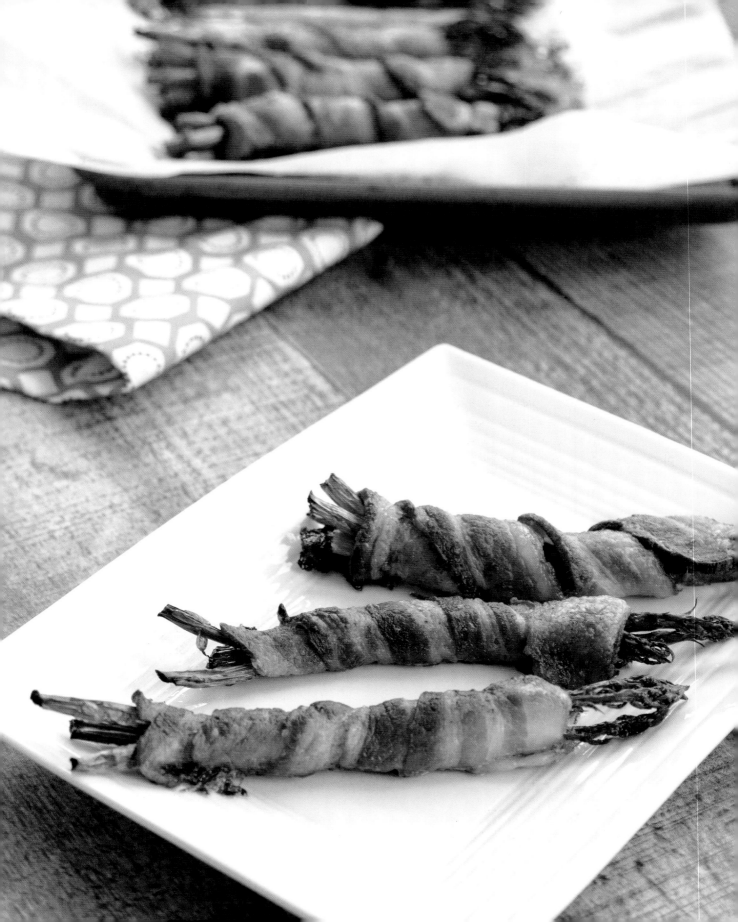

Chapter 10

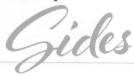

Sides

In the hierarchy of macronutrients (fat, protein, and carbohydrate), vegetables are often last and least on my plate because they are primarily carbohydrates. (See page 46 for a discussion of the lowest-carb produce options.) Because vegetables lack fat and protein, I have created side dish recipes with added fat and, at times, protein so that you can maintain ketogenic ratios in your meals. If you're serving more than one side dish, be sure to pair a higher-carb side with a lower-carb one so that your plate does not become carb-heavy. I often make only one side dish, which saves me time *and* carbs.

I've chosen to include multiple recipes for the same vegetables rather than create recipes that use a lot of different vegetables so that you have a variety of preparations for each vegetable rather than needing to shop for many different vegetables. You can easily turn some of these recipes into main dishes by adding meat or another source of protein.

Zoodles

Zucchini made into noodles is called "zoodles." These veggie noodles provide bulk and texture without the carbs found in traditional pasta. The keys to enjoying zoodles are to allow them to dry out before cooking them and to barely cook them in a skillet with butter or your preferred fat. Cooking them too long will leave you with a plate of mush.

MAKES: **4 servings**

2 medium zucchini (about 12 ounces total)

1 tablespoon unsalted butter

Dash of salt

Dash of ground black pepper

SPECIAL EQUIPMENT:

Spiral slicer

1. Wash and dry the zucchini and cut off the ends. Use a spiral slicer to make long strands of zucchini that look like noodles. Lay the zucchini noodles in a single layer on a sheet of parchment paper and allow to dry for about an hour. You can also use a clean kitchen towel to blot the moisture from the zucchini. While you can skip this step if you're in a hurry, your zoodles will be less watery if you allow them to dry out a bit.

2. Heat the butter in a large skillet over medium-high heat. Add the zucchini noodles and cook until just slightly tender, 3 to 5 minutes. Remove from the heat, season with the salt and pepper, and serve immediately.

Time-Saver Tip:

Zucchini can be spiral-sliced in larger batches and stored in the refrigerator for up to 2 days.

Carb Check:

One medium zucchini weighs about 6 ounces and has roughly 5 grams of total carbs, so it should yield about 2 servings of zoodles. If you eat the zoodles plain, then the carb count isn't bad, but if you add other vegetables and/or tomato sauce, the carbs can add up quickly. For that reason, I like to serve zoodles with Simple Cheese Sauce (page 199), a white sauce like Creamy Alfredo Sauce (page 204), or a red sauce with meat, like Bolognese (page 300).

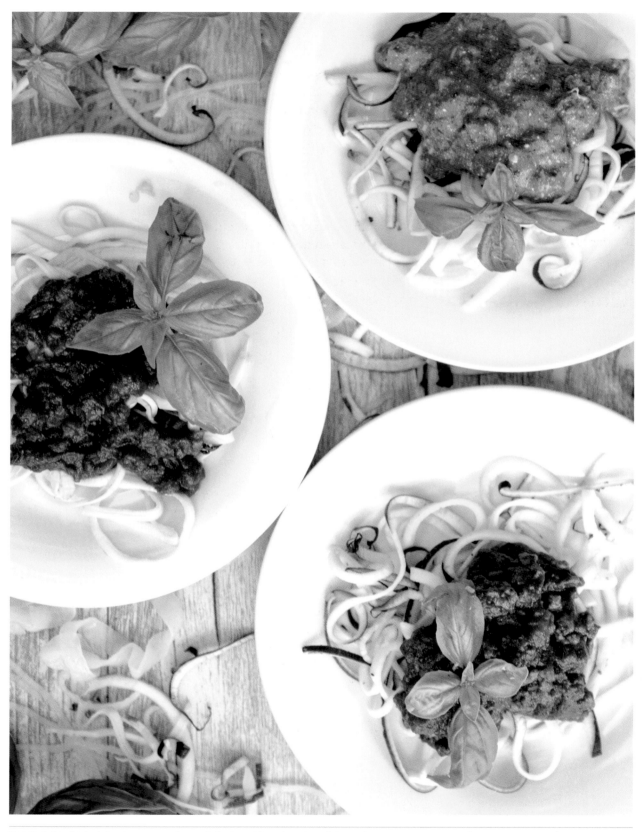

Cabbage Noodles

Of all the veggie noodles that are popular on ketogenic diets, cabbage noodles are my favorite. Carb for carb, they are an even better option than Zoodles (page 340) and Cauli Rice (opposite). What's more, they don't get watery or overly soft. The texture stays al dente, and the flavor is fairly neutral. My family is especially fond of cabbage noodles served under a pile of Swedish Meatballs in Keto Gravy (page 262) or covered in Creamy Alfredo Sauce (page 204), as shown here. They also pair well with Asian dishes.

OPTION

MAKES: 6 servings

1 quart water

½ head green cabbage

2 tablespoons unsalted butter or ghee

1 tablespoon salt

1. Bring the water to a boil in a large pot. While the water is heating, slice the cabbage into ½- to 1-inch-wide strips.

2. Add the cabbage to the boiling water and boil for 7 to 10 minutes, until tender. Drain well. Stir in the butter and salt until the butter melts and thoroughly coats the cabbage. Serve immediately.

3. Store leftovers in the refrigerator for up to 4 days. Reheat in the microwave or on the stovetop with an additional tablespoon of butter.

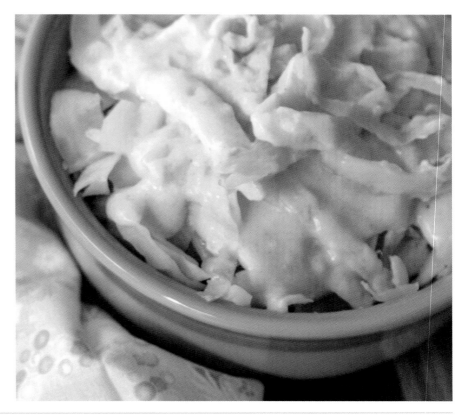

NUTRITION FACTS (PER SERVING):　Calories: 53　|　Fat: 3.9g　|　Protein: 1g　|　Carbs: 4.3g　|　Fiber: 2g

Cauli Rice

To be honest, I'm not a huge fan of cauliflower rice, but I've included it here because it is a staple of low-carb diets that some folks enjoy. The primary reason I dislike it is that it is so easy to overeat. One serving of cauli rice measures ¼ to ⅓ cup, which is a much smaller portion than many of us were used to eating when served white or brown rice. Just remember that you are using cauli rice for texture and as a side, so it should make up a smaller part of your plate than the meat dish you are eating with it.

OPTION

MAKES: 6 servings

1¼ pounds cauliflower florets (about 3 cups)

1 tablespoon unsalted butter or ghee

½ teaspoon salt

¼ teaspoon dried parsley

1. Use a food processor to finely chop the cauliflower until it looks like grains of rice.

2. In a large skillet, melt the butter. Add the riced cauliflower and sauté over medium-high heat until some of the moisture has evaporated and the cauliflower is soft and just warmed. Add the salt and parsley and mix thoroughly. Serve immediately.

3. Store leftovers in the refrigerator for up to 3 days. Reheat in a warm skillet with an additional teaspoon or two of butter.

Carb Check:

Keep an eye on portions. Just ¼ cup of cauli rice equals ½ cup or more of cauliflower florets. It is helpful to weigh the cauliflower before cooking it and to divide the cooked cauli rice into six equal servings for good portion control.

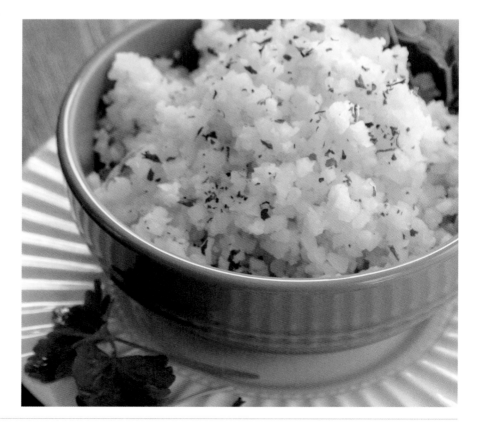

NUTRITION FACTS (PER SERVING): Calories: 23 | Fat: 1.6g | Protein: 0.8g | Carbs: 1.9g | Fiber: 0.8g

Creamy Cauli Mash

No, cauli mash isn't potatoes, and initially I did not love it as much as I used to love mashed potatoes. However, I do love that this dish has a similar creamy texture that I can enjoy while staying healthy. I have three tips for making cauli mash delicious:

- *Remove the excess moisture from the steamed cauliflower.*
- *Be generous when adding butter.*
- *Add a soft cheese that you love. I tend to use whatever soft cheese is in the refrigerator and needs to be used up. Port Salut is my favorite, but I've also tried Havarti, goat cheese, smoked Gouda, and Brie in this dish.*

MAKES: **6 servings**

1¼ pounds cauliflower florets (about 3 cups)

4 ounces cream cheese, Havarti, Port Salut, or your favorite soft/creamy cheese, softened

½ cup (1 stick) unsalted butter, softened

⅓ cup heavy cream

½ teaspoon salt

¼ teaspoon garlic powder

1. Place the cauliflower in a microwave-safe dish and microwave, uncovered, for 4 to 5 minutes, until soft. (Do not add water to the dish before microwaving.) Use a clean kitchen towel or paper towel to squeeze the excess moisture from the steamed cauliflower.

2. Transfer the cauliflower to a blender. Add the cream cheese, butter, heavy cream, salt, and garlic powder and blend until pureed and creamy. Serve warm.

3. Store leftovers in the refrigerator for up to 3 days. Reheat in the microwave or on the stovetop over low heat. Thin the mash with broth or cream, if needed.

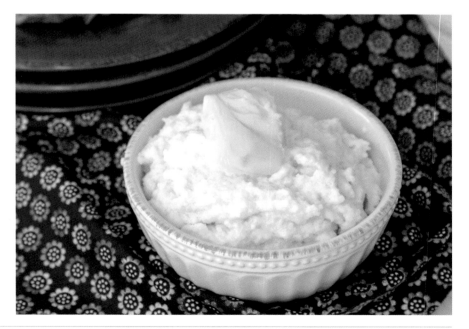

NUTRITION FACTS (PER SERVING): | Calories: 237 | Fat: 24.6g | Protein: 2.5g | Carbs: 3.1g | Fiber: 1.1g

Ranch Cauli Mash
with Bacon

The combination of bacon and my delicious ranch seasoning gives this cauli mash an irresistible flavor. Even my husband, who passes on plain cauli mash, wants his share of this dish. This grown-up mash packs more fat and protein, making it a substantial addition to your plate.

MAKES: 6 servings

1¼ pounds cauliflower florets (about 3 cups)

½ cup (1 stick) unsalted butter, softened

⅓ cup heavy cream

2 ounces cream cheese, Havarti, Port Salut, or your favorite soft/creamy cheese, softened

2 ounces sharp cheddar cheese, shredded (about ½ cup)

¼ teaspoon garlic powder

¼ teaspoon salt

½ cup sour cream

½ cup cooked chopped bacon (7 to 8 slices)

1 tablespoon Ranch Seasoning (page 208)

1 teaspoon dried parsley

1. Place the cauliflower in a microwave-safe dish and microwave, uncovered, for 4 to 5 minutes, until soft. (Do not add water to the dish before microwaving.) Use a clean kitchen towel or paper towel to squeeze the excess moisture from the steamed cauliflower.

2. Transfer the cauliflower to a blender. Add the butter, heavy cream, cheeses, garlic powder, and salt and blend until pureed and creamy. Stir in the sour cream, bacon pieces, seasoning, and parsley. Serve warm.

3. Store leftovers in the refrigerator for up to 3 days. Reheat in the microwave or on the stovetop over low heat. Thin the mash with broth or cream, if needed.

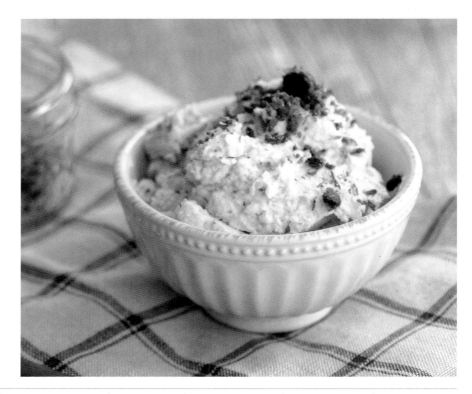

NUTRITION FACTS (PER SERVING): Calories: 316 | Fat: 30g | Protein: 7.4g | Carbs: 4.1g | Fiber: 1.2g

Cauliflower au Gratin

This is one of the dishes that my extended family requests most when we get together to eat. Like my Homecoming Broccoli Salad (page 350), it's become one of my signature recipes that everyone seems to look forward to.

MAKES: 8 servings

4 cups chopped cauliflower

½ cup cooked chopped bacon (7 to 8 slices)

½ cup sour cream

4 ounces cream cheese (½ cup), softened

6 tablespoons (¾ stick) unsalted butter, softened

1½ teaspoons dried minced onions

¼ teaspoon garlic powder

¼ teaspoon salt

Ground black pepper

6 ounces cheddar cheese, shredded (about 1½ cups), divided

1. Preheat the oven to 350°F.

2. Place the cauliflower in a microwave-safe dish. Do not add water. Microwave, uncovered, for 3 to 4 minutes, until crisp-tender (tender but not soft).

3. Place the steamed cauliflower, bacon, sour cream, cream cheese, and butter in a mixing bowl and mix well. Add the dried minced onions, garlic powder, and salt, then season lightly with pepper and mix until incorporated. Stir in 1 cup of the cheddar cheese.

4. Pour the mixture into a 13 by 9-inch baking dish or eight 6-ounce ramekins. Sprinkle the remaining ½ cup of cheese over the top. Bake until golden brown and bubbly, 30 to 35 minutes if using a baking dish or 18 to 20 minutes if using ramekins.

5. Store leftovers in the refrigerator for up to 4 days. Reheat in a preheated 300°F oven for 15 to 20 minutes or microwave until warmed.

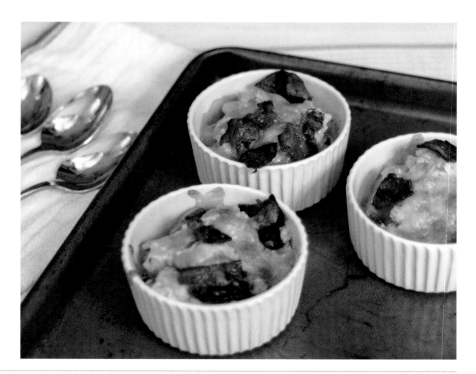

NUTRITION FACTS (PER SERVING):   Calories: 254 | Fat: 23.5g | Protein: 9.6g | Carbs: 3.8g | Fiber: 1.1g

Herb-Roasted Radishes

Some people swear that roasted radishes taste just like roasted potatoes. I will not lie to you; they don't. Roasted radishes taste like radishes, except they are milder than raw radishes and lose some of their bite. Boiling them in salted water before roasting them helps diminish their radish taste, but you aren't likely to fool anyone at the dinner table. Nonetheless, bacon fat, rosemary, and thyme make this a tasty side dish that I hope you will enjoy, without the higher carbs found in roasted potatoes.

MAKES: 2 servings

6 ounces fresh radishes

2 cups water

1½ teaspoons salt, divided

1 tablespoon bacon fat, melted

1 teaspoon dried rosemary leaves

1 teaspoon ground dried thyme

¼ teaspoon ground black pepper

1. Preheat the oven to 375°F. Wash the radishes and trim the tops and bottoms. Slice each radish in half or quarters, depending on size.

2. Bring the water and 1 teaspoon of the salt to a boil in a saucepan. Add the radishes and boil until par-cooked, 6 to 8 minutes. Drain the radishes and use a clean kitchen towel or paper towel to dry them. Toss the radishes into a bowl with the melted bacon fat. Sprinkle with the rosemary, thyme, remaining ½ teaspoon of salt, and the pepper and toss to coat.

3. Spread the radishes on a rimmed baking sheet in a single layer. Roast for 15 to 20 minutes, until lightly browned and tender. Serve immediately.

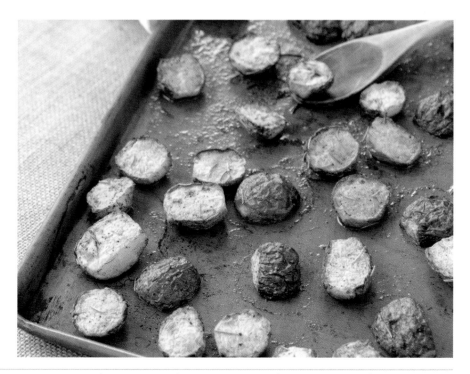

NUTRITION FACTS (PER SERVING): | Calories: 79 | Fat: 7.6g | Protein: 0.8g | Carbs: 4.2g | Fiber: 1.8g

Peppery Roasted Green Beans
with Parmesan

Growing up, I only ever really had green beans one way—boiled nearly to death in a pot with ham, onions, and potatoes. I never dreamed that I could love them prepared any other way. Until I roasted them in bacon fat. Mercy! These beans are best when they are nearly burned, so dry them well before tossing them in the bacon fat and covering them with a generous sprinkle of salt and coarsely ground black pepper. They won't get crispy like french fries, but they make a pretty good substitute.

MAKES: 4 servings

14 ounces fresh green beans, trimmed

1 tablespoon bacon fat, melted

2 teaspoons coarsely ground black pepper

1 teaspoon salt

½ ounce Parmesan cheese, grated or shredded (about 3 tablespoons)

1. Preheat the oven to 400°F.

2. Rinse the green beans and dry them very well. Put the beans in a large bowl and pour the melted bacon fat over them. Sprinkle with the pepper and salt and toss to coat the beans thoroughly.

3. Spread the green beans in a single layer in a 13 by 9-inch baking dish. Roast for 12 to 14 minutes, until the beans begin to get dark brown patches. Remove from the oven and transfer to a serving plate. Sprinkle with the Parmesan cheese and serve warm.

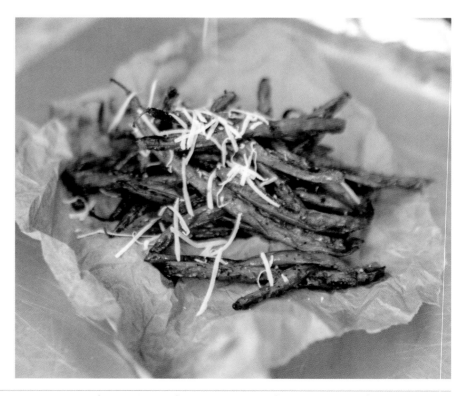

| NUTRITION FACTS (PER SERVING): | Calories: 79 | Fat: 4.7g | Protein: 3.2g | Carbs: 7.2g | Fiber: 3.4g |

Skillet Mushrooms

I've always been a fan of mushrooms, but I've come to adore them in low-carb cooking. The humble, neutral mushroom tends to take on the flavors of what's around it. At the same time, the meaty texture gives substance to a dish or stew. Best of all, at about 3.3 grams of total carbs per 3.5-ounce serving, mushrooms are a low-carb bargain among side dish options. This skillet recipe brings out the best in the mushrooms. I like to serve these mushrooms with steak, burgers, or chicken. Any leftovers are good when tossed into a casserole or stew.

OPTION

MAKES: **4 servings**

2 tablespoons unsalted butter

1 pound mushrooms, sliced

1 teaspoon dried thyme leaves

½ teaspoon salt

1. Heat the butter in a skillet over medium-high heat. Just as the butter begins to melt, add the mushrooms. Allow to cook for 4 to 5 minutes before stirring.

2. Sprinkle in the thyme and cook until the mushrooms are browned on both sides, 12 to 15 minutes. If the mushrooms begin to stick to the pan, add more butter. When the mushrooms have deeply browned edges, sprinkle them with the salt, then remove from the heat and serve.

Substitution Suggestion:

Ghee or bacon fat works well in place of the butter if you are avoiding dairy.

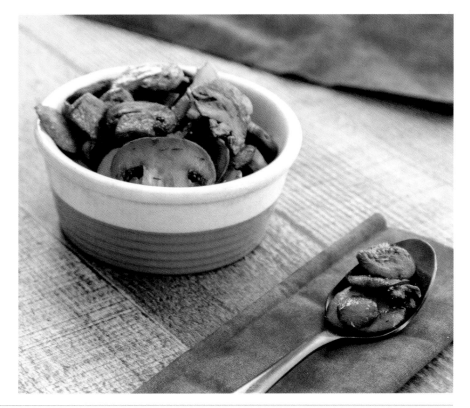

NUTRITION FACTS (PER SERVING):   Calories: 77 | Fat: 6.3g | Protein: 3.6g | Carbs: 4.3g | Fiber: 1.3g

Homecoming Broccoli Salad

There are few recipes that my family always seems to welcome. Broccoli salad is one of them. Even though it is a cold salad, we love it even in the dead of winter. This is one of those recipes that I would put out at any potluck, including a Baptist Homecoming, which is why I call this dish Homecoming Broccoli Salad. In fact, it's such an easy, delicious, and beloved recipe that I selected it for this book's cover. Just trust me!

MAKES: 8 servings

2 medium heads broccoli

¼ cup finely diced onions

½ cup cooked chopped bacon (7 to 8 slices)

6 ounces cheddar cheese, shredded (about 1½ cups)

DRESSING:

1 cup mayonnaise, homemade (page 192) or store-bought

1½ tablespoons apple cider vinegar

2 drops liquid sweetener (optional; see Note)

Dash of salt

Dash of ground black pepper

1. Remove the florets from the heads of broccoli and cut them into bite-sized pieces, then cut the more slender stems into rounds. Discard the thick main stem. (You should get about 8 cups of broccoli floret pieces and sliced stems.)

2. Place the broccoli, onions, bacon, and cheese in a large mixing bowl.

3. In a small bowl, whisk together the ingredients for the dressing until creamy.

4. Pour the dressing over the broccoli mixture and toss well. Refrigerate for at least an hour before serving. Store leftovers in the refrigerator for up to 4 days.

Note:

I add sweetener to this dish to balance the vinegar and to replace the sugar that my grandmother used in her broccoli salad. You can omit it if you prefer.

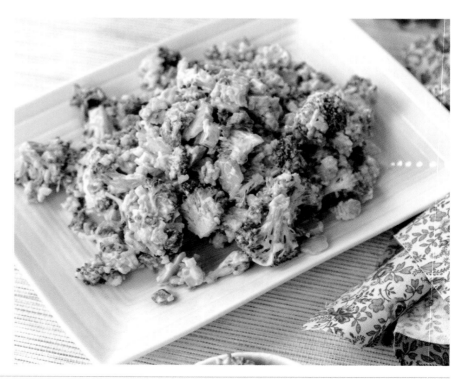

NUTRITION FACTS (PER SERVING): | Calories: 404 | Fat: 38.9g | Protein: 10.7g | Carbs: 6.6g | Fiber: 2.4g

Roasted Broccoli

While I love broccoli, I'm more likely to eat it raw, as in my Homecoming Broccoli Salad (opposite). I really do not enjoy the texture and flavor of steamed broccoli unless it is drowned in cheese sauce (see page 199 for my recipe). But this simple roasting technique transforms broccoli into the perfect side dish, with or without cheese sauce; roasting brings out a depth of flavor that I never knew broccoli could have. It lessens broccoli's cabbagelike taste and gives it a slightly crispy texture. Sometimes the simplest things in life are the best!

MAKES: **8 servings**

1 medium head broccoli

1½ tablespoons bacon fat, melted

½ teaspoon salt

⅛ teaspoon coarsely ground black pepper

1. Preheat the oven to 375°F.

2. Cut the broccoli into large florets and pat dry. In a large bowl, toss the broccoli with the melted bacon fat until lightly coated. Sprinkle with the salt and pepper.

3. Spread the broccoli pieces on a rimmed baking sheet and roast for 12 to 16 minutes, until lightly browned. Serve immediately.

Carb Check:

To increase the fat and protein in this dish, top it with shredded cheese, chopped bacon, and a dollop of sour cream—just like a loaded baked potato!

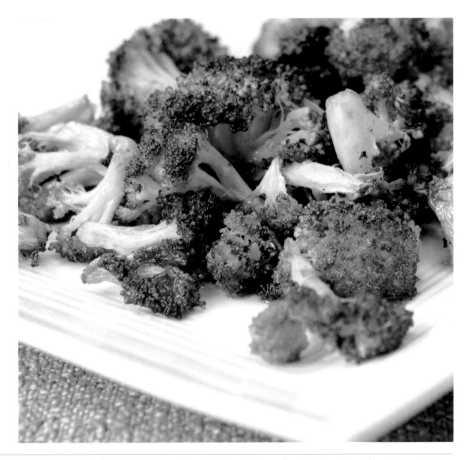

NUTRITION FACTS (PER SERVING):   Calories: 39 | Fat: 2.8g | Protein: 1.3g | Carbs: 3g | Fiber: 1.2g

Parmesan-Baked Tomatoes

The first time I made this dish, my entire family was surprised at how delicious it was. My husband asked, "What did you do to the tomatoes? This is good!" The ingredients are simple, but when they are tossed together, used to top tomatoes, and baked until lightly browned, the result is a sophisticated side dish. This recipe pairs well with any meat.

MAKES: **4 servings**

2 large tomatoes

¼ teaspoon salt

Dash of ground black pepper

2 tablespoons mayonnaise, homemade (page 192) or store-bought

¾ ounce Parmesan cheese, grated or shredded (about ¼ cup)

½ teaspoon Italian seasoning

1. Preheat the oven to 375°F.

2. Slice the tomatoes in half horizontally. Place the halves cut side up on a rimmed baking sheet or in a baking dish.

3. Sprinkle the salt and pepper over the tomato halves. Top each half with ½ tablespoon of mayonnaise. Sprinkle 1 tablespoon of Parmesan cheese over the mayonnaise. Finally, sprinkle the Italian seasoning over the Parmesan cheese.

4. Bake the tomatoes for 15 to 20 minutes, until the cheese is melted and browned. Serve warm.

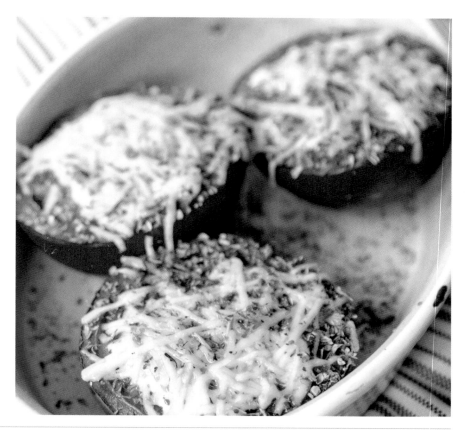

NUTRITION FACTS (PER SERVING): Calories: 237 | Fat: 24.6g | Protein: 2.5g | Carbs: 3.1g | Fiber: 1.1g

Spinach Salad
with Hot Bacon Fat Dressing

This salad gives salad a good name! With more fat and protein than most salads, it is a staple at my house, and it takes only minutes to make if you have hard-boiled eggs on hand. We generally eat this as a main dish or as a side with grilled chicken, steak, or pork. My grandmother's Hot Bacon Fat Dressing is what makes this salad irresistible.

MAKES: **4 servings**

6 cups fresh spinach

2 hard-boiled eggs, peeled and sliced

½ cup coarsely chopped cooked bacon (7 to 8 slices)

1 ounce Parmesan cheese, grated (about ⅓ cup) (optional)

½ cup Hot Bacon Fat Dressing (page 212)

1. Wash the spinach and remove the tough stems. Pat the leaves dry with a clean kitchen towel. Divide the spinach evenly among 4 salad plates.

2. Divide the hard-boiled eggs and bacon evenly among the plates. Sprinkle on the Parmesan cheese, if using. Drizzle with the dressing and serve immediately.

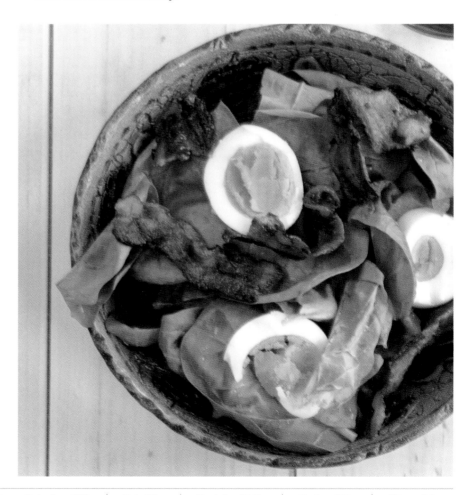

NUTRITION FACTS (PER SERVING):　Calories: 238　│　Fat: 21g　│　Protein: 11.7g　│　Carbs: 2.7g　│　Fiber: 1.1g

Eaux-tato Salad

My mother does not love to be in the kitchen. She cooked for us because she had to, but she would much rather have been sewing or reading. Potato salad is one of her two signature dishes (the other is coleslaw). She made it for every holiday and nearly every potluck. My husband, who was just a boyfriend at the time, once made the mistake of complimenting her potato salad. Not only did she make it every time he came to our house after that, but she always made extra for him to take home.

While I'd always heard that cauliflower makes a reasonably good substitute for potatoes in potato salad, I was pretty sure that it wouldn't be quite the same. I tried it anyway and tested it out on David. I knew I'd been wrong when he responded, "How did you do that?" We like this faux-tato salad even better than the old carby version!

MAKES: 6 servings

3 cups chopped cauliflower florets and slender stems

⅓ cup chopped bell peppers, any color

¼ cup finely chopped onions

2 tablespoons chopped dill pickles

1 cup mayonnaise, homemade (page 192) or store-bought

1 tablespoon prepared yellow mustard

2 drops liquid sweetener

Paprika, for garnish

1. Place the cauliflower in a microwave-safe dish. Do not add water. Microwave, uncovered, for 3 to 4 minutes, until crisp-tender (tender but not soft).

2. Add the bell peppers, onions, and pickles to the dish with the steamed cauliflower and mix well. Add the mayonnaise and mustard and stir until thoroughly combined. Stir in the sweetener, if using.

3. Serve warm or refrigerate for at least an hour before serving. Garnish with a light sprinkle of paprika.

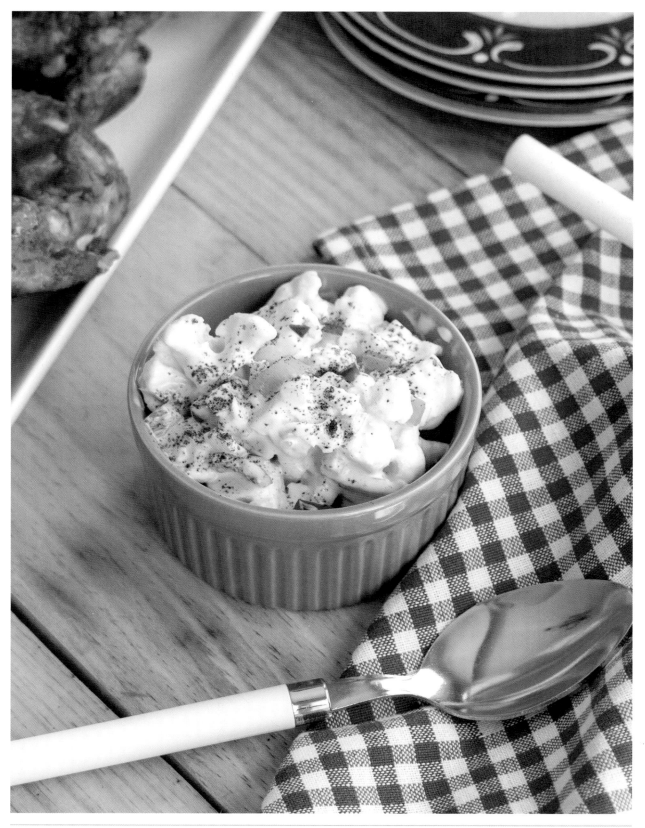

NUTRITION FACTS (PER SERVING):   **Calories: 341** | **Fat: 37.5g** | **Protein: 0.7g** | **Carbs: 1.4g** | **Fiber: 0.3g**

Cucumber, Tomato, and Feta Salad

The magic in this simple summer salad is the spiral-sliced cucumber. Trust me when I say that it is truly worth the extra effort. Spiral slicing the cucumber increases the surface area that absorbs the wonderful Italian dressing poured over it, and you can taste it in every flavorful mouthful. Be sure to peel the cucumber first to lower the carb count. Sometimes I use crumbled goat cheese instead of feta since it has a milder flavor that most people enjoy. Whichever way you choose to make this salad, it is deceptively simple and delicious.

MAKES: 4 servings

ITALIAN DRESSING:

3 tablespoons apple cider vinegar

3 tablespoons olive oil

2 teaspoons granulated sweetener, or 2 drops liquid sweetener

½ teaspoon dried basil

½ teaspoon garlic powder

½ teaspoon onion powder

½ teaspoon ground dried oregano

¼ teaspoon ground dried thyme

Dash of salt

Dash of ground black pepper

SALAD:

1 English cucumber, peeled and spiral sliced

8 grape tomatoes, halved, or 3 Roma tomatoes, quartered

2 tablespoons finely chopped red onions

1⅓ ounces feta cheese, crumbled (about ⅓ cup)

1. In a small bowl, whisk together the ingredients for the dressing; set aside.

2. Put the cucumber, tomatoes, and onions in a large glass bowl. Pour the dressing over the cucumber mixture and toss thoroughly. When the vegetables are well coated with the dressing, gently stir in the feta cheese. Refrigerate for at least 20 minutes before serving.

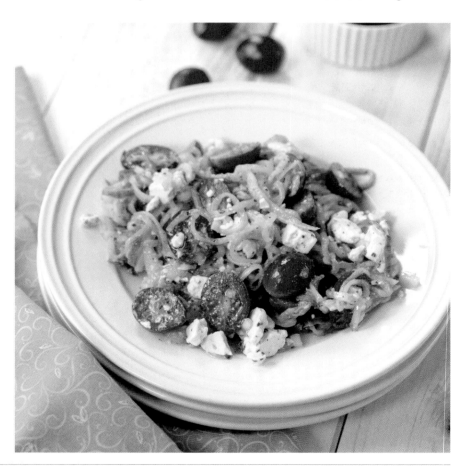

NUTRITION FACTS (PER SERVING):   Calories: 91 | Fat: 13.4g | Protein: 2.5g | Carbs: 4.1g | Fiber: 1.1g

Squash Casserole

The squash casserole that I grew up eating was made with plastic-wrapped cheese slices, cream of something soup, and saltine crackers—oh my! While my keto version contains no crackers or canned soup, it is even more delicious than the traditional version I grew up on, and just as easy to make. I'm not afraid to put this dish on any Southern table. Add cooked chicken or sausage to make it a hearty one-pot meal.

MAKES: **6 servings**

3 cups sliced yellow squash

⅓ cup chopped onions

¼ cup (½ stick) unsalted butter

2 tablespoons water

¼ teaspoon salt

Pinch of ground black pepper

6 ounces cheddar cheese, shredded (about 1½ cups)

⅓ cup mayonnaise, homemade (page 192) or store-bought

⅓ cup sour cream

¾ cup pork dust (ground pork rinds)

⅓ cup cooked chopped bacon (5 to 6 slices) (optional)

1. Preheat the oven to 350°F.

2. In a large saucepan over medium heat, cook the squash and onions in the butter and water until just barely tender, 6 to 8 minutes. Season with the salt and pepper and set aside to cool.

3. In a mixing bowl, combine the cheese, mayonnaise, and sour cream. When the squash mixture is cool, add it to the bowl with the cheese mixture. Stir in the pork dust and bacon, if using, until thoroughly combined. Pour the mixture into a 9-inch square baking dish and bake until browned and bubbly, 30 to 35 minutes.

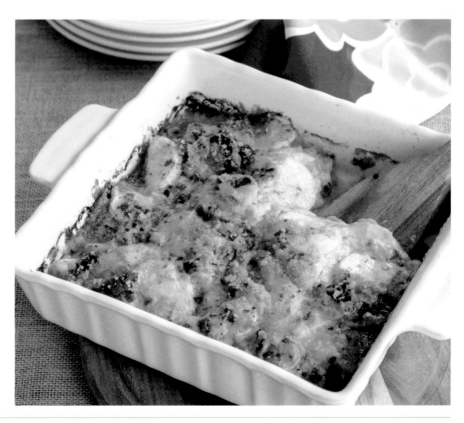

NUTRITION FACTS (PER SERVING): Calories: 452 | Fat: 39.5g | Protein: 20.4g | Carbs: 4.3g | Fiber: 0.8g

Slow-Simmered
Country Green Beans

Green beans are probably the only vegetable meant to be cooked until meltingly soft and tender. I don't know why they are best this way, but they simply are. This is not exactly how my grandmother made them, but it's close. While she used water, I've chosen chicken broth for added flavor and nutrients. She also used ham scraps to season the beans, and you can add those as well if you happen to have some lying around; just be sure to reduce the salt. The key to making slow-simmered country green beans is to reduce the liquid so that all the flavor remains in the pot and isn't drained away. The "pot liquor" is truly the best part of this dish.

OPTION

MAKES: 8 servings

1½ tablespoons bacon fat

2 pounds fresh green beans, trimmed and snapped

4 cups chicken bone broth, homemade (page 186) or store-bought

1 small onion, peeled

1 teaspoon salt

½ teaspoon ground black pepper

2 tablespoons unsalted butter or ghee

1. Melt the bacon fat in a large pot over high heat. Make sure the beans are dry so the fat doesn't spatter when you add them to the pot. When the fat is hot, add the beans. Fry, stirring frequently to coat the beans with the fat, until they turn bright green, 4 to 6 minutes.

2. Add the broth, onion, salt, and pepper. Reduce the heat and simmer, covered, for 30 to 45 minutes, until the green beans are tender.

3. Remove the lid, add the butter, and simmer, uncovered, for another 30 minutes, until the beans are very soft and the pot liquor is reduced to ¼ cup or so. Be careful that the liquid does not simmer dry and scorch. Serve the flavorful pot liquor with the beans.

Substitution Suggestion:

Use 2 ounces of pork side meat instead of bacon fat. Just heat the side meat until some of the fat has rendered. Add the green beans and proceed with the recipe as written. Leave the side meat in the pot and serve it with the beans.

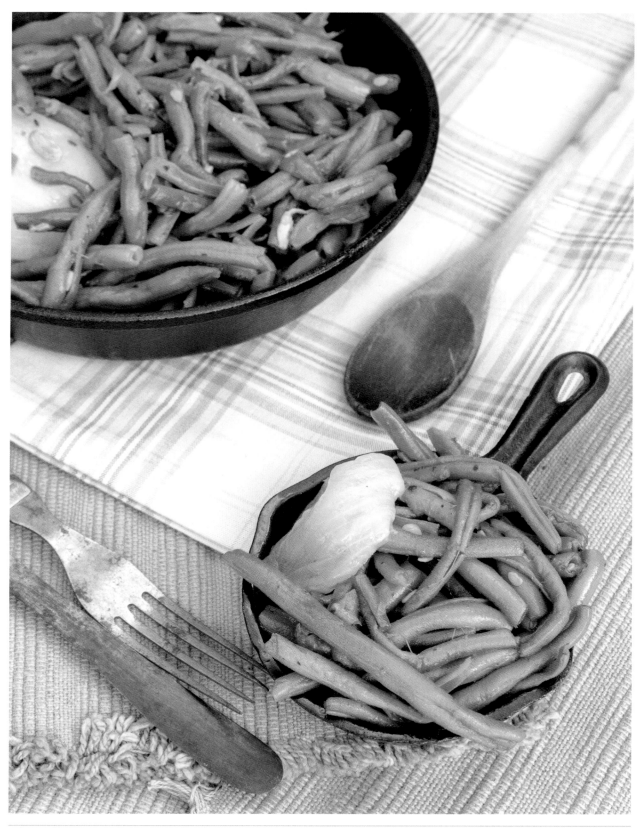

NUTRITION FACTS (PER SERVING):   **Calories: 112** | **Fat: 7.6g** | **Protein: 6.1g** | **Carbs: 7.9g** | **Fiber: 3.8g**

Roasted Mixed Veggies

Roasting veggies really deepens their flavor. I also like that you can toss them in the oven and let them cook while you tend to other things. Because I'm constantly changing up the vegetables I use (I usually toss in whatever is left in the fridge), this dish tastes different nearly every time I make it. Whichever vegetables you choose, just remember to use mostly low-carb ones and to keep the amount of higher-carb ones to a minimum. A total of about 1½ pounds of mixed vegetables will yield six servings.

MAKES: **6 servings**

20 stalks asparagus, trimmed and cut into 1½- to 2-inch pieces

8 ounces mushrooms

5 Brussels sprouts, quartered

1 medium-sized yellow squash or zucchini, sliced

1 medium onion, quartered

1 small green bell pepper, sliced

1 tablespoon coconut oil or bacon fat, melted

1 teaspoon ground dried thyme

¼ teaspoon dried rosemary leaves

½ teaspoon salt

1. Preheat the oven to 425°F. Line a rimmed baking sheet with parchment paper.

2. Pat the vegetables dry with a clean kitchen towel and place them in a large bowl along with the melted coconut oil, thyme, rosemary, and salt. Toss to coat the vegetables with the oil and seasonings.

3. Spread the seasoned vegetables in a single layer on the lined baking sheet. Roast for 25 to 35 minutes, stirring halfway through. The vegetables are done when they are tender and browned.

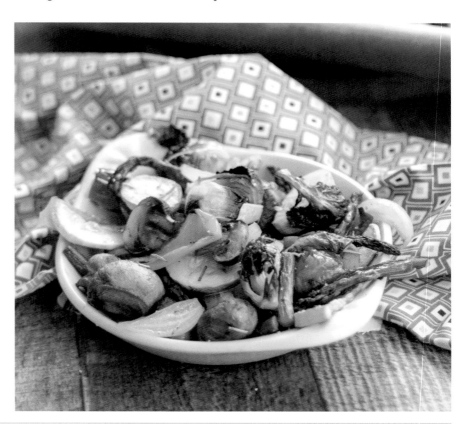

Carb Check:

Be sure to use higher-carb vegetables like onions and peppers sparingly while using plenty of asparagus, mushrooms, and other lower-carb options (see page 46).

NUTRITION FACTS (PER SERVING):   Calories: 61 | Fat: 2.8g | Protein: 3.8g | Carbs: 7.9g | Fiber: 3g

Creamed Brussels Sprouts

This recipe was love at first bite for me! Brussels sprouts have always been a favorite of mine, but I used to eat them with low-fat butter. This recipe breaks all those low-fat rules by serving Brussels sprouts with heavy cream, real butter, and the robust flavor of balsamic vinegar. I like to throw in some bacon as well just because I can!

MAKES: 4 servings

2 cups water

1 pound Brussels sprouts, halved

½ cup heavy cream

2 tablespoons unsalted butter

¼ teaspoon garlic powder

½ teaspoon balsamic vinegar

⅓ cup cooked chopped bacon (5 to 6 slices) (optional)

1. In a 2-quart saucepan, bring the water and Brussels sprouts to a boil over medium heat. Boil until the sprouts are tender, 6 to 8 minutes. Drain well.

2. Return the sprouts to the pan and add the cream, butter, and garlic powder. Simmer over medium-low heat for 10 to 12 minutes, until the cream has thickened. Stir in the vinegar and remove from the heat. Transfer the sprouts to a serving dish and sprinkle with the bacon, if desired.

Time-Saver Tip:

Buy frozen Brussels sprouts instead of starting with fresh ones. If using frozen, skip Step 1. Place the frozen sprouts directly in a saucepan and proceed with Step 2.

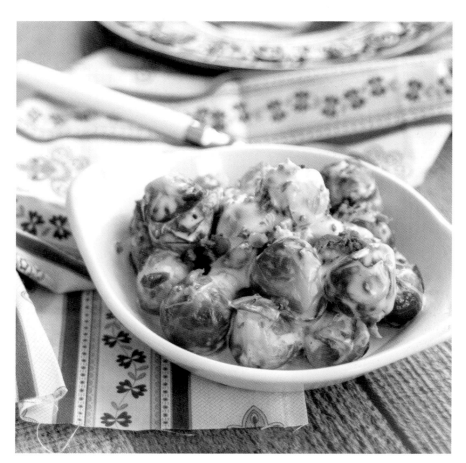

NUTRITION FACTS (PER SERVING): | Calories: 214 | Fat: 11.5g | Protein: 4.8g | Carbs: 8.4g | Fiber: 4.3g

Bacon-Wrapped Asparagus

Asparagus is a good low-carb vegetable, and these bundles look impressive even though they are not difficult to make. Because asparagus can be expensive, we tend to eat it more often in the spring and fall, when prices are more reasonable. This is a great dish to assemble ahead of time: simply complete Step 2 and refrigerate the bundles, then bake just before serving.

MAKES: 4 servings

32 spears asparagus, trimmed

8 slices bacon

1. Preheat the oven to 400°F. Line a rimmed baking sheet with parchment paper.

2. Bundle 4 spears of asparagus and wrap with a slice of bacon. Repeat with the remaining asparagus and bacon, making a total of 8 bundles.

3. Place the bacon-wrapped asparagus bundles on the lined baking sheet and bake for 12 to 15 minutes, until the bacon reaches your desired level of crispness.

Time-Saver Tip:

The bacon will cook faster and more evenly if you place the bundles on a wire rack to cook.

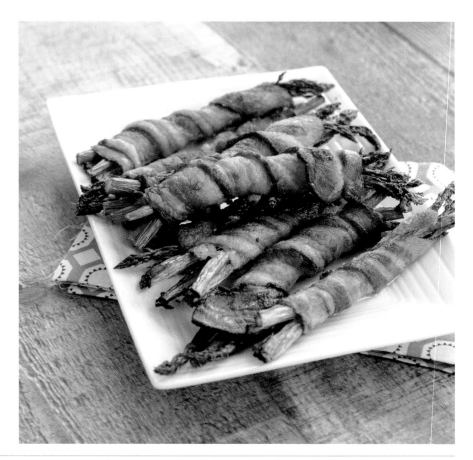

NUTRITION FACTS (PER SERVING): | Calories: 104 | Fat: 7g | Protein: 7.8g | Carbs: 4.2g | Fiber: 2.4g

Roasted Cabbage Steaks

Cabbage steaks are yummy served alongside burgers or fatty rib-eye steaks. We often enjoy them in the winter and then add any leftovers to a pot of soup; their roast-y flavor makes any soup taste better! For variety, I sometimes sprinkle the roasted cabbage wedges with crumbled blue cheese and bacon before serving.

MAKES: **6 servings**

½ head green cabbage

2 tablespoons bacon fat

1 teaspoon salt

½ teaspoon ground black pepper

½ teaspoon red pepper flakes

FOR GARNISH (OPTIONAL):

Crumbled blue cheese

Crumbled cooked bacon

1. Preheat the oven to 400°F.

2. Slice the cabbage into 6 wedges, leaving the core intact. Place the wedges in a single layer on a rimmed baking sheet. Use the back of a spoon or a knife to spread some bacon fat over the top of each cabbage wedge. Sprinkle the salt, black pepper, and red pepper flakes evenly over the wedges.

3. Roast for 15 to 20 minutes, turn, and roast for 15 to 20 more minutes, until the edges are dark brown. If desired, sprinkle the wedges with crumbled blue cheese and bacon before serving.

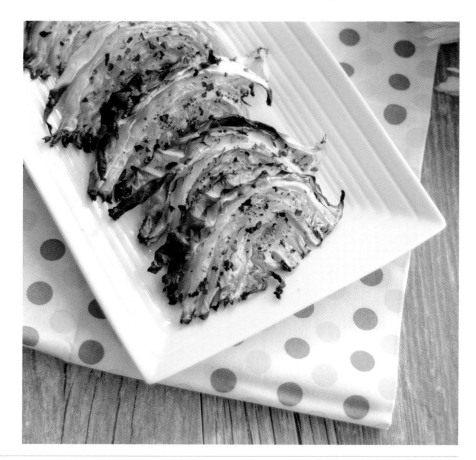

NUTRITION FACTS (PER SERVING):   Calories: 45 | Fat: 5g | Protein: 1.1g | Carbs: 4.5g | Fiber: 2g

Pan-Fried Summer Squash

Fried squash is one of my all-time favorite summertime dishes. My mother and both of my grandmothers would bring in yellow squash straight from the garden, slice it up, dredge it in flour, and cook it in vegetable oil. I used to stand by the stove and eat it hot off the paper towel on which she had placed it. I could eat a pan of squash faster than Mom could fry it! That pan-fried squash was not low-carb, but I discovered that I could pan-fry squash in a similar way without using flour. Who needs flour when we have bacon fat?! The key to making this dish really good is to keep the heat high and to let each side of the squash get really nicely browned.

MAKES: 4 servings

1½ tablespoons bacon fat

3 medium-sized yellow squash or zucchini or a combination, sliced

1 teaspoon dried basil

¼ teaspoon salt

⅛ teaspoon ground black pepper

1. Heat the bacon fat in a large skillet over high heat. Place the squash in the skillet in a single layer and fry for 5 to 6 minutes without turning.

2. Sprinkle the basil, salt, and pepper over the squash. When the bottoms are very well browned, use tongs or a wide spatula to turn the squash and fry on the other side. Do not stir, and turn it as few times as possible. When the squash is browned on both sides, remove from the skillet and serve.

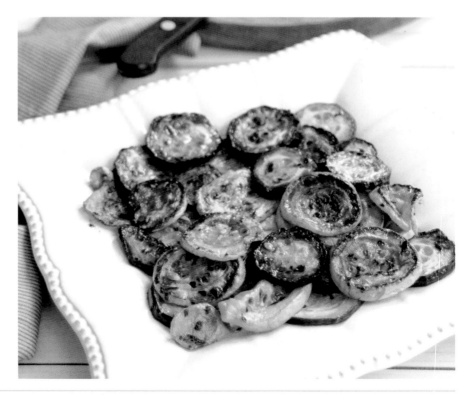

NUTRITION FACTS (PER SERVING):   Calories: 72 | Fat: 5.6g | Protein: 1.8g | Carbs: 5.3g | Fiber: 1.7g

Southern Table Pickles

Summertime dinners always tasted better when my grandmother set these refrigerator pickles on the table. Though it's a simple recipe, the crisp, cool cucumber and the bite of white vinegar and black pepper will perk up your taste buds without heating up the kitchen. These pickles pair well with grilled meats.

MAKES: **4 servings**

1⅓ cups peeled and sliced cucumbers

1 tablespoon whole black peppercorns

¼ white onion, thinly sliced

¾ cup cold water

¼ cup apple cider vinegar

2 teaspoons granulated sweetener

⅛ teaspoon salt

½ cup ice cubes

1. Place the cucumber slices in a small glass mixing bowl. Sprinkle the peppercorns and onion slices over the cucumbers.

2. Mix together the cold water, vinegar, sweetener, and salt. Pour the vinegar mixture over the cucumbers. Add the ice cubes, cover, and refrigerate for 20 to 30 minutes before serving. To keep the cucumbers crisp and cold when serving, nestle the serving bowl inside a larger bowl of ice.

3. Any leftovers can be stored in the refrigerator for up to 3 days, although the cucumbers will not remain crisp and will develop a stronger pickled flavor.

Carb Check:

Be sure to peel the cucumbers; much of the carbohydrate is found in the peel. Eating them unpeeled can add 1.5 grams of total carbs per 3.5-ounce serving!

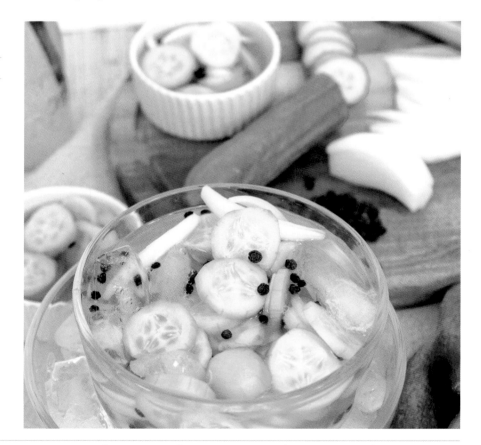

NUTRITION FACTS (PER SERVING): | Calories: 5 | Fat: 1g | Protein: 0.3g | Carbs: 1g | Fiber: 0.3g

Mom's Creamy Coleslaw

This is my mother's recipe. The only things I changed were the sweetener and the yield—my recipe makes a quarter of the amount that hers does. Mom always seemed to serve slaw with hamburgers or with Easter ham. I always enjoyed her version, but I never thought it was special until I took it to my in-laws. My sister-in-law and mother-in-law, both of whom are excellent cooks, asked for the recipe right away. I was almost embarrassed to call it a recipe, but it was a nice reminder that simple can be surprisingly good.

MAKES: **4 servings**

2 cups shredded green cabbage

½ cup mayonnaise, homemade (page 192) or store-bought

2 tablespoons powdered sweetener, or 3 drops liquid sweetener, plus more if needed

1 tablespoon apple cider vinegar

¼ teaspoon poppy seeds

¼ teaspoon salt

⅛ teaspoon freshly cracked black pepper

Place all the ingredients in a mixing bowl and mix well. Cover and refrigerate for at least 20 minutes before serving. Adjust the sweetener to your taste. This slaw keeps well in the refrigerator for up to 4 days.

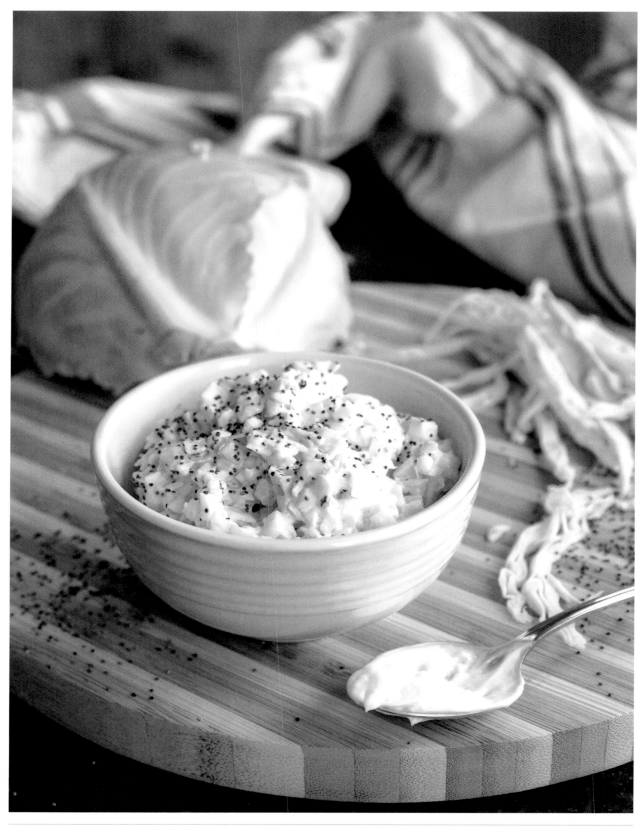

NUTRITION FACTS (PER SERVING):   Calories: 260 | Fat: 28.2g | Protein: 0.9g | Carbs: 2.4g | Fiber: 0.9g

Baked Cauliflower
Mac and Cheese

My daughter has grown up loving macaroni and cheese almost as much as her mother did. About five years before we went low-carb, I finally perfected an old-fashioned baked mac and cheese recipe, and it became somewhat legendary. When I wanted to spoil Grace a little, I made her my baked mac and cheese. We'd been eating low-carb for more than three years before I realized that I could adapt that recipe to keto. The biggest challenges were making the creamy sauce without flour and finding a suitable replacement for the macaroni noodles. When I made this version for the first time, I was a bit nervous about whether Grace would enjoy it. She took a hesitant bite, looked up at me with a big smile, and said, "Mom, you made my mac and cheese!"

MAKES: **8 servings**

4 ounces cream cheese (½ cup)

½ cup (1 stick) unsalted butter

1 cup heavy cream

½ cup sour cream

2 large eggs, beaten

4 cups chopped cauliflower florets and slender stems

1 teaspoon salt

½ teaspoon garlic powder

¼ teaspoon cayenne pepper (optional)

8 ounces sharp cheddar cheese, shredded (about 2 cups)

8 ounces mild cheddar cheese, shredded (about 2 cups)

TOPPING:

1½ ounces Parmesan cheese, grated (about ½ cup)

½ cup pork dust (ground pork rinds)

2 tablespoons unsalted butter, melted

1. Preheat the oven to 325°F.

2. Melt the cream cheese and butter in a large saucepan over low heat. When melted, whisk in the heavy cream, sour cream, and beaten eggs. Be sure to keep the heat low so that the cream doesn't break and the eggs don't curdle. Whisk constantly until the mixture is creamy and smooth and slightly thickened.

3. Place the cauliflower in a microwave-safe dish. Do not add water. Microwave, uncovered, for 3 to 4 minutes, until crisp-tender (tender but not soft).

4. Add the salt, garlic powder, and cayenne pepper, if using. Remove from the heat and stir in the cheddar cheeses and steamed cauliflower. Pour the mixture into a 2-quart oval baker or a 13 by 9-inch baking dish; set aside.

5. Make the topping: In a small bowl, mix together the Parmesan cheese, pork dust, and melted butter. The mixture will be coarse, like sand. Sprinkle the topping evenly over the cauliflower mixture.

6. Bake for 35 to 45 minutes, until the top is golden brown and bubbling. Let cool for at least 10 minutes before serving.

Substitution Suggestions:

Cabbage Noodles (page 342) work well in this dish, too. They are slightly lower in carbs than cauliflower while providing more volume. Boil the cabbage for 5 to 7 minutes, then drain well before stirring into the sauce. I also enjoy using Miracle Noodles' ziti-shaped konjac noodles. They are perfect when baked and contribute very few carbs to the dish.

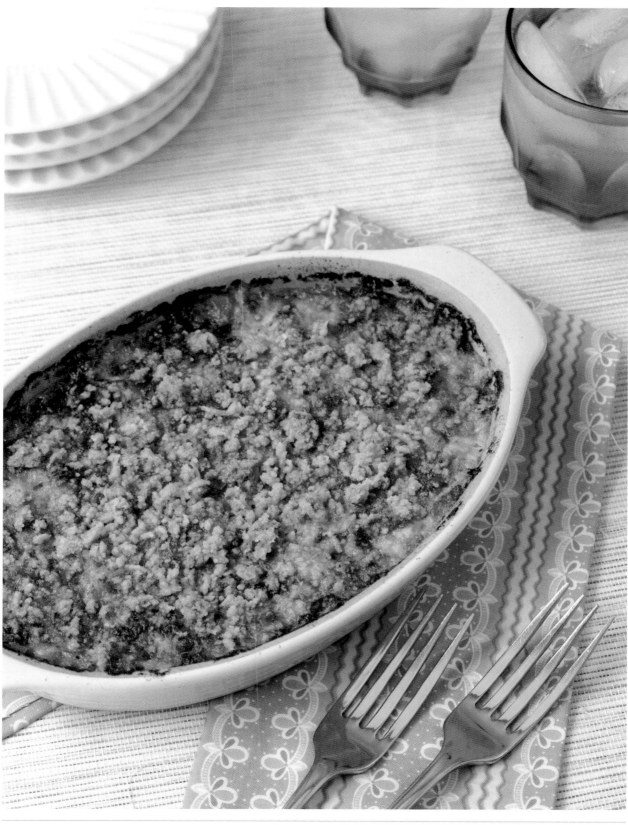

NUTRITION FACTS (PER SERVING): | Calories: 625 | Fat: 58.8g | Protein: 20.9g | Carbs: 4.1g | Fiber: 1.1g

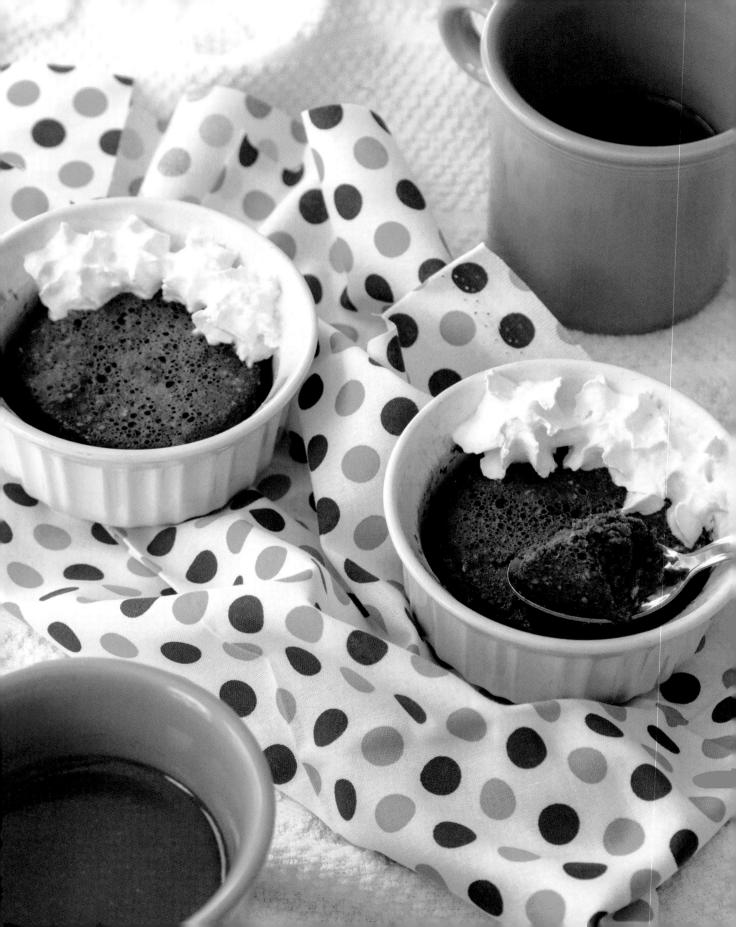

Chapter 11
Break the Glass

The best way to fight cravings is to avoid eating anything sweet. Cravings are like stray critters: if you feed them, they will never go away. Staying satiated and not feeling deprived are the two best ways to prevent cravings. One way to stay satiated is to eat high-fat foods. When you are not physically hungry, you are less likely to eat. If you allow yourself to get overly hungry and then have cravings, you are at a disadvantage in the battle. My tip to avoid feeling deprived is to eat low-carb foods that you truly enjoy.

Nonetheless, if you find yourself white-knuckling your way through cravings and at the brink of disaster, then "break the glass" and try making one of the simple treats in this chapter. The yield of each of these recipes is intentionally small to help with portion control.

Ultra-Creamy Vanilla Ice Cream

Of all the diets I've followed in my life, none of them ever allowed me to eat ice cream—until keto! This low-carb vanilla custard not only allows me to eat ice cream and stay on plan, but also serves as a delicious base that I use to make at least thirty-one flavors. That's my kind of diet! Once you make this rich and delicious homemade vanilla, you will never crave any other brand, because nothing compares to this version. Better yet, it is nearly impossible to overeat this ice cream because its high fat content makes it so filling. Grab a spoon and a very small bowl and you'll see what I mean.

MAKES: **3 cups (½ cup per serving)**

2½ cups heavy cream

¼ cup (½ stick) salted butter

6 large egg yolks, well beaten

½ cup granulated sweetener, powdered

2 teaspoons vanilla extract

¼ teaspoon salt

SPECIAL EQUIPMENT:

Ice cream maker

1. In a heavy saucepan, heat the cream and butter over low heat, stirring with a wire whisk until the butter is melted. Add the beaten egg yolks and continue whisking over low heat until just warmed.

2. Add the sweetener to the cream mixture and whisk until completely dissolved. Continue heating, whisking constantly, until the custard thickens, about 10 minutes. Do not allow the mixture to heat to over 140°F or the eggs will begin to curdle.

3. When the custard coats the back of a wooden spoon or just reaches 140°F on a candy thermometer, remove the pan from the heat. Add the vanilla extract and salt and stir to combine. Transfer the custard to a bowl and place in the fridge until completely chilled.

4. When cool, churn the custard in an ice cream maker following the manufacturer's directions. Serve when it reaches the desired consistency.

5. Store in the freezer for up to 1 month. The ice cream will harden to a solid state in the freezer. Allow it to thaw for about 10 minutes before enjoying.

Time-Saver Tip:

If you are like my daughter and are too impatient to let the ice cream thaw on the counter when it's frozen solid, you can microwave it on low power for 30 to 40 seconds.

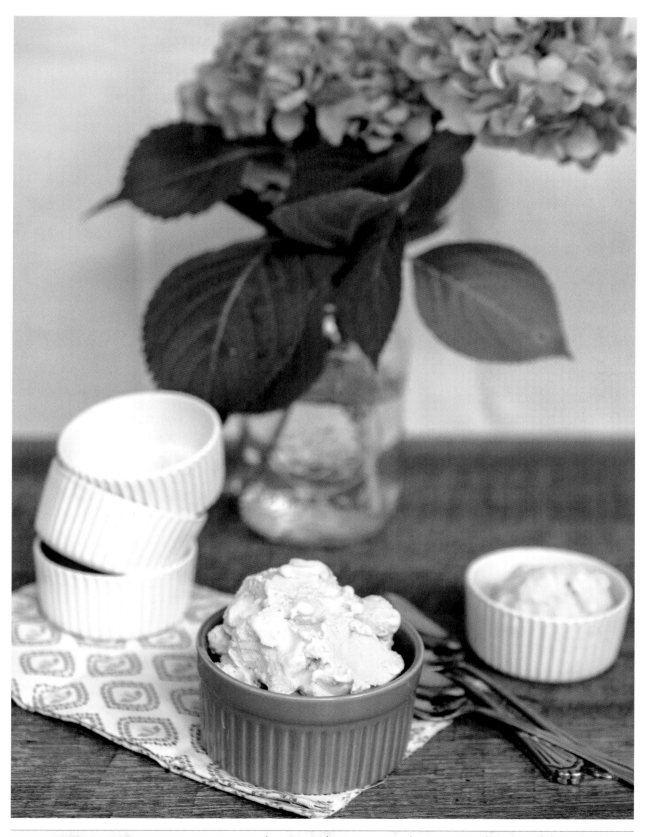

NUTRITION FACTS (PER SERVING): **Calories:** 464 | **Fat:** 48g | **Protein:** 5.6g | **Carbs:** 3.5g | **Fiber:** 0g | **Erythritol:** 24g

Peanut Butter Cookies

These are the cookies that saved my life! In the first two weeks on a ketogenic diet, I had a terrible craving. I made these cookies, took a bite of one, and thought, "If I can eat this and still lose weight, then I can do this for the rest of my life!" That was June 2013, and I still plan to eat this way for the rest of my life.

MAKES: 1 dozen cookies (1 per serving)

½ cup creamy salted peanut butter

¼ cup granulated sweetener

1 large egg

1 teaspoon vanilla extract

½ teaspoon baking powder

⅛ teaspoon salt

1. Preheat the oven to 350°F. Line a baking sheet with parchment paper.

2. Using a hand mixer, mix the peanut butter and sweetener until smooth. Add the remaining ingredients and mix well.

3. Roll the dough between your palms into 1-inch balls and place on a baking sheet, spaced about 2 inches apart. Use your palm to press each ball into a ¼-inch-thick cookie shape. You can drag a fork across the tops of the cookies to make a crisscross pattern if you like.

4. Bake the cookies for 9 to 10 minutes, until browned. Let cool on the baking sheet for a few minutes, then use a spatula to transfer the cookies to a wire rack to cool completely and crisp up. (They will be soft when they first come out of the oven.) Store in the refrigerator for up to 1 week.

Carb Check:

Be sure to check the ingredients in the peanut butter you buy. There should be only two ingredients listed: peanuts and salt. Many brands add some form of sweetener, which would increase the carb count and likely would raise your blood glucose.

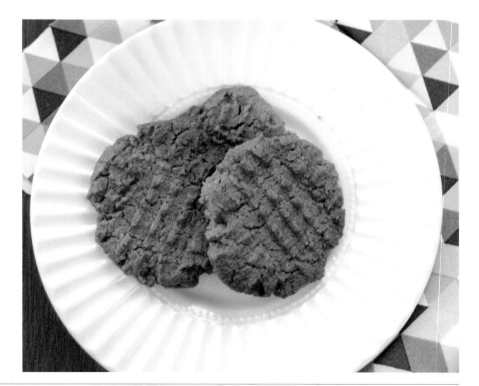

NUTRITION FACTS (PER COOKIE): Calories: 71 | Fat: 5.9g | Protein: 2.9g | Carbs: 2.5g | Fiber: 0.5g | Erythritol: 6g

Lemon Cheesecake Whip

When done right, cheesecake can be an excellent low-carb treat. But a baked cheesecake requires a springform pan, a crust, and time to cure overnight. Some days a low-carb guy or gal needs a quicker option! This cheesecake whip is an easy substitute. Not only does it not need to be baked, but the ingredients, save perhaps the sweetener, are available at any grocery store. If you can use a hand mixer, you can satisfy your sweet tooth with this simple recipe.

1 (8-ounce) package cream cheese, softened

½ cup heavy cream

⅓ cup powdered sweetener

2 tablespoons lemon juice

2 teaspoons vanilla extract

¼ teaspoon salt

Lemon zest, for garnish (optional)

MAKES: 4 servings

Using a hand mixer, whip the cream cheese and heavy cream until smooth and fluffy. Add the sweetener, lemon juice, vanilla extract, and salt and continue whipping until well mixed and smooth. Refrigerate for 20 to 30 minutes before serving. Garnish with lemon zest, if desired.

VARIATION: Lime Cheesecake Whip

Simply replace the lemon juice and zest with lime juice and zest.

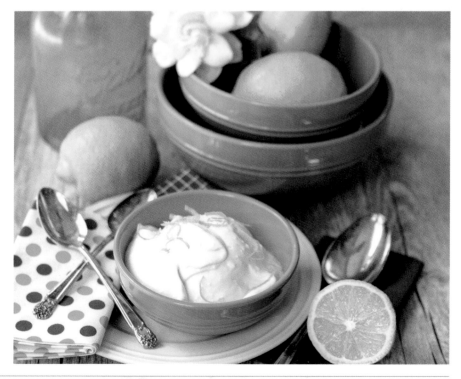

NUTRITION FACTS (PER SERVING):   Calories: 307 | Fat: 30.3g | Protein: 4.4g | Carbs: 3.6g | Fiber: 0g | Erythritol: 24g

Chocolate Minute Muffins

Minute muffins are ideal for a number of reasons. First, this type of recipe typically makes just one or two servings, so portion control is built right in. In addition, they are quick! I mix up the dry ingredients in advance, then add the wet ingredients whenever I want chocolate cake. These muffins really do taste like a treat, but they also make a great breakfast. In fact, I love eating them at work or when I'm staying at hotels because they travel so well. Who doesn't love chocolate cake for breakfast?

A dollop of whipped cream makes these muffins extra special. While the coffee powder is optional, it adds a deeper and richer flavor without adding a coffee taste.

MAKES: 2 muffins (1 per serving)

2 tablespoons unflavored whey protein isolate

2 tablespoons granulated sweetener

2 teaspoons unsweetened cocoa powder

¼ teaspoon baking powder

⅛ teaspoon instant coffee powder (optional)

1 large egg

2 tablespoons unsalted butter, melted but not hot

¼ teaspoon vanilla extract

2 drops liquid sweetener, plus more if needed

Whipped cream, for garnish (optional)

1. Generously grease two 7-ounce ramekins or coffee mugs with butter or coconut oil.

2. Whisk together the whey protein isolate, granulated sweetener, cocoa powder, baking powder, and coffee powder, if using. Add the egg, melted butter, and vanilla extract and mix until smooth. Stir in the liquid sweetener. Taste for sweetness and adjust as desired.

3. Divide the batter between the greased ramekins or mugs. Microwave each for 1 minute. Allow to cool for at least 1 minute before serving. The muffins will firm up as they cool.

Time-Saver Tip:

Mix the dry ingredients in advance and store them in an airtight container in the pantry. When you want a quick treat or breakfast, melt the butter in a microwave-safe mixing bowl, then add the egg, liquid sweetener, and dry ingredients. Stir until smooth, then proceed with Step 3.

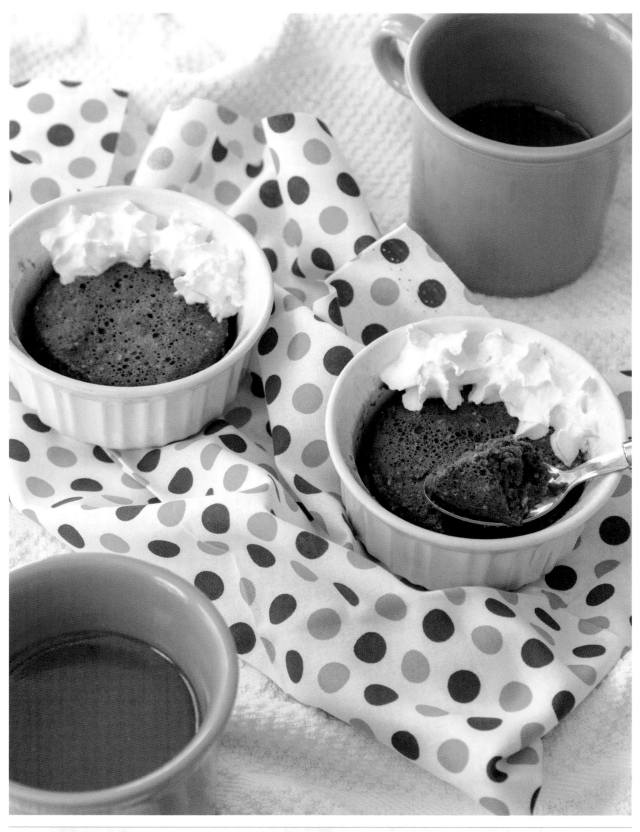

NUTRITION FACTS (PER MUFFIN):   Calories: 194 | Fat: 14g | Protein: 16g | Carbs: 1.4g | Fiber: 0g | Erythritol: 18g

Pumpkin Spice Fluff

"Everything Pumpkin Spice" season officially begins after Labor Day, but, unlike white pants, pumpkin spice stays in style year-round. If you're a pumpkin spice fanatic, this simple treat will satisfy your taste for fall flavors. I remember the first time I served this fluff to my husband. As he dipped his spoon into it a second time, he asked, "Can I really eat this on our diet?" Then he quickly took another bite before I could tell him no. Thankfully, this low-carb treat is a yes!

MAKES: **2 servings**

4 ounces cream cheese (½ cup), softened

½ cup heavy cream

½ cup crème fraîche or sour cream

¼ cup pumpkin puree

⅓ cup granulated sweetener, powdered

1 teaspoon ground cinnamon, plus extra for garnish

½ teaspoon pumpkin pie spice

2 teaspoons vanilla extract

Place the cream cheese and heavy cream in a bowl and use a hand mixer to whip until smooth. Fold in the crème fraîche and pumpkin puree with a rubber spatula. Add the sweetener, spices, and vanilla extract and gently fold in until thoroughly incorporated. Refrigerate for 20 to 30 minutes before serving. Garnish with a sprinkle of cinnamon.

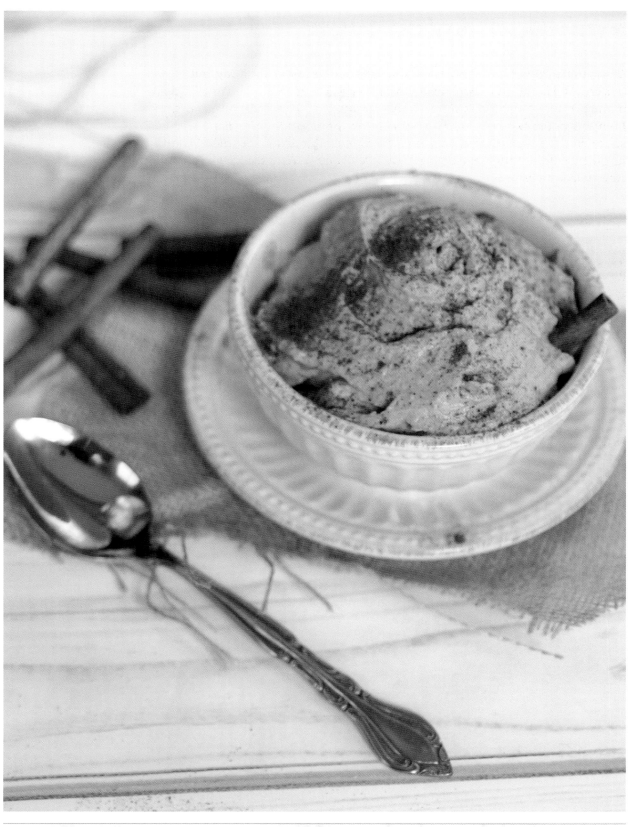

NUTRITION FACTS (PER SERVING):   **Calories:** 648 | **Fat:** 62g | **Protein:** 6g | **Carbs:** 7g | **Fiber:** 1.5g | **Erythritol:** 48g

Whipped Coconut Cream
with Macadamia Nuts

Coconut and macadamia nuts were made to go together. In this dreamy treat, cinnamon and vanilla bring out the best of both flavors. If you're limiting or avoiding dairy, this is a particularly nice option for satisfying your sweet tooth.

MAKES: 4 servings

1 (13.5-ounce) can coconut cream

¼ teaspoon vanilla extract

3 drops liquid sweetener, or 1 tablespoon granulated sweetener

¼ teaspoon ground cinnamon, plus extra for garnish

¼ teaspoon salt

4 ounces macadamia nuts, chopped

Shredded unsweetened coconut, for garnish

1. Place the coconut cream, vanilla extract, sweetener, cinnamon, and salt in a bowl and use a hand mixer to whip until fluffy, about 2 minutes. Stir in the macadamia nuts.

2. Serve immediately or, for a firmer texture, refrigerate for 30 to 45 minutes before serving. Garnish with a sprinkle of cinnamon and coconut.

Carb Check:

Be sure to use coconut cream with no added sweeteners. The only ingredients listed should be coconut, water, and perhaps a stabilizer like guar gum.

Substitution Suggestion:

You can use two cans of full-fat coconut milk to get the equivalent of one can of coconut cream. Turn the cans upside down and place them in the refrigerator to chill for at least 12 hours. When you remove them from the refrigerator, turn them right side up. When you open them, the cream will be at the bottom. Pour off the watery liquid on top and use the cream at the bottom of each can for this recipe.

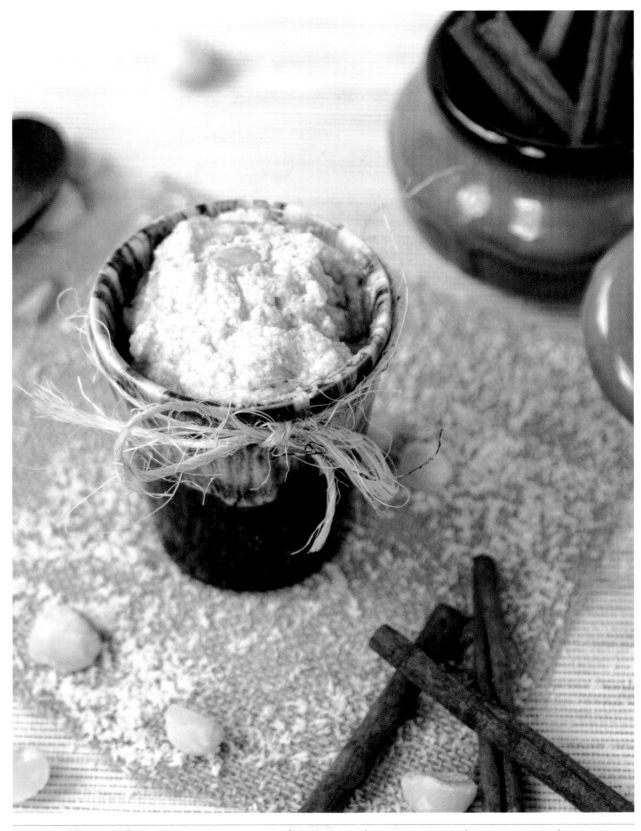

NUTRITION FACTS (PER SERVING):   **Calories:** 344 | **Fat:** 35g | **Protein:** 3.5g | **Carbs:** 6.2g | **Fiber:** 2g

Additional Resources

Fortunately, there are fantastic online resources that can help you learn more about how to eat this way and how to cook wonderful low-carb foods. Whether you want to find recipes, review sample eating plans, understand more about the science, or hear from real people who have had success on keto, you will find it!

As always, when looking at recipes, please make sure to calculate the nutrition information based on the ingredients you use. While I really respect and appreciate each of the food bloggers I've included here, some of them eat more carbs than I am able to eat. Use your best judgment as to what will work well for you.

Here are just a few of the online resources that I recommend.

Information for Beginners

The following sites are either hosted by medical professionals or feature interviews and podcasts with medical professionals. You may find that they contradict each other at times, but those contradictions tend to highlight areas in which more research is needed.

Diet Doctor (www.dietdoctor.com) was founded by Andreas Eenfeldt, a physician in Sweden. He and his team provide a practical, no-nonsense approach to a low-carbohydrate diet. Diet Doctor accepts no ads or sponsors, so the information tends to be neutral and reliable. While much of the content is free, there is a subscription-based service for additional information offered for a nominal monthly fee. In May 2017, I began contributing recipes and blog posts to this site, but I recommended it well before I began working with the team.

Dr. Michael Eades maintains the blog **Protein Power (www.proteinpower.com/drmike/).** Eades is a physician who uses a low-carb diet to treat patients, and his blog is very informative, with practical advice and easy-to-read posts.

Dr. Jason Fung (www. intensivedietarymanagement.com) is a Canadian nephrologist who has used a very-low-carb diet to treat diabetic patients with kidney disease. His writing style is entertaining, and his content is informative.

Zoe Harcombe (www.zoeharcombe.com) is a researcher, author, blogger, and public speaker. She's one sharp cookie, and she was among the first to examine the research base against dietary fat. If Dr. Harcombe says it, I believe her!

Hyperlipid (high-fat-nutrition.blogspot. com) is a blog written by UK veterinarian Petro Dobromylskyj. While this blog is not an easy, casual read, it provides thought-provoking and heavily science-based conversation about metabolism.

Brian Williamson is the mastermind behind **The Ketovangelist (ketovangelist.com).** He has excellent podcasts and a very good blog with solid, practical support.

Jimmy Moore's popular podcast **Livin' La Vida Low Carb (livinlavidalowcarb.com)** features a wide variety of guests, many of whom provide varying viewpoints.

Professor Tim Noakes' banting website **Real Meal Revolution (www.realmealrevolution. com)** has some very good information for folks who are new to eating low-carb and high-fat. Some of the information is fee-based, but much of it is available for free.

Optimizing Nutrition (optimizingnutrition. com) is a blog maintained by Marty Kendall. It focuses on the nutritional impact of foods and macronutrients. While the content is fairly advanced, Kendall writes in a way that makes it easy to understand.

The Poor, Misunderstood Calorie (www. caloriesproper.com) is a blog by Bill Lagakos, who holds a PhD in nutritional biochemistry and physiology. It focuses on obesity, inflammation, and insulin resistance.

Mark Sisson (marksdailyapple.com) is a Paleo, primal, low-carb advocate who focuses on eating whole, real foods. His website is entertaining and informative and covers a wide range of health topics.

Virta Health (blog.virtahealth.com) is a company that not only provides online healthcare but also is making some important contributions to the research literature surrounding low-carb eating. It was started by three of my favorites: Dr. Stephen Phinney, Dr. Jeff Volek, and Dr. Sarah Hallberg. They offer practical and reliable information.

My Favorite Low-Carb Food Bloggers

I am indebted to many of these talented and creative bloggers, not just because they provided delicious low-carb recipes for my journey, but also because through their efforts I learned how to create my own low-carb recipes.

All Day I Dream About Food (www.alldayidreamaboutfood.com)—If anyone can make a great low-carb dessert, it's Carolyn Ketchum. She's an incredible talent in the kitchen. Following her and making many of her recipes taught me a lot about baking for a ketogenic diet.

DJ Foodie (www.djfoodie.com)—While some of his recipes contain more carbs than I can eat in a single meal, DJ Foodie is a culinary genius. Both his blog and his cookbook are excellent. I've relied on his recipes more than once!

I Breathe I'm Hungry (www. ibreatheimhungry.com)—Mellissa Sevigny is another creative genius. Her dessert recipes are excellent, but she also features delicious mains and side dishes. Check out her Meatball Monday selections; you will not be disappointed.

Low Carb Maven (www.lowcarbmaven.com)—Kim is not only amazing in the kitchen, but her photography is exceptional, too. Be sure to pay attention to carbs and portion sizes, but whether you're looking for dinner ideas or an impressive low-carb dessert, she always has excellent ideas.

MariaMindBodyHealth (mariamindbodyhealth.com)—Maria Emmerich and her husband, Craig, adopted two of the cutest little boys ever. Those two very lucky fellas serve as Maria's "test kitchen." Her recipes are reliable and delicious and include a wealth of dairy-free options. She also has several bestselling cookbooks.

Peace, Love, and Low Carb (peaceloveandlowcarb.com)—Kyndra Holley has great recipes. She has had a very public battle with regaining lost weight and has recently recommitted to her goals. Her story is reaching a lot of people.

Ruled Me (www.ruledme.com)—Craig Clarke has been blogging for quite a while. His website offers meal plans and recipes along with helpful information for beginners.

Allergen Index

RECIPES	PAGE	🥛	🥚	🌿	🍲	30 mins or less	🍜
Open-Faced Taco for Two	280	✓				✓	✓
Meatloaf	282		✓				
Big Mac Salad	283	○	✓			✓	
Kristie's Crack Slaw	284					✓	✓
Noodle-less Lasagna	286	✓					✓
20-Minute Skillet Dinner	288	✓				✓	✓
Three-Meat Chili	290	○					✓
Asian-Style Beef and Broccoli	292						✓
Savory Pepper Steak	294						✓
Mississippi Roast	296	✓			✓		✓
Dry-Rubbed Beef Ribs	298						
Bolognese	300					✓	✓
No-Vodka Vodka Sauce	301	✓				✓	✓
Taco Soup	302						
Simple Pulled Pork	304				✓		
Slow Cooker Tender Baby Back Ribs	306				✓		
Pork Chops with Pan Gravy	308					✓	
Simple Roasted Pork Tenderloin	310						
Taco Bake	312	✓				✓	✓
Skillet Pizza	314	✓					✓
Whole Roasted Chicken	316				✓		
Pickle-Brined Chicken Tenders	318	✓	✓				
Parmesan-Crusted Roasted Chicken Thighs	320	✓	✓				
Chicken Philly Cheesesteak Casserole	322	✓	✓				✓
Broccoli Cheddar Ranch Chicken Soup	324	✓				✓	✓
Lemon Mushroom Chicken	326	✓					
BBQ Chicken	327						
Chicken Salad	328		✓				✓
Shredded Mexican Chicken	329	✓			✓		✓
Moo Goo Gai Pan	330						✓
Skinny Chicken Fried "Rice"	332		✓				✓
Chicken Broccoli Alfredo	333	✓				✓	
Baked Salmon with Creamy Dill Sauce	334	✓	✓			✓	
Lemon Pepper Flounder	335	○				✓	
Sautéed Lemon Garlic Shrimp	336	○				✓	
Tuna Salad	337		✓			✓	✓
Zoodles	340					✓	
Cabbage Noodles	342	○				✓	
Cauli Rice	343	○				✓	
Creamy Cauli Mash	344	✓				✓	
Ranch Cauli Mash with Bacon	345	✓				✓	
Cauliflower au Gratin	346	✓					
Herb-Roasted Radishes	347					✓	
Peppery Roasted Green Beans with Parmesan	348	✓				✓	
Skillet Mushrooms	349	○				✓	
Homecoming Broccoli Salad	350	✓	✓			✓	
Roasted Broccoli	351					✓	
Parmesan-Baked Tomatoes	352	✓	✓			✓	
Spinach Salad with Hot Bacon Fat Dressing	353		✓			✓	
Faux-tato Salad	354		✓			✓	
Cucumber, Tomato, and Feta Salad	356	✓				✓	
Squash Casserole	357	✓	✓				
Slow-Simmered Country Green Beans	358	○					
Roasted Mixed Veggies	360						
Creamed Brussels Sprouts	361	✓				✓	
Bacon-Wrapped Asparagus	362						
Roasted Cabbage Steaks	363						
Pan-Fried Summer Squash	364					✓	
Southern Table Pickles	365					✓	
Mom's Creamy Coleslaw	366		✓			✓	
Baked Cauliflower Mac and Cheese	368	✓	✓				
Ultra-Creamy Vanilla Ice Cream	372	✓	✓				
Peanut Butter Cookies	374		✓			✓	
Lemon Cheesecake Whip	375	✓				✓	
Chocolate Minute Muffins	376	✓	✓			✓	
Pumpkin Spice Fluff	378	✓				✓	
Whipped Coconut Cream with Macadamia Nuts	380			✓		✓	

Recipe Index

The Basics

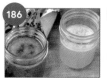
186
Beef or Chicken
Bone Broth

188
Baked Bacon and
Rendered Bacon Fat

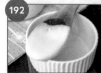
190
Kristie's Ketchup

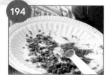
192
Mayonnaise

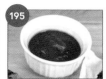
194
Eastern NC
BBQ Sauce

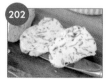
195
Classic BBQ Sauce

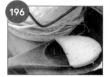
196
White BBQ Sauce

197
Tartar Sauce

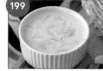
198
Cocktail Sauce

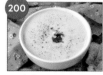
199
Simple Cheese
Sauce

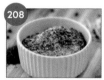
200
Chile con Queso

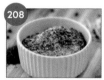
202
Lemon-Herb
Compound Butter

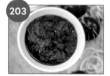
203
Marinara Sauce

204
Creamy Alfredo
Sauce

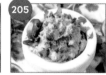
205
Guacamole

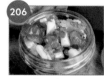
206
Simple Salsa Fresca

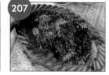
207
Taco Seasoning

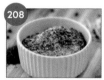
208
Ranch Seasoning

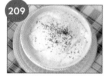
209
Ranch Dressing

210
Parmesan
Peppercorn
Dressing

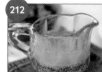
211
Thousand Island
Dressing

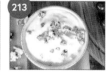
212
Hot Bacon Fat
Dressing

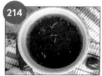
213
Blue Cheese
Dressing

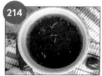
214
Basic Vinaigrette

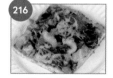
216
The Sullivans'
KeDough
Pizza Crust

218
Unsweetened
Iced Tea

Breakfast

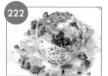
222
Minute Mug Omelet

224
Breakfast Sausage

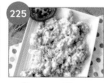
225
Sausage Gravy

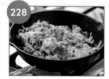
226
Sausage and Goat
Cheese Skillet Scramble
with Spinach and
Sun-Dried Tomatoes

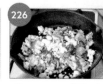
228
Pizza Skillet
Scramble

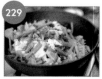
229
Spring Veggie
Skillet Scramble

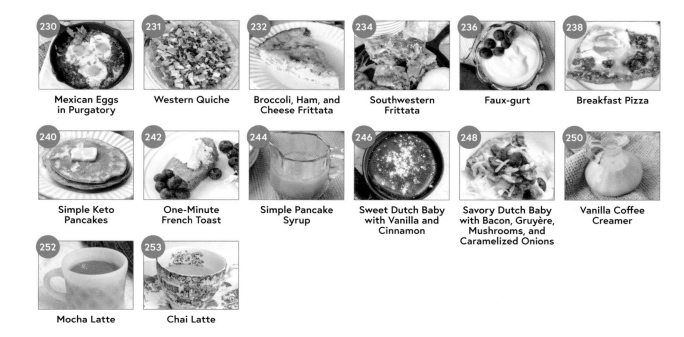

230 Mexican Eggs in Purgatory

231 Western Quiche

232 Broccoli, Ham, and Cheese Frittata

234 Southwestern Frittata

236 Faux-gurt

238 Breakfast Pizza

240 Simple Keto Pancakes

242 One-Minute French Toast

244 Simple Pancake Syrup

246 Sweet Dutch Baby with Vanilla and Cinnamon

248 Savory Dutch Baby with Bacon, Gruyère, Mushrooms, and Caramelized Onions

250 Vanilla Coffee Creamer

252 Mocha Latte

253 Chai Latte

Small Bites

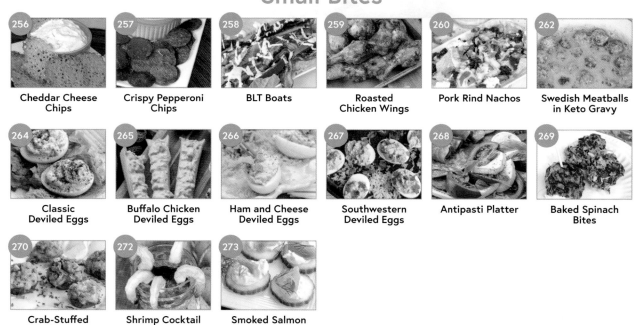

256 Cheddar Cheese Chips

257 Crispy Pepperoni Chips

258 BLT Boats

259 Roasted Chicken Wings

260 Pork Rind Nachos

262 Swedish Meatballs in Keto Gravy

264 Classic Deviled Eggs

265 Buffalo Chicken Deviled Eggs

266 Ham and Cheese Deviled Eggs

267 Southwestern Deviled Eggs

268 Antipasti Platter

269 Baked Spinach Bites

270 Crab-Stuffed Mushrooms

272 Shrimp Cocktail

273 Smoked Salmon Cucumber Bites

Mains: Beef

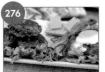
276

Burgers—Six Ways

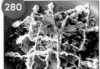
280

Open-Faced
Taco for Two

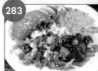
282

Meatloaf

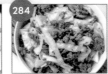
283

Big Mac Salad

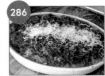
284

Kristie's Crack Slaw

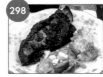
286

Noodle-less
Lasagna

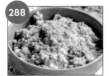
288

20-Minute
Skillet Dinner

290

Three-Meat Chili

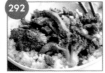
292

Asian-Style
Beef and Broccoli

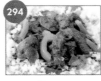
294

Savory
Pepper Steak

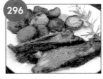
296

Mississippi Roast

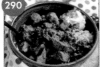
298

Dry-Rubbed
Beef Ribs

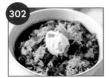
300

Bolognese

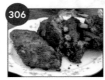
301

No-Vodka
Vodka Sauce

Mains: Pork

302

Taco Soup

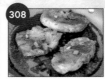
304

Simple Pulled Pork

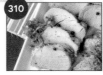
306

Slow Cooker Tender
Baby Back Ribs

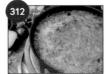
308

Pork Chops
with Pan Gravy

310

Simple Roasted
Pork Tenderloin

312

Taco Bake

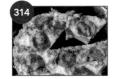
314

Skillet Pizza

Mains: Poultry

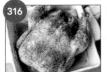
316

Whole Roasted
Chicken

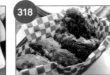
318

Pickle-Brined
Chicken Tenders

320

Parmesan-Crusted
Roasted Chicken
Thighs

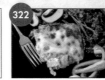
322

Chicken Philly
Cheesesteak
Casserole

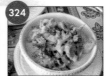
324

Broccoli Cheddar
Ranch Chicken Soup

326

Lemon Mushroom
Chicken

327

BBQ Chicken

328

Chicken Salad

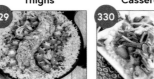
329

Shredded Mexican
Chicken

330

Moo Goo Gai Pan

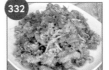

332

Skinny Chicken
Fried "Rice"

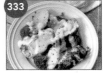
333

Chicken Broccoli
Alfredo

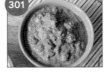
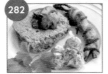

Mains: Seafood

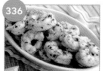

334
Baked Salmon with Creamy Dill Sauce

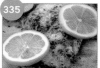

335
Lemon Pepper Flounder

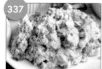

336
Sautéed Lemon Garlic Shrimp

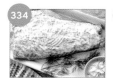

337
Tuna Salad

Sides

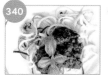

340
Zoodles

342
Cabbage Noodles

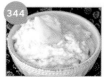

343
Cauli Rice

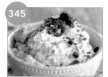

344
Creamy Cauli Mash

345
Ranch Cauli Mash with Bacon

346
Cauliflower au Gratin

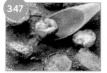

347
Herb-Roasted Radishes

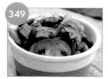

348
Peppery Roasted Green Beans with Parmesan

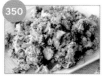

349
Skillet Mushrooms

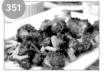

350
Homecoming Broccoli Salad

351
Roasted Broccoli

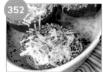

352
Parmesan-Baked Tomatoes

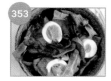

353
Spinach Salad with Hot Bacon Fat Dressing

354
Faux-tato Salad

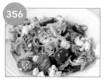

356
Cucumber, Tomato, and Feta Salad

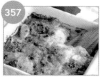

357
Squash Casserole

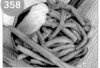

358
Slow-Simmered Country Green Beans

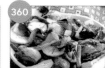

360
Roasted Mixed Veggies

361
Creamed Brussels Sprouts

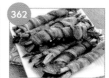

362
Bacon-Wrapped Asparagus

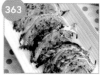

363
Roasted Cabbage Steaks

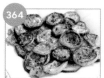

364
Pan-Fried Summer Squash

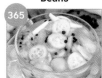

365
Southern Table Pickles

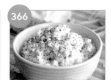

366
Mom's Creamy Coleslaw

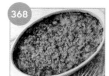

368
Baked Cauliflower Mac and Cheese

Break the Glass

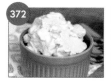

372
Ultra-Creamy Vanilla Ice Cream

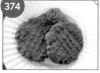

374
Peanut Butter Cookies

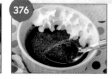

375
Lemon Cheesecake Whip

376
Chocolate Minute Muffins

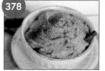

378
Pumpkin Spice Fluff

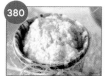

380
Whipped Coconut Cream with Macadamia Nuts

General Index

With Gratitude

This book would not have happened without the hard work and contributions of a lot of special people.

To my family, thank you so very much for enduring every missed minute of family time as I worried over recipes and photos of recipes and whether Day 4 should be Day 11 or whether Day 22 was the right message for the reader. Grace and Jonathan, I know that you can't understand my passion for this, but one day I hope that you are proud of my work and that you recognize the individual contributions you made. David, while I don't deserve your love, patience, or dedication, I pray each day that you never figure that out. Thank you for being an amazing partner, father, and dishwasher. To my mom, thanks for giving me a childhood that gave me room and encouragement to never stop trying. To my brother, Stewart, who said, "Why don't you put those videos on YouTube?"

To the amazing friends who are admins and moderators of my Facebook group, you are the most dedicated, hardworking volunteers I have ever known. Your heart for others is unmatched. Thank you for every single minute you give back to others so that they can enjoy the better health that you have found. Your love, support, and commitment to the group allowed me the time and gave me the encouragement to complete this book. You are my people. You have my back. I love you guys.

To Jenny Lowder, thank you for every Friday, Saturday, and Sunday that you worked with me from sunup to sundown to photograph every recipe. You climbed ladders, lay on your tummy, and crouched on your knees to get the very best shots. Thank you for your commitment to this project.

To Dr. Eric Westman and Gary Taubes, thank you for writing your own books. You changed my life before we even met. To Dr. Westman, I am so grateful to have met you and to have the opportunity to work with you to support others. Your work on behalf of "the least of these" is changing lives well beyond the walls of your own examination rooms. Your work is also changing the lives of other medical professionals who are finally listening because you didn't stop working.

To the team at Victory Belt, thank you for your work in bringing this book together. To Pam and Holly, you never forget a detail, even when I do. Your attention to detail, concise edits, and careful consideration for precise recipe directions made this a better book. To Erich and Lance, thanks for your patience and for talking me off the ledge a few times. Hayley and Bill, you've got a gift! To Susan, thanks for your guidance.

To my real-life friends who were there for the before pictures, thank you for being lifetime friends. Gwen, Susan, and Allison, very few people are lucky enough to have even one person who loves them for a lifetime. I have all three of you! From kindergarten introductions to weddings to babies to the darkest days, you have always been a part of my life. Regardless of what value the scale assigned to me, you somehow saw the real value in me.

To my colleagues at Sandhills Community College, thank you for your support, patience, taste-testing, and encouragement to pursue my passion.

To the Diet Doctor team that I've been so fortunate to join, you guys stretch and challenge me, and I love it! I adore each of you and the work you do. Andreas, Kristin, Jill, Giorgios, Simon, Emoke, Inger, and Bjarte, let's keep empowering people to change their lives.